HEALTH AND HUMAN DEVELOPMENT

THE ASTONISHING BRAIN AND HOLISTIC CONSCIOUSNESS

NEUROSCIENCE AND VEDĀNTA PERSPECTIVES

HEALTH AND HUMAN DEVELOPMENT

Joav Merrick - Series Editor

National Institute of Child Health and Human Development,
Ministry of Social Affairs, Jerusalem

Adolescent Behavior Research: International Perspectives
Joav Merrick and Hatim A. Omar (Editors)
2007. ISBN: 1-60021-649-8

Complementary Medicine Systems: Comparison and Integration
Karl W. Kratky
2008. ISBN: 978-1-60456-475-4 (Hardcover)
2008. ISBN: 978-1-61122-433-7 (E-book)

Pain in Children and Youth
Patricia Schofield and Joav Merrick (Editors)
2008. ISBN: 978-1-60456-951-3

Challenges in Adolescent Health: An Australian Perspective
David Bennett, Susan Towns, Elizabeth Elliott and Joav Merrick (Editors)
2009. ISBN: 978-1-60741-616-6 (Hardcover)
2009. ISBN: 978-1-61668-240-8 (E-book)

Behavioral Pediatrics, 3rd Edition
Donald E. Greydanus, Dilip R. Patel, Helen D. Pratt and Joseph L. Calles, Jr. (Editors)
2009. ISBN: 978-1-60692-702-1 (Hardcover)
2009. ISBN: 978-1-60876-630-7 (E-book)

Health and Happiness from Meaningful Work: Research in Quality of Working Life
Søren Ventegodt and Joav Merrick (Editors)
2009. ISBN: 978-1-60692-820-2

Obesity and Adolescence: A Public Health Concern
Hatim A. Omar, Donald E. Greydanus, Dilip R. Patel and Joav Merrick (Editors)
2009. ISBN: 978-1-60456-821-9

Poverty and Children: A Public Health Concern
Alexis Lieberman and Joav Merrick (Editors)
2009. ISBN: 978-1-60741-140-6

Living on the Edge: The Mythical, Spiritual, and Philosophical Roots of Social Marginality
Joseph Goodbread
2009. ISBN: 978-1-60741-162-8

Alcohol-Related Cognitive Disorders: Research and Clinical Perspectives
Leo Sher, Isack Kandel and Joav Merrick (Editors)
2009. ISBN: 978-1-60741-730-9 (Hardcover)
2009. ISBN: 978-1-60876-623-9 (E-book)

Rural Child Health: International Aspects
Erica Bell and Joav Merrick (Editors)
2010. ISBN: 978-1-60876-357-3 (Hardcover)
2010. ISBN: 978-1-61324-005-2 (E-book)

Children and Pain
Patricia Schofield and Joav Merrick (Editors)
2009. ISBN: 978-1-60876-020-6 (Hardcover)
2009. ISBN: 978-1-61728-183-9 (E-book)

Conceptualizing Behavior in Health and Social Research: A Practical Guide to Data Analysis
Said Shahtahmasebi and Damon Berridge
2010. ISBN: 978-1-60876-383-2

Chance Action and Therapy: The Playful Way of Changing
Uri Wernik
2010. ISBN: 978-1-60876-393-1 (Hardcover)
2011. ISBN: 978-1-61122-987-5 (Softcover)
2011. ISBN: 978-1-61209-874-6 (E-book)

Adolescence and Chronic Illness. A Public Health Concern
Hatim Omar, Donald E. Greydanus, Dilip R. Patel and Joav Merrick (Editors)
2010. ISBN: 978-1-60876-628-4 (Hardcover)
2010. ISBN: 978-1-61761-482-8 (E-book)

Adolescence and Sports
Dilip R. Patel, Donald E. Greydanus, Hatim Omar and Joav Merrick (Editors)
2010. ISBN: 978-1-60876-702-1 (Hardcover)
2010. ISBN: 978-1-61761-483-5 (E-book)

International Aspects of Child Abuse and Neglect
Howard Dubowitz and Joav Merrick (Editors)
2010. ISBN: 978-1-60876-703-8 (Hardcover)
2010. ISBN: 978-1-61122-049-0 (Softcover)
2010. ISBN: 978-1-61122-403-0 (E-book)

Positive Youth Development: Evaluation and Future Directions in a Chinese Context
Daniel T.L. Shek, Hing Keung Ma and Joav Merrick (Editors)
2010. ISBN: 978-1-60876-830-1 (Hardcover)
2010. ISBN: 978-1-61668-376-4 (E-book)
2011. ISBN: 978-1-62100-175-1 (Softcover)

Positive Youth Development: Implementation of a Youth Program in a Chinese Context
Daniel T.L Shek, Hing Keung Ma and Joav Merrick (Editors)
2010. ISBN: 978-1-61668-230-9 (Hardcover)
2010. ISBN: 978-1-61209-091-7 (E-book)

Pediatric and Adolescent Sexuality and Gynecology: Principles for the Primary Care Clinician
Hatim A. Omar, Donald E. Greydanus, Artemis K. Tsitsika, Dilip R. Patel and Joav Merrick (Editors)
2010. ISBN: 978-1-60876-735-9

Understanding Eating Disorders: Integrating Culture, Psychology and Biology
Yael Latzer, Joav Merrick and Daniel Stein (Editors)
2010. ISBN: 978-1-61728-298-0 (Hardcover)
2011. ISBN: 978-1-61470-976-3 (Softcover)

Advanced Cancer Pain and Quality of Life
Edward Chow and Joav Merrick (Editors)
2010. ISBN: 978-1-61668-207-1 (Hardcover)
2010. ISBN: 978-1-61668-400-6 (E-book)

Bone and Brain Metastases: Advances in Research and Treatment
Arjun Sahgal, Edward Chow and Joav Merrick (Editors)
2010. ISBN: 978-1-61668-365-8 (Hardcover)
2010. ISBN: 978-1-61728-085-6 (E-book)

Environment, Mood Disorders and Suicide
Teodor T. Postolache and Joav Merrick (Editors)
2010. ISBN: 978-1-61668-505-8

Social and Cultural Psychiatry Experience from the Caribbean Region
Hari D. Maharajh and Joav Merrick (Editors)
2010. ISBN: 978-1-61668-506-5 (Hardcover)
2010. ISBN: 978-1-61728-088-7 (E-book)

Narratives and Meanings of Migration
Julia Mirsky
2010. ISBN: 978-1-61761-103-2 (Hardcover)
2010. ISBN: 978-1-61761-519-1 (E-book)

Self-Management and the Health Care Consumer
Peter William Harvey
2011. ISBN: 978-1-61761-796-6 (Hardcover)
2011. ISBN: 978-1-61122-214-2 (E-book)

Sexology from a Holistic Point of View
Soren Ventegodt and Joav Merrick
2011. ISBN: 978-1-61761-859-8 (Hardcover)
2011. ISBN: 978-1-61122-262-3 (E-book)

Principles of Holistic Psychiatry: A Textbook on Holistic Medicine for Mental Disorders
Soren Ventegodt and Joav Merrick
2011. ISBN: 978-1-61761-940-3 (Hardcover)
2011. ISBN: 978-1-61122-263-0 (E-book)

Clinical Aspects of Psychopharmacology in Childhood and Adolescence
Donald E. Greydanus, Joseph L. Calles, Jr., Dilip P. Patel, Ahsan Nazeer and Joav Merrick (Editors)
2011. ISBN: 978-1-61122-135-0 (Hardcover)
2011. ISBN: 978-1-61122-715-4 (E-book)

Climate Change and Rural Child Health
Erica Bell, Bastian M. Seidel and Joav Merrick (Editors)
2011. ISBN: 978-1-61122-640-9 (Hardcover)
2011. ISBN: 978-1-61209-014-6 (E-book)

Rural Medical Education: Practical Strategies
Erica Bell, Craig Zimitat and Joav Merrick (Editors)
2011. ISBN: 978-1-61122-649-2 (Hardcover)

Advances in Environmental Health Effects of Toxigenic Mold and Mycotoxins
Ebere Cyril Anyanwu
2011. ISBN: 978-1-60741-953-2

Child and Adolescent Health Yearbook 2009
Joav Merrick
2011. ISBN: 978-1-61668-913-1 (Hardcover)

Public Health Yearbook 2009
Joav Merrick
2011. ISBN: 978-1-61668-911-7 (Hardcover)

Child Health and Human Development Yearbook 2009
Joav Merrick
2011. ISBN: 978-1-61668-912-4 (Hardcover)

Alternative Medicine Yearbook 2009
Joav Merrick (Editor)
2011. ISBN: 978-1-61668-910-0 (Hardcover)

The Dance of Sleeping and Eating among Adolescents: Normal and Pathological Perspectives
Yael Latzer and Orna Tzischinsky (Editors)
2011. ISBN: 978-1-61209-710-7 (Hardcover)

Child and Adolescent Health Yearbook 2010
Joav Merrick (Editor)
2011. ISBN: 978-1-61209-788-6 (Hardcover)

Child Health and Human Development Yearbook 2010
Joav Merrick (Editor)
2011. ISBN: 978-1-61209-789-3

Public Health Yearbook 2010
Joav Merrick (Editor)
2011. ISBN: 978-1-61209-971-2

Living on the Edge: The Mythical, Spiritual, and Philosophical Roots of Social Marginality
Joseph Goodbread (Editor)
2011. ISBN: 978-1-60741-162-8 (Hardcover)
2011. ISBN: 978-1-61122-986-8 (Softcover)

Alternative Medicine Yearbook 2010
Joav Merrick (Editor)
2011. ISBN: 978-1-62100-132-4 (Hardcover)
2011. ISBN: 978-1-62100-210-9 (E-book)

The Astonishing Brain and Holistic Conciousness: Neuroscience and Vedanta Perspectives
Vinod D. Deshmukh
2011. ISBN: 978-1-61324-295-7 (Hardcover)

Translational Research for Primary Healthcare
Erica Bell and Joav Merrick (Editors)
2011. ISBN: 978-1-61324-647-4 (Hardcover)

Drug Abuse in Hong Kong: Development and Evaluation of a Prevention Program
Daniel T.L. Shek, Rachel C.F. Sun and Joav Merrick (Editors)
2011. ISBN: 978-1-61324-491-3 (Hardcover)

Human Development: Biology from a Holistic Point of View
Søren Ventegodt, Tyge Dahl Hermansen and Joav Merrick (Editors)
2011. ISBN: 978-1-61470-441-6 (Hardcover)
2011. ISBN: 978-1-61470-541-3 (E-book)

Our Search for Meaning in Life
Søren Ventegodt and Joav Merrick (Editors)
2011. ISBN: 978-1-61470-494-2 (Hardcover)
2011. ISBN: 978-1-61470-519-2 (E-book)

Understanding Eating Disorders: Integrating Culture, Psychology and Biology
Yael Latzer, Joav Merrick and Daniel Stein (Editors)
2011: ISBN: 978-1-61470-976-3 (Softcover)

HEALTH AND HUMAN DEVELOPMENT

THE ASTONISHING BRAIN AND HOLISTIC CONSCIOUSNESS

NEUROSCIENCE AND VEDĀNTA PERSPECTIVES

VINOD D. DESHMUKH

Nova Science Publishers, Inc.
New York

Library of Congress Cataloging-in-Publication Data

The astonishing brain and holistic consciousness: neuroscience and Vedanta perspectives / Vinod D. Deshmukh.
p. ; cm.
Includes bibliographical references and index.
ISBN 978-1-61324-295-7 (hardcover)
1. Holistic medicine. 2. Consciousness. 3. Psychology and religion. I. Deshmukh, Vinod D. II. Title.
[DNLM: 1. Holistic Health. 2. Brain--physiology. 3. Consciousness. 4. Nervous System Physiological Phenomena. 5. Religion and Psychology. W 61]
R733.A87 2011
181'.48--dc22

2011011451

Published by Nova Science Publishers, Inc. † New York

OTHER BOOKS PUBLISHED BY THE AUTHOR

Noninvasive Measurement of Regional Cerebral Blood Flow in Man
Vinod D. Deshmukh and John Stirling Meyer (1978)
SP Medical & Scientific Books
Spectrum Publications, New York, NY

Presence: The Key to Mental Excellence (1990)

The Last Leaf: A Collection of Poems and Essays (1993)

A Poet's Walk: A Collection of Poems, Essays, and Photographs (2002)

Poet's Vision: A Collection of Original Poems, Essays, and Photographs (2005)

The Front Cover: The holistic conscious energy of a Blue Heron

The cover photograph of a Blue Heron was taken by the author on the St. Johns River, in Jacksonville, Florida. The author was very lucky to capture this amazing posture of an Blue Heron, in conscious readiness just before his take-off. One can see that he had gathered all of his conscious energy, in perfect synergy, synchrony and harmony. His whole body looked like a living arrow, a perfect vector, aimed at the infinite matrix of the clear blue sky. It was as if the finite form was leaping toward the infinite formless. What a wonder it was to see such a perfect example of physical~mental attentiveness, followed by a holistic engagement in its current action. His very presence and the ready posture was a great wonder of the moment! He was a living example for presence, wisdom and the art of holistic living in harmonious communion with Nature.

The Back Cover: Author's oil painting of a beautiful Lily pond, from Vellore, India

"When a single flower blossoms,
The whole garden smiles!"

(A short poem by the author, written on September 9th 2003)

DEDICATION

This book is dedicated to the memory of my beloved father, Shri Dhundiraj Govind Deshmukh. He was my first teacher and mentor in Vedānta as well as in the art of living. He had a great passion and curiosity for all sciences and philosophies of both the East and the West. He was always thoughtful, caring and compassionate. He lived his life with equanimity *Sthitaprajña* and wisdom. He used to teach us about the nature of Brahman by explaning many of his favorite Upaniṣadic quotations like:

सर्वं खल्विदं ब्रह्म तज्जलानिति शान्त उपासीत ||३१:१४:||

"All this is verily *Brahman*. That (*tat*) from which the phenomenal existence emerges (*ja*); That in which it merges (*li*); and That in which it breathes (*an*). One should meditate on It with serenity."

Chāndogya Upaniṣ ad (3:14:1).

तदेजति तन्नैजति तद्दूरे तद्वन्तिके | तदन्तरस्य सर्वस्य तदु सर्वस्यास्य बाह्यतः ||

It, the *Brahman*, moves. It moves not. It is far. It is close. It is within all. It is beyond all. *Īśavāsyopaniṣ ad* (5).

In 1961, when I was studying for my final MD examination at BJ Medical College, Pune, India, I was clearly overwhelmed by the amount of work and study that I had to do to prepare for the examination. From my letters, my father sensed my anxiety and fear. He wrote back to me saying, "Vinod, fear not the outcome. Just do your best and remember that the Great Divine Energy is always with you, *Iṣ warī Śakti tujhyā pāṭ hīśī āhe.* ईष्वरी शक्ति तुझ्या पाठीशी आहे. That blessing still resonates in my heart and gives me strength. This book is a humble tribute to him.

This book is dedicated to the memory of my beloved mother, Shrimati Leelabai Dhundiraj Deshmukh. She was always kind, gentle and loving. She did not hate anyone and never uttered a harsh word about anyone. She lived a simple, quiet life, ever devoted to her family and God. Her gentle smile still brightens my *heart*.

This book is also dedicated to the memory of my beloved younger sister, Sau. Meena Madhav Chandekar, MA (Psycholgy). Meena was gentle, kind and loving, just like her mother. She lived a simple, loving and caring life, devoted to her family and God. She was a dedicated student of Vedānta. She loved *Jñāneṣ warī, Dāsabodha* and the spiritual poetry or *Abhanga* of many Marathi Saints, like *Śri Jñāneṣ war, Tukārām* and *Mīrabai*. She recited her favorite *Abhanga* for us, during our last telephone conversation, shortly before her unexpected death.

ठेविले अनंते तैसेचि रहावे, चित्ती असो द्यावे समाधान,
वाहिल्या उद्वेग दुखःचि केवळ, भोगणे ते फळ संचिताचे,
तुका म्हणे घालू तयावरी भार, वाहू हा संसार देवापायी.

"One should live, in the way the "Infinite Being" intended for us to live. Let the "*heart*" always be serene. Carrying the burden of anger, fear or guilt, makes one suffer even more. What one has to endure in life is the fruit of one's own past actions. Tuka says it is better to surrender one's ego and lay down the burden of this worldly life, at the feet of God."

CONTENTS

List of Original Poems by the Author

List of Figures

LIST OF AUTHOR'S ARTICLES QUOTED IN THE BOOK

1. Deshmukh, VD. Presence as a new mode of human attention. Society for Neuroscience Abstracts, 1982 November:8.
2. Deshmukh VD. Oscillatory Neural Ectoderm (ONE): the "ONE" hypothesis for human holo-encephalon and behavior. Medical Hypotheses 1987, 23: 107-108.
3. Deshmukh VD. Mental Excellence. Self-published and registered with the Library of Congress: 1988.
4. Deshmukh VD. A chain of supra-segmental neuro-oscillatory circuits: A human brain theory. Clinical Electroencephalography, 1988, 19(1): 7-13.
5. Deshmukh, VD: Presence: The Key to Mental Excellence. Jacksonville, Florida: Sunanda V Deshmukh, MD; 1990.
6. Deshmukh VD. Neurophysiological Interpretation of Ida, Pingala, and Sushumna. Neurology India, 1991; 39:125-31.
7. Deshmukh VD. Limbic-autonomic arousal: its physiological classification and review of the literature. Clinical Electroencephalography 1991, 22(1):46-60.
8. Deshmukh VD. Physiological classification of sleep-wake states: based on tri-vesicular (3V) model of the brain. Clinical Electroencephalography 1991, 22(4):225-235.
9. Deshmukh VD. Cascading morpho-regulatory energy and the biological form: Theory and Reality. Medical Hypotheses 1991, 35: 59-67.
10. Deshmukh VD. 1994. The quiescent brain and consciousness. Poster presentation in the conference on "Toward a Scientific Basis for Consciousness," Tucson, Arizona April 12-17, 1994.
11. Deshmukh, VD. Turiya: The fourth state of consciousness and the STEP model of self-consciousness. Journal of Interdisciplinary Crossroads 2004 Dec:1, 3, 551-60.
12. Deshmukh VD. Ipseity, Atman and consciousness. In the Proceedings of the Fifth International Conference of World Association of Vedic Studies. Washington, DC: 2004 July; 9–11.
13. Deshmukh VD. Neuroscience of Meditation. TSW Holistic Health and Medicine. 2006:1, 275-89.
14. Deshmukh VD. The Multistream Self: Biophysical, Mental, Social, and Existential. TheScientificWorldJOURNAL: 2008;(8):331-41.
15. Deshmukh VD. Introduction to Vedānta. In Tattva: An International online monthly magazine for Hindu youth 2009. Available from: URL: www.hinduyuva.org/tattva.
16. Deshmukh VD. Functional Brain Model: A Nested Hierarchical and Parallel Organization during Development and Evolution. Journal of Alternative Medicine Research 2010:1(1) 5-13.

17. Deshmukh VD. Vedic Psychology: A Science of Wisdom. J Altern Med Res 2011;3(1): 29-43.
18. Deshmukh VD. The Energy~Being Perspective in Neurophysics and Vedanta. In print as proceedings of a conference by the Center for Indic Studies, University of Massachusetts, Dartmouth.

FOREWORD

Professor Gururaj Mutalik

तत्वज्ञानं सुविज्ञानं पूतं च तव पुस्तकं ।
काव्य लालित्य युक्तं च मननीयं बुधैः सदा ॥

Tatvajñānaṁ suvijñānaṁ putuṁ ca tava pustakaṁ |
Kāvya lālitya yuktaṁ ca mananīyaṁ budhaiḥ sadā ||

Your book is rich with sacred philosophy and science.
Being filled with thoughtful and beautiful poetry,
It should always be pondered upon by the wise.

We are living in extraordinary times. Science and Technology led by physics and molecular biology has made significant inroads into our understanding of nature and natural laws. Quantum mechanics, Einstein's General theory of relativity and the current version of the mother of all theories – The M theory are offering lot of food for thought for the human quest toward understanding of the nature of reality. Theoretical physicists, a breed at the cutting edge of science are forced rather uncomfortably to grapple with the concept of consciousness, which is the cornerstone of all observation and measurement on which all modern theories of the nature of reality depend. Indeed, physics and philosophy, once on a non-concordant parallel trajectory, seem to converge rapidly in their common quest for understanding reality. Neurology as a branch of medicine dealing with the brain is uncovering many mysteries surrounding cognition, insight and consciousness, although we may just be studying grains of sand on a vast ocean beach!

It is at such an exciting moment that Dr. Vinod Deshmukh, blessed with a scientific understanding of modern neurology and equally adept in understanding the metaphysical interpretation of Vedantic teachings, has penned this thought-provoking book, "The Astonishing Brain and Holistic Consciousness." A holistic approach as repeatedly emphasized in his writing is the metaphysical key that can unlock many mysteries. The Challenge in metaphysics, as indeed in life, is to be able to perceive the unity and holistic dimension of the Universe, and configure the woods and not mistake the trees for the entity.

This book will be read and appreciated by all those who are willing to venture boldly beyond the self-limited frontiers of conventional thinking, that seem to believe, that it is the sole privilege of experimental sciences to unravel the mysterious universe and beyond. The book attempts to open our eyes into other avenues of comprehension. In this context it is pertinent to observe that in the Vedic culture of ancient India, these fundamental questions have been dealt with for several thousand years in the best traditions of "*Jijñāsā*," जिज्ञासा or the spirit of enquiry, often, with uncanny insights.

The icing on this delicious cake served by the author is the elegant and inspired poems, which, showcase many abstract concepts and ideas, that prose may sometime inadequately articulate.

Dr. Deshmukh deserves our appreciation and thanks for this insightful work.

Gururaj Mutalik, MD, FAMS
Dean and Professor of Medicine(Emeritus) BJ Medical College, Pune, India
Former Director WHO liaison office to the United Nations, NEW YORK, NY, USA
and Former CEO International Physicians for the Prevention of Nuclear War
(IPPNW-recipient of Nobel Prize for Peace -1985).

FOREWORD

Professor Subhash Kak

The problem of consciousness, and how it arises in the brain, is at the frontiers of both science and philosophy. According to one view, brain and mind are identical, and mind is merely the sum total of the activity in the brain. Opposed to this is the viewpoint that although mind requires a physical structure, it ends up transcending that structure.

Although the view that the brain is like a machine became influential as computers assumed a larger role in society, the limitations of this view are clear from the findings in psychology and neuroscience related to individuals with anomalous abilities. Idiot savants, or simply savants, perform spectacularly at certain tasks. Anomalous performance has been noted in the areas of mathematical and calendrical calculations, music, art, mechanical ability, memory, and unusual sensory discrimination or "extrasensory" perception. The abilities of these savants and of mnemonists cannot be understood in the framework of a machine-like mind.

Further evidence that the brain is more than a machine is provided by the phenomenon of neuroplasticity. Although it is most dramatic in the case of patients who have suffered strokes or other injury, in which the brain is able to rewire itself, it is a part of the normal behavior of the brain.

Human intelligence has aspects that cannot be equaled by computers. Machines fall short on two counts as compared to brains. Unlike brains, machines do not self-organize in a recursive manner, and whereas machines are based on classical logic, Nature's intelligence may depend on non-classical processes.

It is safe to say that modern science has been unsuccessful in describing the phenomenon of consciousness. Many scientists have long argued that any effort to bring consciousness within the framework of science is doomed to failure because it is not associated with any objectively quantifiable variable. But then what do we make of the Vedic texts of India that claim to be ātmavidyā, "science of self" or "consciousness science?" The most ancient of these is the cryptic Ṛgveda. But prose commentaries, called the Brāhmaṇas and the Upaniṣads, which appeared in the centuries following the Vedas, provide a framework to decode its narrative, establishing its central concern with consciousness.

In the Vedic view, reality, which is unitary at the deepest level, is called *Brahman* (neuter gender). Brahman engenders and, paradoxically, transcends the mind/matter split. It is identical to consciousness at the cosmic scale and it informs individual minds.

Since language is linear, whereas the unfolding of the universe takes place in a multitude of dimensions, language is limited in its ability to describe reality. Because of this limitation, reality can only be experienced and never described fully. All descriptions of the universe lead to logical paradox, and Brahman is the category transcending all oppositions. According to the Vedic view, it is impossible to develop a language-based "theory of consciousness." But consciousness may be experienced intuitively and its phenomenal traces may be understood using science.

According to the Vedas, knowledge is classified in two ways: the higher or unified and the lower or dual. The higher knowledge concerns the perceiving subject (consciousness), whereas the lower knowledge concerns objects. The higher knowledge is obtained through intuition, and the lower knowledge represents science. In addition, *darśana* is philosophy where the problem of self is taken together with some aspect of outer reality. There is a complementarity between the higher and the lower, each being necessary to define the other. This complementarity mirrors the one between mind and body. Vedānta is a *darśana* that goes into the heart of the problem of consciousness. These insights were obtained by sages through deep introspection.

Dr Vinod Deshmukh has in his book, *The Astonishing Brain and Holistic Consciousness*, brought together the latest results from neuroscience and correlated them with insights on consciousness from the Vedic tradition. This book makes important contribution to the philosophy of neuroscience and it makes Vedānta accessible to those who are not able to read its original texts.

The Astonishing Brain correlates Yogic phenomena to particular neuroscientific processes. This is a pioneering contribution that opens the door for other neuroscientists to examine the enormous literature of Vedānta. This path of inquiry has the potential of not only furthering a deeper understanding of the brain but also of the nature of reality.

Dr Deshmukh is that rare individual who is equally comfortable in the worlds of medicine and the Vedas. He has assembled nuggets from diverse Vedāntic texts and provided their Sanskrit original together with translation so that the scholars can better understand the material. This book will be valuable to scholars and laypersons alike.

Professor Subhash C Kak, PhD
Regents Professor and Head of Computer Science Department,
Oklahoma State University, Stillwater, OK 74078, USA

PREFACE: A JOURNEY TO MY *SELF*

Vinod D Deshmukh *

How did I come to write this book?

In 1955, after my high school graduation, a friend asked me, "What is your ambition in life? What do you want to become?" My answer was: "*Malā malā bhetāyaca āhe*, मला मला भेटायचं आहे; I want to meet my Self; I want to know my Self." This has been a lifelong journey to my "Self."

As a second year medical student, I happened to read in the college library, Dr Wilder Penfield's classic book "*Epilepsy and the Functional Anatomy of the Human Brain*." His pioneering work on electrically stimulating the human brain, in fully conscious patients with epilepsy, inspired me and fired my interest in the study of brain and mind. At that time, there was no neurosurgeon or a neurologist practicing in Pune, who could guide me in my search.

Therefore, after graduating from B. J. Medical College, Pune, India in 1962, I went to see Dr Ginde in Mumbai, who was one of the only four neurosurgeons, practicing in India at that time. Based on his advice, I completed three years of residency in General Surgery and obtained Master of Surgery and Fellowship in General Surgery degrees, from the University of Mumbai in 1966. Then, upon recommendation of another neurosurgeon, Dr S. N. Bhagavati, I went to do Neurosurgery residency, under the guidance of Mr. Wylie McKissok, at the National Hospital for Nervous Diseases, Queen Square, London, UK, in 1967-68.

After doing one year of Neurosurgery training, I realized that I was more interested in the relationship of brain and mind and in the functional neurosurgery for Epilepsy, rather than general neurosurgery, which I had found to be rather mechanical. Unfortunately, at that time, there was no opening in the residency program with Dr Penfield, at the Montreal Neurological Institute. But, I still cherish his encouraging letter to me to pursue Neuroscience.

Later, I received training in Clinical Neurophysiology, Neurology and Psychiatry and also did three years of research in brain blood flow and obtained the PhD degree, from the University of Glasgow, in 1972. Since then, I have worked in various academic positions as well as in private practice, in UK and USA. I have published over sixty research papers in

---

* Mailing address: 3600 Rustic Lane, Jacksonville, Florida 32217; Email: vinod38@aol.com

peer-reviewed Neuroscientific journals. I worked as a tenured Associate Professor of Neurology at the University of Florida from 1984-1996. In 2007, I retired from my Neurology practice, in St. Augustine, Florida. Finally, during the last 3 years, I have found the necessary time, energy and peace of mind to complete writing this complex book that I have been thinking about for many years. This has been my lifelong dream. It is fulfilling to see this effort come to fruition.

I found out that the answer to my original question of 1955, about the nature of my Self depended upon my own mindset and my perspective of Self. I can view myself as a vulnerable, mortal, human being, or a mindful, individual person, or an incredible, Holistic Energy-Being, which includes all that is.

Interestingly, my answer is similar to the classic answer found in the Indian Mythological literature. As Śri Hanuman expressed his feelings towards Lord Rāma as follows:

देहभावेन दासोऽस्मि | जीवभावेन त्वदंशक: ||
आत्मभावेन त्वमेवाहं | इति मे निश्चिता मतिः ||

"When I consider myself as the physical body, Dehabhāva देहभाव, I am your servant; when I consider myself as a living person, Jīvabhāva जीवभाव, I am an integral part of you; but, when I consider myself as the self-existent, holistic being, Ātmabhāva आत्मभाव, I am You. This is my firm conviction."

This book has been an attempt to build a bridge, Setubandhaḥ सेतुबंधः between Vedānta and Neuroscience. It is also a bridge between the Eastern and Western mindsets, philosophies and natural sciences.

When I wrote this book, I did not have a specific audience in my mind. It was for anyone who happens to be interested in deeper understanding of the Self and wishes to learn more about the inter-relationship between the brain and mind. It is about the science and art of meditation. The book also includes twenty five of my original poems.

The book, as the title suggests, is aimed at neuroscientists to learn more about Vedānta and for Vedāntins and the general readers to learn more about Neuroscience. It is an integration of many intellectual fields. It is not just a technical, science book or a lengthy philosophical treatise. It includes both, a detailed Neuroscientific basis for consciousness as well as the Vedic intuitive insights into the nature of consciousness. It is also about the art of purposeful life.

I have used three languages, English, Sanskrit and Marāṭ hi, because I wanted the text to be authentic with original quotations. Some of the expressions in Sanskrit and Marathi are unique and very difficult to translate accurately into English. However, I have tried to translate all Sanskrit and Marāṭhi quotations in English, including their transliterations.

It is my sincere wish that many people will enjoy reading this book and find it useful in their personal search for the meaning of life. Hopefully, it will spark a new vision, greater creativity, promote deeper Self-understanding, and allow for the blossoming of Self-contentment and an enduring peace of mind.

Vinod D Deshmukh, MBBS, MS, FCPS, PhD
Associate Professor (Emeritus)
Department of Neurology
University of Florida
Jacksonville, Florida, USA

ACKNOWLEDGMENTS

First of all, I would like to thank Prof. Joav Merrick, Professor of Child Health and Human Development, at the Ben Gurion University, Beer-Sheva, Israel. He encouraged me to write a proposal for this book to Nova Science Publishers of New York. He has served as the editor-in-chief in this series of publications on “Health and Human Development.” He has continued to guide me professionally throughout this lengthy process of writing a complex book.

I am very grateful to Prof. Gururaj Mutalik, Dean and Professor of Medicine (Emeritus) BJ Medical College, Pune, India, who wrote a concise foreword to this book, with his original Sankrit poem. Now, I know that he is not only a great teacher of Medicine, but also a Vedic scholar and a Sanskrit poet. I appreciate his clear discussions on many topics of common interest.

I wish to thank Prof. Subhash Kak, Regents Professor and Head of Computer Science Department, Oklahoma State University, Oklahoma, for his generous and prompt advice and help in accurate Sanskrit transliterations. He is not only a well known Vedic scholar, who has published extensively in this field, but also a good friend. He was kind enough to write a foreword based on his expertise in Vedanta, Computer Science and Neuroscience.

I am grateful to many of my colleagues and friends, with whom I had discussions and who wrote reviews or comments about the manuscript: Kenneth M. Heilman, MD, the James E. Rooks Jr. Distinguished Professor of Neurology, at the University of Florida School of Medicine, Gainesville, Florida, Henry J Mankin, MD, Edith M. Ashley Professor of Orthopedics Emeritus, Harvard Medical School, Boston, Massachusetts, Lothar Schafer, PhD, Wertheim Professor of Physical Chemistry, at the University of Arkansas, Antonio de Nicolas, PhD, Professor Emeritus, SUNY at Stony Brook, New York. Professor Bal Ram Singh, PhD, Director of Center for Indic Studies, at University of Massachusetts, Dartmouth, Prof. Kazanas, Athens, Greece, Dr Jana Whiddon PhD, Psychologist, Lakeland, Florida, Dr Doree Lynn PhD, practicing Psychologist, Washington, DC.

My regards to Swami Shantananda of Shānti Temple, Montrose, Philadelphia, for interesting dicussions on Vedanta and for his writing a beautiful review. My appreciation for Dr. Prem Sharma PhD a scholar of Vedic Literature and a good friend from Jacksonville, Florida, who suggested a title for the front cover photo: “A leap from finite to Infinite.” He also suggested readings from some of rare Upaniṣ ads.

My regards and gratitude to Dr Madhav Nagarkar, PhD, of Pune, India, for his appreciation of my poems and philosophical essays. I appreciate his insight into Vedānta Philosophy and Meditation. He read the manuscript meticulously, especially the Sanskrit text, and provided valuable suggestions. He encouraged me to complete this project, and was happy to see this bridge, Setubandhaḥ सेतुबंधः between Vedānta and Neuroscience.

Much appreciation for our three sons, Abhijit V. Deshmukh, MD, Ashwin V. Deshmukh, MD, and Rahul V. Deshmukh, MD, for their enthusism and suggestions about this book. I hope that it will help them in their own Life's journey.

Finally, I cannot say enough about my beloved wife, Sunanda V. Deshmukh, MD, for her loving and caring support and participation in this dream project. She carefully reviewed and discussed the whole manuscript and made many valuable suggestions. As a matter of fact, on this long journey of mutual interest, she has been a true soulmate, who walked with me for the past 50 years, with equal interest and enthusism, in both Vedānta and Neuroscience.

INTRODUCTION

एकंज्योतिः बहुधा विभाति |

Ekaṁ jyotiḥ bahudhā vibhāti.
One flame, one energy, shines in infinite ways, in many forms and processes.

The holistic energy is the whole energy, Pūrṇ aśaktiḥ पूर्णशक्तिः. Holistic consciousness is is Pūrṇ acaitanya पूर्णचैतन्य, an all-inclusive awareness of the currently situated body-mind-being of an individual person or a living organism. Holo or holos means whole, Pūrṇ a पूर्ण, complete or total. Holism, [1], is Pūrṇ atā पूर्णता, a theory that the universe and especially living nature is correctly seen in terms of interactive wholes, as all living organisms, that are more than the mere sum of their parts. It is related to and concerned with wholes or with complete systems, rather than with the analysis and treatment of the parts. It holds, that a system or an organism, is a coherent unified whole, that cannot be fully explained in terms of individual parts or characteristics. The system or an organism may have properties, in addition to those of its parts, as a completely new entity or phenomenon. For example, a water molecule has entirely new properties of wetness, fluidity and clarity, as compared to the properties of water's elements, namely, hydrogen and oxygen gases. Thus, an analysis or understanding of the parts does not provide a full understanding of the whole. The Webster's third new international dictionary defines "holism" as the philosophic theory that the determining factors in nature are wholes, such as organisms, which are irreducible to the sum of their parts and that the evolution of the universe is the record of such activity in the making of these wholes.

Holistic medicine [2] is a branch of medicine that deals with the prevention and treatment of diseases, and focuses on the whole person – including physical, mental, social, spiritual and environmental aspects – rather than on disease symptoms alone. The life mission theory states that "everybody has a purpose of life. Happiness comes from living this purpose and succeeding in expressing the core talent in one's life. To do this, it is important to develop as a person into what is known as the natural condition, a condition where the person will know himself (or herself) and use all his/her efforts to achieve what is most important for him/her."

Holistic psychology is a perspective that psychological phenomena must be studied as a whole, and that individuals are biological, psychological, and sociocultural totalities that cannot be fully explained in terms of individual components or characteristics. Holistic ecology views humans and their environment as a single natural system.

Holistic field, Pūrṇ akshetra पूर्णक्षेत्र, of consciousness, Caitanya चैतन्य, is the total awareness of an individual at the present moment. It is an all-inclusive eco-systemic consciousness of physical, mental, social, spiritual and environmental events at a given moment. "Caitanyam *Ātmā* चैतन्यं आत्मा, the energy~being~awareness is one's supreme self," says Śiva Sūtras.

The field-space or life-space, in the field theory of Kurt Lewin [3], is the totality of possible events for one person, at a particular time, that is, a person's possible options together with environment that contains them. The life-space is a representation of the environmental, biological, social and psychological influences that define one person's unique reality at a given moment in time. Contained within the life-space are positive and negative valences, which are, forces or pressures on the individual to approach a goal or move away from a perceived danger. Lewin assumes that a person is a complex energy-system. The kind of energy that performs psychological work is called psychical energy. Lewin's field theory emphasizes: i) behavior is a function of the total field that exists at the time, when the behavior occurs, b) analysis begins with the situation as a whole, from which are differentiated component parts, and iii) the concrete person, in a concrete situation, can be represented mathematically.

Another term used for holistic consciousness is "Superconsciousness." The American Psychological Association APA dictionary of psychology defined superconscious as i) a term for transpersonal awareness. ii) In certain eastern traditions, with variations in Buddhism, Hinduism and Taoism, a state in which the individual attains highest knowledge, freedom from pain and suffering, and a perfect spiritual insight, because the mind is free from (reactive) passions and (unrealistic) desires. At their most profound level, the practices of Meditation and Yoga may be directed toward the ultimate achievement of the superconscious state.

To me, superconsciousness is a unique integrative and spontaneous mode of conscious being. It is calm and clear, undistracted, blissful presence. It is an optimal alertness with the highest form of conscious energy, clarity, and calmness. It is a global, undirected, undistracted, effortless, spontaneous, vigilant attentiveness. It is an ideal, loving and caring presence, a present-mindedness, [4, 5], or mindfulness, Śamathā~Vipassanā (The symbol ~ signifies complementarity throughout this book), Buddhist's terms in Pali and probably Śamatā~Vipaśyanā शमता विपश्यना in Sanskrit (my personal interpretation).

Gunaratana, [6], described some of the characteristics of Vipassanā or mindfulness. My personal interpretation is that the word Vipassanā came from two roots, Vi or Viśeṣ eṇ a meaning in a special way and Passanā or Paśyanā means perceiving, observing, or witnessing. The ten characteristics of mindfulness are that it is i) presymbolic, ii) preverbal, prethought, soft-focused, fluent moment of pure awareness, iii) mirror-like, accurately reflecting what is presently happening, iv) unbiased and nonjudgemental observation, v) impartial watchfulness, vi) bare attentiveness without thinking, vii) presence or present-moment awareness, viii) nonegoistic alertness, ix) witnessing the passage of changing experience from moment-to-moment, witness awareness, Sākshībhāva साक्षीभाव and x) participatory observation.

J. Krishnamurti, [7], described it as a choiceless awareness and holistic observation: "One has to look at life, not the American life or the Asiatic life, but life as a whole; holistic observation; an observation that is not a particular observation; it is not one's own observation, but the observation that comprehends the totality, the holistic view of life." Such awareness is choiceless, because when there is absolute mental clarity, there is no need to think, deliberate or choose. The right behavioral decision is obvious to such a watchful mind. Such holistic observation may be called Pūrṇ adṛ ishtiḥ पूर्णदृष्टि:.

In the Vedic tradition, it has been described as the Blissful, Conscious Being, Sat~Cit~Ānanda सच्चिदानन्द. The word Sat सत् means being, existing, occuring, happening, being present, living-being, sentient being, enduring, real, actual, true, good, right, beautiful, wise, honest, essence, strong, energy, the self-existent Reality, the Truth or the universal Spirit of Brahman. Cit चित् means essential, existential awareness or consciousness-as-such. Ānanda आनन्द is spontaneous, unconditional bliss. It is characterized by cheerful serenity, Praśānti प्रशान्ति, vigilant mindfulness, Vipaśyanā विपश्यना, and a wise, calm and caring presence, Prajñā प्रज्ञा. In it an individual attains a clear understanding and an insight into his or her true nature, which is intimately embedded in Nature or Reality. One develops natural wisdom with a loving and caring attention, friendliness maitri मैत्री, compassion, karuṇ ā करुणा, and cheerfulness muditā मुदिता, toward the natural Reality as a whole. One develops freedom from egoistic thoughts, feelings of fear, anger, hostility, lust and greed. One is free of unrealistic expectations, mental pain and suffering. One is naturally calm, composed, and blissful in the present Reality-at-large. One is at-ease with self and at-home in the World. It is an inspired, creative, and altruistic way of living in the present actuality, with an everfresh sense of wonderment, Āṣ charyṁ आश्चर्य or Vismayaḥ विस्मय:, curiosity and blessedness, Dhanyatā धन्यता.

Traditionally, in Hinduism, Buddhism, and Taoism, various practices of meditation and Yoga are prescribed for the achievement of such an ideal, natural state of being. Such a superconscious state is so distinctive that it has been called the fourth state of consciousness Turīya तुरीय; the other three states being deep sleep, dream sleep state, and wakeful consciousness. The unique superconscious experience of Turīya has been well described in the Direct Self-Realization, Aparokshānubhūti अपरोक्षानुभूति, by Ādi Śaṅ karāchārya. Since such Self-experience is ineffable, it has been described mostly in negative terms as follows:

ब्रह्मैवाहं समः शान्तः सच्चिदानन्द लक्षणः | निर्विकारो निराकारो निरवद्योऽहमव्ययः ||
निरामयो निराभासो निर्विकल्पोऽहमाततः | निर्गुणो निष्क्रियो नित्यो नित्यमुक्तोऽहमच्युतः ||
निर्मलो निश्चलोऽनन्तः शुद्धोऽहमजरोऽमरः | नाहं देहो हि असद्रूपो ज्ञानं इति उच्यते बुधैः ||

I am truly the Absolute Energy~Being~Awareness, which is equanimous, serene, existential, conscious, blissful, non-changing, unformed, flawless, non-dissipating, healthy, non-symbolic (real), non-wavering, pervasive, attributeless, restful, enduring, steady, pure, immovable, infinite, sacred, non-aging, imperishable. I am not merely this represented, body-image. This is the true Self-knowledge expressed by the wise. [8].

Śri Ramaṇ a Maharṣ i summarized his philosophy of Existence and the Self as the *Heart* or the Source of our mind as follows:

हृदय कुहर मध्ये केवलं ब्रह्ममात्रं, हिअहमहम् इति साक्षात् आत्मरूपेण भाति|

हृदि विश मनसा स्वं चिन्वता मज्जता वा, पवन चलन रोधातात्मनिष्ठो भव त्वं||

"Within the sanctum of the *heart*, *Brahman* alone exists. "I…I"-feeling pulsates and shines as the *Ātman* itself. Enter your "*heart*" yourself, by self-inquiry, or ego-mergence. By quieting breathing, (and mentation), abide blissfully in your true Being~Self."

Śri Ramaṇ a Maharṣ i further explained the nature of the *heart* or the self as follows: "The Self is the Heart. The Heart is self-luminous. Light of consciousness arises from the Self and reaches the brain, which is the seat of the mind. The world is seen with the mind that is by the reflected light of the Self. It is perceived with the aid of the mind. When the mind is illumined, it is aware of the world. When it is not so illumined, it is not aware of the world. If the mind is turned in, toward the source of light, objective knowledge ceases and Self alone shines forth as the (luminous) Heart." [9].

Gautam Buddha made the following statement, when explaining to the monks the state of Nirvaṇ a: "There is, monks, an unborn, unbecome, unmade, and unconditioned. If, monks, there were no unborn, unbecome, unmade, and unconditioned, no escape (freedom) would be discerned from what is born, become, made, and conditioned. But because there is an unborn, unbecome, unmade, and unconditioned, therefore an escape (freedom) is discerned from what is born, become, made, and conditioned." [10]. Here, the death or Nirvaṇ a निर्वाण is referred to as the extinction of a conditioned, egoistic mind.

In Buddhism, self-monitoring[1] from moment-to-moment is emphasized. There are four aspects of self-monitoring: i) Awareness and contemplation on the body's current state, Kāyānupāsanā कायानुपासना. Kāyānupāsanā includes self-monitoring of body-posture, breathing, bodily activities, body's appearance, transience of bodily elements, body's vulnerability and death. ii) Awareness and contemplation on present feelings, Vedanānupāsanā वेदनानुपासना, iii) Awareness and contemplation on the menta stream and thoughts, Cittānupāsanā चित्तानुपासना and iv) Awareness and contemplation on the Universal Reality and the Cosmic laws, Dhammānupāsanā धम्मानुपासना.

THE PROCESS

Burning is a process,
And not a thing.

1 Bhikkhu Bodhi, ed. Teachings of the Buddha in the Buddha's Words: An Anthology of Discourses from the Pali Canon. Boston: Wisdom Publications, 2005:263.

A candle burns.
The fuel in a jet engine burns.
Atoms collide and
Transform into energy.
$E=MC^2$
Is the essence of
Energy transformation.

Life is a metabolic process,
And not a thing.

All organisms, amoeba to human,
Are parts of the Life-process.
Human behavior is
An expression of the human brain.

Self is a process,
And not a thing.

Our orientation, to person, place and time,
Is a due to complex brain processes.
With it, we weave the dynamic duality
Of ego-in-the-World.

Universe is a dynamic process,
And not a thing.

It includes galaxies and all that exists.
Universe is
The ultimate creative process,
And metaphorically,
The Ultimate Verse!

Vinod D Deshmukh
August 29, 2001

SANSKRIT AND MARĀTHI ALPHABET WITH TRANSLITERATION[1]

Vowels a अ ā आ i इ ī ई u उ ū ऊ ṛ ऋ ḷ ऌ e ए ai ऐ o ओ au औ

Anusvāra ṁ अं

Visarga ḥ अः

Consonants

Guttarals ka क kha ख ga ग gha घ ṅa ङ

Palatals ca च cha छ ja ज jha झ ña ञ

Cerebrals ṭa ट ṭha ठ ḍa ड ḍha ढ ṇa ण

Dentals ta त tha थ da द dha ध na न

Labials pa प pha फ ba ब bha भ ma म

Semivowels ya य ra र la ल va व

Sibilants sa स as in *sun*

śa श palatal sibilant pronounced like the soft s of *Russian*

ṣa ष cerebral sibilant as in *shun*

Others kṣa क्ष tra त्र jña ज्ञ ḷa ळ

Aspirate ha ह

---

[1] Based on: i) Radhakrishnan S. The Principal Upaniṣads. New Delhi, India: HarperCollins Publishers India; 1994: 13, ii) Kak SC. The Prajñā-Sūtras: Aphorisms of Intuition. New Delhi, India: D. K. Printworld; 2003: xi and iii) de Nicolas AT. Meditations through the ṚgVeda: Four Dimensional Man. Boulder, CO and London, UK: Shambhala; 1978. xi-xii.

AUM ॐ the symbol of *Brahman*

Chapter 1

The Sound of Silent Energy

Śānta Śaktiḥ शान्तशक्तिः Anāhata Nāda अनाहत नाद

ब्रह्मग्रंथेर्भवेद्भेदो ह्यानन्दः शून्यसंभवः ।
विचित्रः क्वणको देहे अनाहतः श्रूयते ध्वनिः ||४:७०||

When the great puzzle, or the knot of *Brahman*, is understood and solved, then, a unique, blissful sound spontaneously emerges out of the great *Emptiness*, and is clearly heard.

Hatha Yoga Pradīpikā,[1] हठयोग प्रदीपिका

When the mind is relatively free of inner chatter or talk and thoughts, in a relatively quiet place like an empty concert hall, a library, an old church, a temple, a mountain top, or a quiet forest, one may hear a fine, spontaneous, background, sound of inner silent energy and peace. This sound of silent energy has been likened variously to the humming of bees, ripples on the surface of water, a distant waterfall, a fine background instrument like a high frequency bell or drum, or a finely running, electric motor. One may hear this sound-energy especially, during meditation, when the mind remains at-ease with itself, not anchored to any object or thought, and being really still, silent and serene. This is especially true if one is sitting in a quiet room, with eyes and ears covered, and one pauses breathing momentarily and remains completely still, silent and serene. This sound of inner peace and silent energy is a reliable cue for a quiet, speechless mind, with meditative awareness and minimal mental content, memory and thoughts. Such a silent, meditative awareness is associated with a feeling of boundless energy and a sense of timeless, blissful being. A truly silent Mind listening to the great Silent Energy is a nondual state; Silence listening to Silence, is truely an indescribable wonder!

Śri Jñāneṣ wara श्री ज्ञानेष्वर described beautifully, the ineffability of such a unique experience of the great Silence, in his book, Amṛ itānubhava[2] अमृतानुभव, in the following Marathi verse:

[1] Pancham Sinh, translator. The Hatha Yoga Pradīpikā. 3rd ed. New Delhi, India: Munshiram Manoharlal Publishers; 1980. And Akers BD, translator. The Hatha Yoga Pradīpikā. Woodstock, NY: YogaVidya.com LLC; 2002.

म्हणोनी माझी वैखरी | मौनाचेंही मौन करी ||
हे पाणियावरी मकरी | रेखिलिया ||१७||

That is why my speech remains speechless, in the great Silence. Because, describing it, is like drawing a fish on the surface of water. (It serves no purpose).

Traditionally, this spontaneous, blissful, existential sound of the holistic silent energy-being is called Anāhata Nāda अनाहत नाद or Sadānand Nada सदानन्द नाद (my new term), which has been well described in the Hatha Yoga Pradīpikā हठयोग प्रदीपिका. Here are a few quotations from that source:

शक्तिमध्ये मनःकृत्वा शक्तिं मानस मध्यगाम् |
मनसा मन आलोक्य धारयेत्परमं पदम् ||४:५३||

Center the mind in the holistic energy and that energy in the mind. Observe the mind with the mind, and then, dwell in that highest conscious state.

सर्व चिन्ता परित्यज्य सावधानेन चेतसा |
नाद एव अनुसंधेयो योग साम्राज्यमिच्छता ||४:९३||

One, who aspires to master the art and science of yoga, should let go of all mental activities, worries and thoughts, and be aware of the intrinsic sound of the silent energy, with an attentive mind.

तावदाकाश संकल्पो यावद्शब्दः प्रवर्तते |
निःशब्दम्तत्परम् ब्रह्म परमात्मेति गीयते ||४:१०१||

The idea of a mental space or an experiential field exists, as long as there is a verbal thought or an object, occupying the mind. When the mind stays empty and free of inner voices and thoughts, one reaches the highest, nonverbal state of *Ātman~Brahman* sthiti.

यत्किंचिन्नाद रूपेण श्रूयते शक्तीरेव सा |
यस्तत्वान्तो निराकारः स एव परमेश्वरः ||४:१०२||

One hears sound-energy only, whenever any form of sound is heard. One, who is beyond all forms and phenomena, is the Supreme Being.

सदा नादानुसंधानात् क्षीयन्ते पापसंचया :|

---

[2] Joga NR. Sārtha Śri Amṛ itānubhava by Śri Jñāneshwara. Pune, India: Yaśawant Prakāśan; 2004, 7th ed; 10:17.

निरंजने विलीयते निश्चितम्चित्त मारुतौ ||४:१०५||

Unhealthy thoughts, memories and habits are dissipated by constantly dwelling on the intrinsic, sound of silent energy. Breathing and mental activity definitely merge in the spotless, silent Awareness.

This description of the transcendental, inward sound of the essential Mind is similar to the description of an inner, spontaneous sound that one hears when the mind is inwardly silent with no inner speech or thought. It is known as Anāhata Nāda अनाहत नाद in the Yogic literature as well, and it is well described by Ādi Śankaracharya in Nādānusandhān नादानुसंधान, a section of Yogatāravali[3] योग तारावली.

Śri Ramaṇ a Maharṣ i[4] remained blissfully silent most of the time. People were touched and healed by his great, serene Silence. This is what he said about language and Silence: "Language is only a medium for communicating one's thoughts to another. It is called in only after thoughts arise; other thoughts arise after the 'I-thought' rises; the 'I-thought' is the root of all conversation. When one remains without thinking, one understands another by means of the universal language of Silence. Silence is ever-speaking; it is a perennial flow of language; it is interrupted by speaking. These words obstruct that mute language. There is electricity flowing in a wire. With resitance to its passage, it glows as a lamp or revolves as a fan. In the wire it remains as electric energy. Similarly also, Silent Energy is the eternal flow of language (energy) obstructed by words."

The fact that this holistic energy flows for ever, like a great river has been beautifully expressed in Vijñāna Bhairava[5] विज्ञान भैरव:

अनाहते पात्रकर्णे अभग्न शब्दे सरिद् द्रुते |
शब्द ब्रह्मणि निष्णातः परं ब्रह्माधिगच्छति ||३८||

One who is deeply versed and steeped in Anāhat Nāda attains to *Brahman*. This Anāhata Nāda is *Brahman* in the form of sound energy. This is vibrating inside (all) spontaneously. This can be heard only by the ear that has been trained, and made competent by Yoga. This energy goes on sounding uninterruptedly, and it rushes headlong like a (rapid) river.

Swāmi Chinmayānanda[6] expressed this divine Peace and Silence as follows: "You can experience at this moment a Godly Peace and a Divine Silence descending upon you, wrapping your heart in folds of a Supreme Joy. Remain in that position as long as you can. This state of Silence, at its highest intensity, is a state of transcendence of the the mind and the intellect. It will take some time for the individual to master it, because of his habit of

3 Varadānand-Bhārati S. Ātmānusandhān: Parāpuja and Yoga-Tārāvali. 3rd ed. Pune, India: Śri Rādhā-Dāmodhar Pratiśthāna; 2003.
4 Ramanan VS. ed. Talks with Śri Ramaṇ a Maharṣ i. Tiruvannamalai, India: Sri Ramaṇ aśramam; 2010:210.
5 Singh J. Vijñāna-Bhairava or Divine Consciousness: A Treasury of 112 types of Yoga. Delhi, India: Motilal Banarasidas Publishers; 1999: 36.
6 Chinmayānanda S. Meditation and Life. Chennai, India: Chinmaya Publication; 1962:124-125.

thinking – his habit of entertaining thought currents always in the mind. As soon as he comes to that state of no-thought, he automatically and unconsciously initiates for himself new thread of thoughts to follow! The longer the interval that one can create between the moment one has "stopped" chanting and the moment when the first thought current enters, the more shall one experience the positive quality and the vitality of the seemingly empty existence. With reference to the endless thought currents and their non-stop rumbling disturbances, the mental atmosphere at this moment is "empty." But, with reference to the positive Spirit and the life in the Spirit, this state is not an empty "non-existence," but it is the all-full existence, Paripūrṇ a Sat परिपूर्ण सत्.

Swami Iśwarānanda[7] expressed the power of silence: "Silence supports sound. Before the beginning of sound, there is silence and when the sound ceases to be, there is silence. Unless you are silent, you can't listen. In the seat of meditation, you try to listen to silence. Silence is not mere absence. If you are looking for sound, you will find silence is absence of sound. If you seek silence, you do not see any absence; you discover only a presence, which has no particular characteristic. It just *is*. Your true self is like silence. It is complete presence."

The Buddhist Suraṅ gama Sūtra[8] सुरंगम सूत्र emphasized the value of transcendental and intuitive listenting inward. "How sweet and mysterious is the Transcendental Sound of Avalokiteṣ wara![9] It is the pure Brahman Sound, or Nāda Brahma नादब्रह्म. It is the subdued murmur of the sea-tide settling inward. Its mysterious Sound brings liberation and peace to all sentient beings, who in their distress are calling for aid; it brings a sense of permanency to those, who are truly seeking the attainment of Nirvaṇ a's Peace… All the Brothers in the Great Assembly, and you too, Ānand, should reverse your outward perception of hearing, and listen inwardly for the perfectly unified and intrinsic sound of your own Mind-Essence, for as soon as you attain perfect accomodation, you will have attained to the Supreme Enlightenment."

J. Krishnamurti expressed his observations of this spontaneous, inner silence. "Sound plays an extraordinary part in our lives: the sound of thunder, a flute playing in the distance, the unheard sound of the universe; the sound of silence; the sound of one's own heart beating; the sound of a bird and the noise of a man walking on the pavement; the waterfall. The universe is filled with sound. This sound has its own silence; all living things are involved in this sound of silence. To be attentive is to hear this silence and move with it." (From Letters to the Schools vol II, p 30).

J. Krishnamurti elaborated: "When you realize that there is no method, no system, that no mantram, no teacher, nothing in the world that is going to help you to be quiet, when you realize the truth that it is only the quiet mind that sees, then the mind becomes extraordinarily quiet. It is like seeing danger and avoiding it; in the same way, seeing that the mind must be completely quiet, it is quiet. Now the quality of silence matters… a mind that has limitless space and that quietness, that stillness, has no centre as the `me', the `observer,' is quite

7 Iśwarānanda S. Appreciating the Presence. In Tejomayānada S, Shantānanda S, eds. Living in the Present. Langhorne, PA: Chinmaya Publications; 2008: 43-46.

8 Goddard D, ed. A Buddhist Bible. Boston, MA: Beacon Press; 1994:257-260.

9 A form of Lord Buddha Amitābha with eleven faces, thousand eyes and hands to help the suffering sentient beings. He or She hears the Sound that illumines the world. He is endowed with great compassion and wisdom, Maha-karuṇ ā and Prajñā. Kohn MH, translator. The Shambhala Dictionary of Buddhism and Zen. Boston, MA: Shambhala; 1991: 14-15.

different. In that silence there is no `observer' at all; that quality of silence has vast space, it is without border and intensely active; the activity of that silence is entirely different from the activity which is self-centered. If the mind has gone that far (and really it is not that far, it is always there if you know how to look), then perhaps that which man has sought throughout the centuries, God, Truth, the immeasurable, the nameless, the timeless, is there – without your invitation, it is there. Such a man is blessed; there is truth for him and ecstasy." (From The Flight of the Eagle by J. Krishnamurti).

Swāmi Paramānanda[10] expressed the value of observing inner silence and peace. He made an observation that inner silence and peace can be attained through absence of thought as well as through fullness of thought. "In that hour of silent co-ordination, when of all our faculties are in perfect tune, we realize that we are part of the cosmic Being. It is in this hour, we find the fullness of our Life, for then our little life has become united with the great Life, and our little mind with the cosmic Mind. Only at such moments, when the finite and the Infinite are so commingled, does our mind stand apart in speechless Silence and unspoken Wonder."

The therapeutic value, of whole-hearted listening and inner silence, are well recognized in modern psychology and psychotherapy. As an advice to novice counselors, Christine Longaker[11] said: "You must listen with your whole being, not just your ears. Listen with your body, your heart, your eyes, your energy, your total presence. Listen in silence, without interrupting."

Michael Hutton[12] described a spontaneous subtle sound that one may hear. "One could also practice noticing the silence of newly falling snow, or that on a mountain top, or in a deep forest, or in the depths of the sea. There is the sound of silence, of the late night, or predawn hours, before the world awakens to a new day. When we are truly in silence, we open not only our hearing, but our curiosity as well: what is there? ... We may become aware of the subtle sound current, which is often there, a very quiet vibration, which may be background vibration of the Earth. Listening to silence, is truly one of the great spiritual practices, in which we tune into a deeper level of Being and experience."

TEMPLE OF SILENCE

In the temple of Silence,
The Deity is Silent.
The devotees and their prayers are silent
Because they know

That saying any word would break
The wonder of this natural Silence.

---

10 Paramānanda S. Silence as Yoga. Cohasset, MA: Vedanta Centre, Inc; 1974: 25-26.

11 Longaker C. Listening with presence, awareness and love. In Brady M. ed. The wisdom of listening. Boston, MA: Wisdom Publications; 2003:7-23.

12 Hutton MS. Listening to the Land. In Brady M. ed. The wisdom of listening. Boston, MA: Wisdom Publications; 2003: 243-257.

In the temple of Infinite Space,
The Deity is still.
The devotees are also still,
Because they know
That any movement would disturb
The wonder of this natural Order.

In the temple of Serenity,
The Deity is serene.
The devotees are also serene
Because they know
That any negative emotion would nullify
The beauty of this natural Bliss.

This temple of Silence is within us.
Its door is always open.
If we can be naturally
Silent, Still and Serene,
Even for a moment,
Then, the great Wonder
Will reveal itself,
From within!

Vinod D Deshmukh

April 30, 2005

Chapter 2

HOLISTIC ENERGY~BEING~AWARENESS चिदात्मशक्ति: PERSPECTIVE

Holistic Energy, Pūrṇ aśaktiḥ पूर्णशक्ति: Holistic Being, Pūrṇ ātman पूर्णात्मन्

Holistic Awareness, पूर्ण चित्

शक्तिः शक्तात्पृथक् नास्ति | तद्वद्दृष्टेः न चाभिदा ||

The energy is not different from the person, who possesses it, because they cannot be experienced separately.

Subodha Pañcadaśi[1] सुबोध पञ्चदशी

According to the energy-matter perspective of Śaktism, the Absolute is, on the one hand, unchanging, unqualified and formless, potential energy and on the other hand, dynamic, qualified, and actualized matter, with endless forms and processes. Śiva शिव and Śaktiḥ शक्ति: represent these two aspects of the Absolute Reality respectively. These two principles, namely, Śiva and Śaktiḥ are inseparable from each other and together they form one integral Reality of the whole Universe. It is interesting to note that this ancient concept of interconnectedness between energy and matter, Śiva and Śaktiḥ or Puruṣ a and Prakṛ iti, is subjectively not different from Einstein's fundamental equation, $E = MC^2$ in modern physics.

The holistic Energy-Being is also called Parāśaktiḥ and Paramātman as described in the following verse from the Vijñāna Bhairava.[2]

शक्ति शक्तिमतोर्यद्वत् अभेदः सर्वदा स्थितः |

अतः तत्धर्म धर्मित्वात्पराशक्तिः परमात्मनः ||१८||

---

[1] Vishnu Waman Bapat (Translator & Publisher). Subodha Pañcadaśi by Vidyāranya Muni. Pune, India: 1922:651-654.

[2] Singh J. Vijñāna-Bhairava or Divine Consciousness: A Treasury of 112 types of Yoga. Delhi, India: Motilal Banarasidas Publishers; 1999: 16.

Since there is never any difference between the Energy, Śaktiḥ and the possessor of energy the Being, Śaktimataḥ शक्तिमत:, hence, the primal Energy Śaktiḥ is endowed with the same attributes as those of the primal Being, Ātman. Therefore, being non-different from Paramātman, the highest being, Bhairava, She is known as Parāśaktiḥ, the highest Energy, Bhairavi.

In Vīra वीर (Strong, Courageous) Śaivism, the conscious energy was called Citśaktiḥ चित्शक्ति: and the unconscious energy was named as the Acitśaktiḥ अचित्शक्ति:. Śri Caitanya[3] (1486-1533 A.D.) described three forms of holistic energy: i) the essential, Psychic or Swarūpaśaktiḥ स्वरूपशक्ति:, the intrinsic energy Antaraṅ gā Śaktiḥ अन्तरङ्गा, or the Transcendental Energy, Parāśaktiḥ परा, ii) Jīvaśaktiḥ जीव or Taṭ asthāśaktiḥ तटस्था, the standing energy of being still, silent, serene, and iii) Mayāśaktiḥ माया or Bahiraṅ gā Śaktiḥ बहिरङ्गा for the experience of the manifestated, external world.

J. Krishnamurti described the highest form of conscious energy as apogee (apo: far from + ge: earth), meaning ego-free, selfless, spontaneous, conscious energy. "The highest form of this energy, the apogee, is the state of mind when it has no idea, no thought, and no sense of direction or motive – that is pure energy. And that quality of energy cannot be sought after." [11].

Śri Aurobindo personified the Superconscious Energy as the divine Mother or Mahāśaktiḥ महाशक्ति:, who had four personalities or qualities in the form of: i) self-knowledge and wisdom, Maheṣ warī महेष्वरी, ii) strength and creativity Mahākālī महाकाली, iii) harmony and beauty, Mahālakshmī महालक्ष्मी, and iv) perfection in skills and knowledge, Mahāsaraswatī महासरस्वती. [12].

A living organism is essentially, a biophysical signal-transformer or converter. A signal is the complex of biophysical energy-matter-information. Such transformative or metabolic activity is a fundamental property of all Life, living organisms or beings. A living organism's neurobiological energy can manifest in many forms: i) the neuromuscular-motor energy for physical and biomechanical work, ii) the vocal-phonetic energy for speech, cognition and verbal communication, iii) the neuro-physiological, metabolic energy for visceral processes, like respiration, digestion, Prāṇ aśaktiḥ प्राणशक्ति:, iv) the conscious and preconscious mental mental energy, Mananaśaktiḥ मननशक्ति: or Citśaktiḥ चित्शक्ति:, iv) the spontaneous energy energy of essential, self-aware being, Swayaṁ Jyotiḥ स्वयंज्योति:, and v) the explosive energy, Sphotaśaktiḥ स्फोटशक्ति: of the universe and vi) the Kuṇ ḍ alini Śaktiḥ कुण्डलिनिशक्ति[4] which continuously creates and supports all Life on Earth and elsewhere in the universe. It is also called the incomprehensible Energy, Acintyaśaktiḥ अचिन्त्यशक्ति: or

3 Sinha KP. The Self in Indian Philosophy. Calcutta, India: Punthi Pustak; 1991:121-164.

4 The subject of Kuṇ ḍ alini Śaktiḥ is complex and controversial. I have given an explanation with references in a later chapter.

Brahmaśaktiḥ ब्रह्मशक्तिः. Brahman, as a cosmic, tranformative Energy-Being is beautifully described in the Bhagvad Gītā: IV: 24.

ब्रह्मार्पणं ब्रह्महविः ब्रह्माग्नौ ब्रह्मणा हुतं |
ब्रह्मैव तेन गन्तव्यं ब्रह्मकर्मसमाधिना ||

The dynamic, existential, cosmic process is *Brahman*. The energy-matter-information or the fuel offered to the sacred fire, in the devotional worship, Yajña यज्ञ, is *Brahman*. The person or the agent, making the devotional offering, is *Brahman*. The sacred fire, the transformative energy, is *Brahman*. One, who realizes this holistic, cosmic process, realizes *Brahman* itself. (From Bhagvad Gītā भगवद्गीता ४:२४).

In this sense, all of our transient, phenomenal experiences continuously dissipate in the living, matrix or the field of our conscious awareness. This is the wonder of true conscious living, which we need to learn and appreciate, at each moment.

स्पन्दशक्तिश्च वातेषु दाढ्र्यशक्तिः तथोपले |
द्रवशक्तिः तथांभसु दाहशक्तिः तथानले ||१६||
शून्यशक्तिः तथाकाशे नाशशक्तिः विनाशिनि |
यथा अण्डे अन्तर्महासर्पो जगदस्ति तथात्मनि ||१७||
फल पत्र लता पुष्प शाखा विटप मूलवान् |
ननु बीजे यथा वृक्षः तथेदम् ब्रह्मणि स्थितम् ||१८||

This quote is from Subodha Pañcadaśi सुबोध पञ्चदशी. Its translation: "The wind has vibrational-sound energy; a rock has the potential energy of inertia; water has energy of fluidity; fire has heat energy; sky has the energy of an empty space or vaccum; destruction-creation has transformative, dissipative energy. Just as the embryo of even a huge python is contained in a tiny egg, the whole experiential world is contained within me, the Ātman. Just as a tiny seed, potentially contains a giant fig tree, with fruits, leaves, vines, flowers, branches and roots, similarly, all of this existence is contained in Brahman.

During a quiet meditative state, one can feel this holistic, experiential energy~being~awareness field. It is the essential, existential, ground-energy, with infinite qualities and aspects. Complete description of this infinite, holistic energy~being~awareness or Sat~Cit~Ānanda सच्चिदानन्द is humanly impossible. In brief, it may be symbolized by:

A still body, a silent mind, serene feeeling and an infinite conscious space,
It is the very Source of all Self-Healing Energy (SHE),
The Pūrṇ aśaktiḥ पूर्णशक्तिः~Pūrṇ ātman पूर्णात्मन्~Pūrṇ acit पूर्ण चित्

I find it helpful to use the following twelve adjectives for the holistic energy~being~awareness चिदात्मशक्तिः for better understanding and a reminder of this unique, ineffable state during daily prāṇ āyāma and meditation:

Pūrṇ a (Holistic reality)	Śūnya (Empty awareness)	Spanda[5] (Pulsating body)
Prāṇ a (Breath-energy)	Rasa (Satisfying taste)	Amrita (Nectar content)
Mouna (Silent mind)	Acala (Unmoving eyes)	Śānta (Serene feeling)
Akhaṇ da (Indivisible reality)	Ananta (Infinite energy)	Acintya unthinkable truth

These adjectives only point to the great holistic Reality, but one has to experience and feel It, in one's own energy~being. This amazing, ineffable, primordial, foundational, holistic energy has been described using many adjectives like the Holistic Pūrṇ aśaktiḥ पूर्णशक्तिः, the Self Ātmaśaktiḥ आत्मशक्तिः, the Primal Ādiśaktiḥ आदिशक्तिः, the Divine Śivaśaktiḥ शिवशक्तिः, the Still-Silent Taṭ asthā Śaktiḥ तटस्थाशक्तिः, the Essential Swarūpaśaktiḥ स्वरूपशक्तिः, the Transcendental Parāśaktiḥ पराशक्तिः, the Existential Brahmaśaktiḥ ब्रह्मशक्तिः, the Infinite Anantaśaktiḥ अनन्तशक्तिः, and the Incomprehensible Acintyaśaktiḥ अचिन्त्यशक्तिः!

The self-healing holistic Energy is i) the rock-bottom or the ground of all of our physical, physiological, behavioral and mental energies and activities; ii) no transient phenomena like any action, movement, a word or a thought can affect or alter It; iii) It is like a living, pilot flame, that is spontaneously and continuously burning, enrgizing and self-organizing; iv) It manifests in infinite ways, in all life-forms and processes; v) It is spontaneous, self-integrating, multi-modal, and multi-dimensional; vi) It can take various energy-forms like the biomechanical, biochemical, neuro-electromagnetic, behavioral, psychic, mental and conscious energies; vi) an organism-in-environemnt or a person-in realtiy is a unified field of this holistic Energy; vii) all of our conscious and subconscious experiences depend on this holistic Energy; viii) it is, through the holistic Energy-Being perspective, that we can liberate ourselves from the limited, petty, selfish, ignorant, fear-driven, habitual and egoistic mental tendencies and lifestyles. SHE is the wonder of all wonders. We can feel her enduring and ever fresh presence and verify this truth, in our own energy~being, in our innermost "*heart*," at any moment. The holistic Energy-Being is always there, only if we knew how to "BE" in the present moment. As Śri Ramaṇ a Maharṣ i said, "All that we have to do is just BE; and not be this or that."

---

5 Spanda means spontaneous pulsating or throbbing of life. It is the Divine creative pulsation. It is the throb of ecstacy of the Divine I-Consciousness (Vimarśa). It is the throb of Śiva's absolute freedom or swātantrya. It is the primal creative quivering or vibration. It is movement as it were. It reminds me of David Bohm's term, "Holo-movement." To me, it is high-frequency creative energy~awareness like a scanning or strobe light. In the brain, it would be high-frequency electromagnetic activity like the gamma waves and higher, typically seen during vigilant attentiveness. Spanda also means pulse, which can be sensed during meditation. See Singh J. Spanda-Kārikās: The Divine Creative Pulsation. Motilal Banarasidass Publishers, Delhi, India. 1980. Reprint 2009: xvi-xviii.

The voluntary act of this complete ego-surrender to the Infinite, the Universal Energy reminds me of a beautiful short Marathi poem by a well known saint, Tukārāma. Here is his poem and its translation:

ठेविले अनन्ते तैसेचि रहावे, चित्ती असो द्यावे समाधान,
वाहिल्या उद्वेग दु:खचि केवळ, भोगणे ते फळ संचिताचे,
तुका म्हणे घालू तयावरी भार, वाहू हा संसार देवापायी.

One should live, in the way the "Infinite Being" intended for us to live. Let the "*heart*" be serene always. Carrying the burden of anger, fear, conflicts and worries, makes one suffer even more. What one has to endure in life are the fruits of one's own past actions and thoughts. Tuka says it is better to surrender and lay down the burden of this worldly life, at the feet of God.

During quiet meditation, one has a feeling of conviction that this entire observable phenomenon is not me; "(this is) not me, not me," Neti, Neti नेति, नेति. I am the intrinsic, spontaneous, self-existent, self-content, and self-aware psychic Being, the holistic Self, Pūrṇ ātman पूर्णात्मन् or the primal Being Ādipuruṣ a आदिपुरुष. The holistic energy and being are two aspects of the same primal Reality, which is Nitya, Nirmal Swarūpa नित्य निर्मल स्वरूप.

Vedānta described four stages of this existential, mystical union between the holistic Energy Pūrṇ aśaktiḥ पूर्णशक्तिः the holistic Being, Pūrṇ ātman पूर्णात्मन् and Pūrṇ acit पूर्ण चित्. These four statges are i) being in the same existential field, Sālokya सालोक्य, ii) being closest to one's essential Being, Sāmipya सामिप्य, iii) being of the same form or essence, Sārupya सारुप्य, and iv) being united with the Energy-Being itself, Sāyujya सायुज्य.[6]

Ādi Śankarāchārya has beautifully expressed such mystical union in his collection of verses called Brahma Jñānāvali[7]. The following is the last verse concluding the essential, existential union of Energy-Being:

अन्तर्ज्योतिः बहिर्ज्योतिः प्रत्यक्ज्योतिः परात्परः |
ज्योतिर्ज्योतिः स्वयंज्योतिः आत्मज्योतिः शिवोऽस्मिहम् ||१९||
आदि शङ्कराचार्य; ब्रह्मज्ञानावली

I am the intrinsic energy, the extrinsic energy, the existential energy, the transcendental energy. I am the energy of energy, the self-effulgent energy, and the self-energy. I am Lord Śiva, the God of absolute auspiciousness and perfect goodness.

6 From Ādi Śankaracharya's "Śivananda Lahari."

7 Ādi Śankarāchārya. Brahma Jñānāwali. In Chinmayānanda S. Meditation and Life. Chennai, India: Chinmaya Publication; 1962: 131-136.

THE LETTER 'S'

Slow, but
Steady flow and the momentary
Stillness of a
Soft breath;

Spontaneous, and
Speechless,
Sweet
Song of
Silence;
Spacious, undistracted,
Spherical and effortless awareness;

It is the
Spectacular
Source and
Sink of conscious experience, and the
Sense of my
Situational
Self.

So resourceful is
The letter 'S' on this
Slippery
Slope of
Serenity, with cascading
Streams of
Sights,
Sounds, and
Silence! What a wonderful
Surprise this is!

Vinod D Deshmukh
July 31, 2009

Chapter 3

EVOLUTIONARY ENERGY

KUṆḌALINI ŚAKTIḤ कुण्डलिनि शक्तिः

FROM UNCONSCIOUSNESS TO HOLISTIC CONSCIOUSNESS

तमसो मा ज्योतिर्गमय।

TAMASO MA JYOTIRGAMAYA

LEAD US FROM THE UNCONSCIOUS TO HOLISTIC CONSCIOUSNESS

A Journey from the Collective Unconscious to the Collective Conscious: A New Understanding and Interpretation

Introduction and Review

Historically, Kuṇ ḍ alini has been understood to be the unconscious, automatic, or spontaneous, neuro-behavioral energy of an organism. It is a dormant and multi-dimensional bio-energy in all animals and human beings. The concept of Kuṇ ḍ alini and the oscillatory neural centers of energy called, Cakra चक्र, in Sanskrit have been a great mystery for many centuries. This ancient system of bio-energy is being widely used for health promotion, disease prevention, personal growth, and as a path to Self-realization and Self-mastery. It has been described in details in the ancient Sanskrit literature dating back to at least 800 BC. Earlier, during the Vedic-Upanishadic period in India, it was passed on, through generations by oral tradition.

It is currently practiced as Kuṇ ḍ alini Yoga, Prāṇ āyāma, and dhyānaṁ or meditation, which involve Self-regulation and Self-mastery of breathing and all egoistic mental activity. These concepts of bio-energy, Prāṇ āyāma, yoga, and meditation are now coming into the main stream of Alternative, Complimentary, Integrative medicine and Mental Health [13, 14]. Certain Kuṇ ḍ alini Yoga techniques are being evaluated for specific psychiatric disorders, couple therapy and personal growth [15]. Dr. C. G. Jung gave four lectures on the Psychology of Kuṇ ḍ alini Yoga in 1932, which have been recently published [16].

Energy is the capacity to do work. The neurobiological energy is an organism's capacity to do physiological, physical and mental work. It is what an organism is capable of doing. Neuromuscular energy achieves physical work, whereas attentional energy achieves cognitive and mental work. Animal behavior, including cognition and mentation, is what an organism does. The intrinsic state of an organism is defined by its current molecule-energy-information content, its affective state, and the environmental input or context. In a broad sense, neurobehavioral energy is the creative force of an organism in the natural world.

The Sanskrit word Kuṇ ḍ alini means potential bio-energy, which is in a circular or spiral, winding form, like a conch shell or a coiled-up snake. Cakra means a whirlpool of bio-energy similar to an electromagnetic field or an oscillatory neural network [17 - 20]. Several books on the subject of Kuṇ ḍ alini and Cakra are currently available [21 - 27].

इह स्थाने चित्तं निरवधि विनिधायात्मसंपूर्णयोगः |
कविर्वाग्मि ज्ञानी स भवति नितरां साधकः शान्तचेतः ||
त्रिकालानां दर्शि सकलहितकरो रोगशोकप्रमुक्तश्चिरन्जीवी |
जीवी निरवधिविपदां ध्वंसहंसप्रकाशः ||३१||

Śat-Cakra-Nirūpaṇ a[1]

He/she who have attained complete knowledge of the *Ātman~Brahman* by constantly dwelling his mind, Citta, on this Lotus, becomes eloquent and wise, and such a great sage enjoys uninterrupted peace of mind. He perceives three periods of time, past, present and future, and becomes a compassionate benefactor of all. He is free from disease and sorrow and lives a long life. He lives like Hamsa, Antarātmā, the destroyer of fears and dangers.

From this and other verses in Śat Cakra Nirūpaṇ a, one can see that by practicing Kuṇ ḍ alini Yoga, one develops special knowledge, skills and virtues like deep Self-understanding, enduring meditative awareness with a steady peaceful mind, mindful presence and benevolence towards all. Being a compassionate benefactor to all is similar to Buddha's great compassion, Mahakaruṇ ā, for all living beings. One also becomes free of mental pain, suffering and disease. One lives a long healthy life, free of psychological stress and fears.

The six Kuṇ ḍ alini Cakra or energy-centers have been described in the ancient text of Yogakuṇ ḍ alyupaniṣ ad[2], योगकुण्डल्युपनिषद्

षट् चक्राणि परिज्ञात्वा प्रविशेत्सुखमण्डलम् |
मूलाधारं स्वाधिष्ठानं मणिपूरं तृतीयकम् ||९||
अनाहतं विशुद्धिं च आज्ञाचक्रं च षष्ठकम् |
आधारं गुदमित्युक्तं स्वाधिष्ठानं तु लैङ्गिकम् ||१०||
मणिपुरं नाभिदेशं हृदयस्थमनाहतम् |
विशुद्धिः कण्ठमूले च आज्ञाचक्रं च मस्तकम् ||११||

1 Arthur Avlon (Sir John Woodroffe). The Serpent Power: The Secrets of Tantric and Śaktic Yoga including the translation of Śat Cakra Nirūpaṇ a and Padukā-Pañcaka. New York: Dover Publications, Inc. 1974: 390.

2 Sharma S. ed. 108 Upaniṣ ad: Sādhanā Khaṇ ḍ a. Mathura, India: Yuga Nirmāṇ a Yojanā; 2005:195-209.

By knowing and experiencing the six Cakra, one enters the sphere of great Bliss. The six Cakras are named, in the ascending order, as Mūlādhāraṁ, Swādhiṣ ṭ hānaṁ, Maṇ ipūraṁ, Anāhataṁ, Viśuddhiṁ, Ājñā Cakra. Mūlādhāraṁ Cakra is located in the perineum; Swādhiṣ ṭ hānaṁ Cakra is located around genitals; Maṇ ipūraṁ Cakra is located in the umbilical region; Anāhataṁ Cakra is located in the region of heart, in the chest; Viśuddhiṁ Cakra is located in the throat region, related to the larynx and Ājñā Cakra is located in the forehead, between eyebrows.

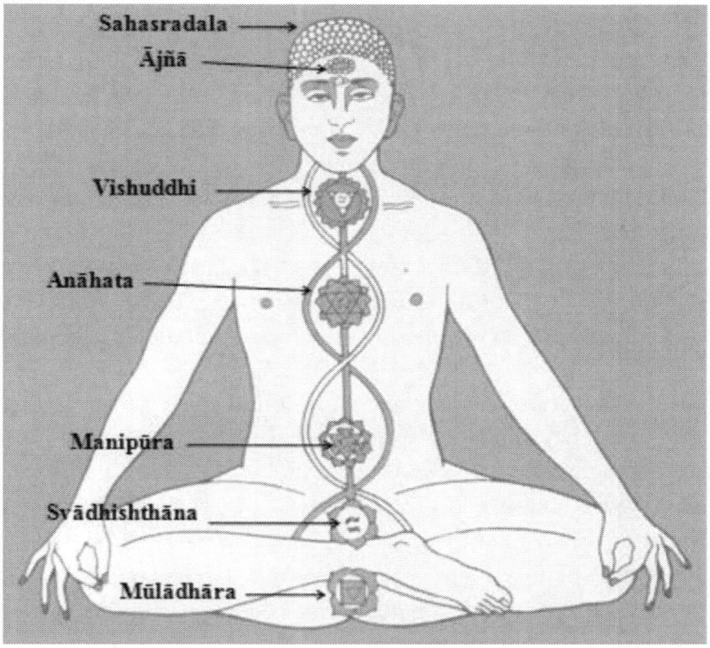

Figure 1. A diagram[3] of the approximate locations of the six Kuṇ ḍ alini Cakra as described in the ancient Upaniṣ adic text. These Cakra are symbolic representations of the functional neuromagnetic energy circuits. (Please see the neurophysiological interpretation below).

Jung CG, in his series of lectures in 1932, on "The Psychology of Kuṇ ḍ alini Yoga," briefly described each of the six Kuṇ ḍ alini Cakra or energy-centers. He emphasized that the rise of Kuṇ ḍ alini is a process of becoming Conscious. Mookerjee has described seven Cakrās in details. Shannahoff-Khalsa has interpreted the Cakrās from the psychological perspective. The following is a brief synopsis based on all of these references, without too many symbolic details:

i. *Mūlādhāra Cakra* is the ground or foundation, and it represents the energy of the Earth. The activity in this center is unconscious, latent and dormant. Its symbol is an elephant, which represents a living organism or a sentient being. The lotus of this Cakra has four petals. The sense of smell (tanmātrā) is experienced here. This Cakra is primarily for organism's survival.

3 This diagram is a modified figure based on plate 1 in Arthur Avlon (Sir John Woodroffe). The Serpent Power: The Secrets of Tantric and Śaktic Yoga including the translation of Śat-Chakra-Nirupaṇ a and Padukā-Panchaka. New York: Dover Publications, Inc. 1974.

ii. *Swādhiṣ ṭ hāna Cakra* is the second energy center, representing the energy of water or fluids. It corresponds with the water-sphere and rules the bladder (and kidneys). It is the seat of desire and error. The symbol of this Cakra is an acquatic monster, like a crocodile. The lotus of this Cakra has six petals. It governs the functions of taste and the vital breath prāṇ a. This Cakra represents sexuality and reproduction.

iii. *Maṇ ipūra Cakra* is the third center representing light and heat energy. It is located in the navel region. It is the place of fire of desire, motivation and mental vacillation due to being cought in the pairs of opposites like to approach or to avoid, to do or not to do. These opposites generate conflicting emotions and passions. Anger can be controlled by concentrating on this Cakra. It is also symbolic of the life-force of the meat-eating, corporeal human being. The lotus of this Cakra has ten petals. It is related to the functions of sight and light. This Cakra is for the ego, its power and territory.

iv. *Anāhata Cakra* is the fourth center representing air and vibrational energy. It is related to the heart and compassion. It represents prāṇ a or vāyu-śakti. This is the seat of puruśa or the conscious human being. It is at this level that the human being starts becoming conscious. The symbol of this Cakra is Kalpataru tree, which fulfills all human desires. The lotus of this Cakra has twelve petals. This Cakra is associated with the element of air and the experience of touch. It symbolizes compassion and love for others.

v. *Viśuddhi Cakra* is the fifth center representing sound energy. It is located in the throat or larynx and it is the source of speech and spirituality. It is the gateway for great liberation, through which a person leaves the world of conflict in the form of pairs of opposites. Ākāśa represents the fullness of the archetypes. It involves the renunciation of the transient world of images and becoming conscious of the eternal things. The lotus of this Cakra has sixteen petals. This Cakra is related to hearing, speaking and the experience of sound and Silence. This is the basis for creative, verbal expression and communication.

vi. *Ājñā Cakra* is the highest corporeal center representing conscious mental activity. It is situated between the eyebrows. It is for knowledge, understanding and command. Ātman shines here like a quiet flame. It is the seat of Mahat or the mind and Prakṛiti or Nature. It controls various states of meditation and commands one's personality. Its deity is the inseparable Śiva~Śaktiḥ , the pair of Cosmic Unity, whose Self-luminous Consciousness is all-pervading, all-transcending and all-unifying. It is associated with various cognitive functions of the mind. The lotus of this Cakra has two large petals, like hemispheres. In this Cakra, the undivided and indivisible existence manifests as two for the sake of one creation. This center is for rising above polar dualities and to receive intuition and clairvoyant abilities.

vii. *Sahasradala Cakra* is symbolized by the lotus of thousand petals representing witness consciousness or mindful presence. It is seated at the top or vertex of the head. "This Cakra synchronizes all colors, encompasses all senses, and all functions, and is all-pervading in its power…It is the center of quintessential consciousness, where integration of all polarities is experienced and the paradoxical act of transcendence is accomplished in passing beyond ever-changing Samsāra and emerging from time and space." The lotus of this Cakra has thousand petals. This Cakra is for clear thinking, saintly intelligence and concern for the highest good of all. It represents the experience of universal connectedness and holistic consciousness.

Interestingly, Mr. Guḷ awaṇ i in his book, described five forms of Kuṇ ḍ alini Śaktiḥ, energy or fire, Pañcāgniḥ पञ्चाग्नि: or Pañcajyotiḥ पञ्चज्योति: i) Mūlāgniḥ मूलाग्नि: the source fire, heat or thermal energy, ii) Vaḍ awāgniḥ वडवाग्नि: the sound-vibrational, acoustic and protonic energy, iii) Pārthiwāgniḥ पार्थिवाग्नि: the mechanical energy, iv) Vidyutāgniḥ विद्युताग्नि: the energy of lightning and bio-electromagnetic energy, and v) Sūryāgniḥ सूर्याग्नि: the solar, photic or photonic energy from the Sun.

Rele defined Kuṇ ḍ alini Yoga as a science of physical and mental discipline of a particular form, by which an individual establishes a conscious control over his autonomic nervous system, so as to get in tune with the Infinite. He interpreted the Cakra as the neural plexuses of the autonomic nervous system, which is a limited perspective. However, he made a good observation that some of the Kuṇ ḍ alini yogic practices tend to cause sympathetic over-stimulation, resulting in various symptoms described in the historical literature. In fact such symptoms are well described by Mr. Guḷ awaṇ i.

Shannahoff-Khalsa has done considerable research on the neurophysiology of an ultradian rhythm called, the nasal cycle. In brief, the nasal cycle is i) a marker for the ultradian rhythm of alternating cerebral hemispheric activity during wakefulness and sleep. When airflow dominates through the right nostril, greater activity is seen in the left cerebral hemisphere and vis-a-versa, ii) a marker for the dynamic lateralization of the autonomic nervous system function, iii) right nostril breathing correlates with dream REM sleep, and the left nostril breathing correlates with deep non-REM sleep, iv) greater airflow through the right nostril correlates with behavioral activity, whereas, greater airflow through the left nostril correlates with behavioral quiescence, v) the hypothalamus integrates and regulates the behavioral rest-activity cycle, vi) unilateral nasal breathing tends to stimulate the sympathetic activity on the same side and the cerebral hemispheric activity on the opposite side; these effects are integrated and mediated through the hypothalamus.

Deshmukh [28, 29] had also published experimental research work on the oro-nasal breathing cycle and the classification of limbic-autonomic arousal, behavioral activation and the sleep-wake states.

Saraswatī proposed that the activity of the reticular formation in the brainstem may be the neural mechanism for general and autonomic arousal associated with the awakening of Kuṇ ḍ alini. He also described an interesting concept of not only the ascent of, but also, the descent of Kuṇ ḍ alini. With the full descent of Kuṇ ḍ alini, one may go through a non-dual indescribable experience of Samādhi, with a mystical union of Śiva~Śakti or Puruṣ a~Prakṛ iti.

The concept and experience of ascent as well as descent of Kuṇ ḍ alini have been beautifully described in a poetic form by Śri Jñāneshwar in Jñāneṣ warī[4].

ते कुंडलिनी जगदंबा | जे चैतन्य चक्रवर्तीची शोभा |
जिया विश्वबिजाचीया कोम्भा | साउली केली ||६:२७२||

4 Dandekar SV. Editor. Sārtha Jñāneṣ wari (Marathi). Pune, India: Y G Joshi; 1953.

Kuṇ ḍ alini is the Universal Energy, Mother of the Universe. She is the splendor of the Supreme Consciousness. She shadows and nurtures the seed of all Existence.

सहस्रदळाचा मेघु। पियूषे वर्षोनी चांगु।
तो मूळवरी वोघु। आणूनियां ॥१८:१०३९॥

The calming shower of the blissful energy from the thousand-petal, Sahasradala Cakra, reaches to the primal Mūlādhāra Cakra.

Śri Jñāneṣ wara also described some of the signs and symptoms of the ascent of Kuṇ ḍ alini. Such an enlightened person becomes highly inspired and creative. His/her gaze becomes steady. His breathing becomes spontaneously slow and may pause briefly. The mind is totally turned inward and becomes merged in the Self. One feels happy and blessed. One may hear spontaneous sounds of Silence. The body gets energized as if by lightening. The body is completely relaxed and still like a tree. One discovers many new ways of doing Yoga, Prāṇ āyāma, Mudra, hand postures, dance, music, poetry, reciting, novel phonations, spontaneous singing, speaking, and new intuitive ideas. One may see one's favorite images of God or Goddess. One may develop clairvoyant abilities. One may solve complex problems by great intuitive insights. But, every sage does not necessarily have all of these experiences. What matters is the deep Self-understanding, primal feeling, compassion for all and the direct experience of Self-realization and an unshakable conviction of this Truth-within.

NEUROPSYCHOLOGICAL INTERPRETATION OF KUṆḌALINI

It is proposed that the concept of ascent (and descent) of Kuṇ ḍ alini from Muladhara to Sahasradala Cakra represents the journey of human evolution. The human mind evolves through four major stages of development, growth and maturation: i) Collective unconscious, ii) Individual unconscious, iii) Individual conscious, and iv) Collective conscious. In an individual human being, these four stages of evolution are also represented by the sleep-wake cycle, namely, i) Unconscious, non-REM[5] sleep, ii) Partially conscious, dream REM sleep, iii) Partially conscious, individual, egocentric wakefulness, and iv) fully conscious, Holistic Awareness. With this neuropsychological model, one can understand both the ascent as well as the descent of this primal, neuro-behavioral energy, Kuṇ dalini.

During the first "Collective Unconscious" phase, living organisms are non-conscious and tend to function in self-organized groups, like bacterial colonies, colonies of bees, schools of fish, flocks of birds and herds of animals like wildebeests. Sometimes, even a group of people may behave in such a blind, non-conscious way, especially during periods of panic, danger and wars.

During the second phase of "Individual unconscious," the process of individuation begins. This is evident in infancy and early childhood. This period of human life is dominated by REM sleep and a fair amount of day-dreaming. During this phase, one develops some

[5] REM: Rapid Eye Movements.

subconscious individual memories and habits, including our sense of embodiment, gender identity and core personality.

During the third phase of "Individual conscious," an organism or a human being becomes more conscious and self-aware. He/she is less dreamy and more realistic. But the conscious mind is dominated by personal, autobiographical memories, self-image, self-identity, egoistic power, dominance and territorial defences. Individual life is a constant struggle to prove oneself, to aspire and to achieve, and to feel disappointed, when unsuccessful. It is a life of choosing between polarities, like pain-pleasure, happiness-sadness, good-evil, me-others, mine-yours, life-death etc.

During the fourth stage of "Collective Conscious," one matures and grows out of such polarized thinking, conflicting emotions and divisive personal perspectives. One experiences and appreciates the wonderful connectedness and the unity of all Life and Existence. One discovers the Holistic Consciousness and the holistic nature of Reality-at-large. One is not overly concerned about oneself. One becomes considerate, wise and compassionate with a genuine concern, care and love for all living beings. It is being a friend and a benefactor of all beings and Nature, Sakala hitakaraḥ सकलहितकर:

One realizes that one is the world, and the world is me. As J Krishnamurti said, "You are the World." Vedānta says: "You are *That*," Tattvamasi तत्त्वमसि. You are the Holistic Energy. Śri Ramaṇa Maharṣi said that once you have realized the Truth of Unity, Ekatvaṁ एकत्वं, "There are no 'others'." Almost every world religion teaches this golden rule of universal brotherhood and the ethics of reciprocity. The famous teaching of Jesus, "Love thy neighbor, as you would love thyself." There are statements similar to this one, in almost every world religion. What matters most is our own innermost feeling and the mindful, compassionate behavior.

The application of this model to the four stages of sleep-wake cycle has been discussed at length in many sections of this book. The fourth stage of full Holistic Consciousness would be similar to Turīya, Samādhi, Nirvāṇa or the Ground Consciousness.

This four-stage model also reminds me of Maslow's (and others) Conscious Competence Theory[6] or "The Four Stages of Learning."

1. Unconscious Incompetence: The individual neither understands nor knows how to do something, nor recognizes the deficit, nor has a desire to address it.
2. Conscious Incompetence: Though the individual does not understand or know how to do something, he or she does recognize the deficit, without yet addressing it.
3. Conscious Competence: The individual understands or knows how to do something. However, demonstrating the skill or knowledge requires a great deal of conscious effort and concentration.
4. Unconscious Competence: The individual has had so much practice with a skill that it becomes "second nature" and can be performed easily (often without concentrating too deeply). He or she may or may not be able to teach it to others, depending upon how and when it was learned.

6 See www.wikipedia.org.

After all, the whole purpose of Yoga and meditation is to learn and to excel in the art of healthy and happy living, Yogaḥ Karmasu Kaushalam. It is the great skill of nondual presence or holistic attentiveness, with awareness undivided by space-time-person-object. Maslow[7] described some of the characteristics of such "B-values" as wholeness, perfection, completion, justice, aliveness, richness, simplicity, beauty, goodness, uniqueness, effortlessness, playfulness, truth and self-sufficiency.

NEUROPHYSIOLOGICAL INTERPRETATION OF KUṆḌALINI

The ascent and descent of Kuṇ ḍ alini are related to the activation or inhibition of the brainstem-reticular-diencephalic-limbic, arousal and calming systems. There are specific areas in the brainstem and subcortex that mediate conscious arousal as well as calmness including wakefulness and sleep (please see Appendix 1 for a brief review of the Functional Neuroanatomy).

There is a reciprocal relationship between the prefrontal executive cortex, the great integrator, and the brainstem-diencephalic arousal systems. The prefrontal executive network can activate as well as inhibit the central arousal systems. There is a circular relationship between the prefrontal executive cortex and the brainstem-diencephalic arousal systems. These brainstem-diencephalic arousal systems involve specific neurotransmitters that activate or inhibit the cerebral cortex.

Three neurotransmitter systems are of special relevance. The mesolimbic dopaminergic system mediates behavioral energy-impulse, motivation and pleasure. This system is activated by natural activities like sports, creative arts and meditation, but it can also be stimulated by psycho-stimulant drugs like amphetamine and cocaine, with temporary pleasure, but, they can cause many side effects including drug addiction. The cluster of neurons called substantia nigra, in the midbrain, release dopamine. The septal nuclei and nucleus accumbens are part of the neural network at the cortical level that mediates pleasure and satiety.

The second neurotransmitter system that can mimic some of the psychoactive states and impulsive creativity is the midline serotoninergic system, mediated by the chain of raphe nuclei. Some of the hallucinogenic drugs acting through this system include Lysergic acid or LSD. Patients suffering from depression may lack central serotonin and/or noradrenalin. Antidepressant drug use usually increases these levels of neurotransmitters and relieve depression.

The third neurotransmitter system that has been associated with behavioral arousal and impulsive creativity is the central noradrenergic system with Locus Coeruleus as the cluster of neurons that release the neurotransmitter noradrenalin. Release of noradrenalin is associated with novelty, surprise, danger, excitement and learning.

The fourth major neurotransmitter system is that of Acetyl Choline, which is involved in many general fuctions, but more specifically for memory processing. There is known deterioration of cortical cholinergic neurons in Alzheimer's disease.

---

7 Maslow AH. Toward a Psychology of Being. New York, NY: Van Nostrand Reinhold Company; 1968:83.

These four neurotransmitters, namely dopamine, serotonin, noradrenalin, and Acetyl Choline affect all functions of the cerebral cortex, and the conscious as well as the unconscious mental activities.

Some of the key points of these neuropsychological and neurophysiological interpretations of Kuṇ ḍ alini are:

i) Kuṇ ḍ alini is clearly a global, holistic phenomenon, affecting every aspect of our unconscious as well as conscious mind and body.
ii) This unique phenomenal experience is mediated through central neural networks like the brainstem-diencephalic-limbic arousal system and the multimodal thalamo-cortical system, rather than just the peripheral autonomic plexuses, which have been previously mentioned.
iii) The ascent and descent of Kuṇ ḍ alini can be understood as the general activation and/or inhibition of the brainstem, subcortex and the cortex, with multi-dimensional, physiological and mental effects.
iv) The number of petals of the seven lotuses of Kuṇ ḍ alini Cakra, grow, in an ascending order, from 4, 6, 10, 12, 16, and then 2 hemispheres, and finally the 1000 petals. One interpretation of these petals is that their number represent an ascending order of human body's energy frequency spectrum. The action-inaction, activation-inhibition or rest-activity cycles are well known in neurophysiology. At the lower spinal level, the frquency of alternative states is slower as compared to the rapid changes at higher cortical levels. At the highest cerebral cortical level, the electro-encephalographic (EEG) frequencies can reach upto 600 or even 1000 Hertz or cycles per second. Buzsaki[8] has described a multi-oscillator hierarchical system in the cerebral cortex. The collective activity of cortical neuro-oscillators can vary in frequency from 0.05 Hz to 600 Hz. EEG frequencies follow non-linear, fractal dynamic process. He has also provided a mathematical equation that seems to fit the observed frequencies of the cerebral electromagnetic energy-spectrum.
v) The somatic motor-sensory components of these seven energy centers, are represented in the cerebral cortical sensory-motor gyri, representing the homunculus. The homunculus is the representational image of an upside-down "dwarf man" on the surface of both cerebral hemispheres. Homuncular reprentation is somatotopic, in the sense that the amount of neural space devoted to a part of the body e.g., hand, depends upon its use and location. Somatotopic organization is evident at many levels of the central nervous system, including spinal cord, cerebellum, thalamus and the cerebral cortex. In the homuncular map, there are regions dedicated to tongue, lips, mouth, swallowing, salivation, vocalisation, eyes, head, shoulders, arms, hands, chest, abdomen, pelvis, genitals and perineum. There is a similiarity and a functional corrspondence between the homuncular map and the symbolic functional representations of the six Kuṇ ḍ alini Cakras. Many of the voluntary and intentional practices of Yoga Meditation and skillful breathing exercises, called Prāṇ āyāma, are

8 Buzsaki G. Rhythms of the Brain. New York, NY: Oxford University Press; 2006: 111-135.

mediated through these wide-speard neural networks, extending from the cerebral cortex to the spinal cord via the pyramidal system and its connections. When some of these skills are over-learned, then their performance can become subconscious, effortless, egoless, spontaneous and natural. It can become a way of holistic being and living.

Chapter 4

Core Concepts of Neuroscience and Vedānta

Brain is the organ of self-conscious mind.
Mind is a function of the brain.

Society for Neuroscience defined the core concepts of neuroscience as follows: i) the nervous system controls and responds to body functions and directs behavior. The brain is the body's most complex organ, ii) Neurons communicate using both electrical and chemical signals, iii) Brain structure and function are determined by both genes and environment throughout life. Genetically determined neural circuits are the foundation of the nervous system, iv) Life experiences change the nervous sytem, v) the brain is the foundation of mind. Intelligence arises as the brain reasons, plans, and solves problems, vi) the brain makes it possible to communicate knowledge through language, vii) the human brain endows us with a natural curiosity to understand how the world works, viii) Fundamental discoveries promote healthy living and treatment of diseases.

Vedānta is an ancient philosophy of life, based on direct intuitve experience and inspirations of exceptionally gifted and enlightened Vedic seers. These amazing insights and wisdom were recorded in the four Vedās, 108 Upaniṣ ads, Brahma-Sūtra, Bhagavad-Gītā, and Pātañjali's Yoga-Sūtra. Since, Vedānta is an authentic way of life, there have been many subsequent examples of enlightened individuals, who have expressed their insights, in their own words like Ādi Śankarāchārya's direct experience, Aparokshānubhūti अपरोक्षानुभूति, Jñāneṣ wara's blissful experience, Amṛ itānubhava अमृतानुभव, and Rāmadāsa's Dāsabodha दासबोध. Some of the more recent visionaries from India include Śri Ramakrishna Paramahansa, Śri Vivekānanda, Śri Aurobindo, Śri Ramaṇ a Maharṣ i, and J Krishnamurti.

It is important to realize that Buddhism emerged, as a reformed philosophy and a way of life, from the original matrix of the Vedic Hinduism. There are more similarities than differences between the two philosophies of life. Neuroscience has now accepted the Buddhist way of mindfulness meditation, as an effective method to achieve mental health and spiritual wellbeing. Significant research is being done to study the effects of meditation on various brain networks, mental functions, and human behavior.

Is it possible to integrate and understand the holistic consciousness, from both neuroscience and Vedānta perspectives? My personal answer is "Yes." But, in order to achieve such understanding and a personal conviction, we have to learn, and experience, the essential truths from both disciplines. This book is an attempt to achieve such a monumental integration. Of course, the ultimate understanding depends upon our own, actual mind-set, experience and our perspective of Self-in-the-World.

The Transparent Mind

After a long period of maturation,
An orange ripens
And becomes truly sweet.
One day, it suddenly falls,
Effortlessly.

After a long period
Of growth and development,
An overloaded mind,
Suddenly becomes light and transparent,
As if, it has just disappeared,
Without any effort, thought or recall;
With no regrets, rehearsals or expectations.

What remains is
The slowly aging human organism,
Functioning wisely,
In an ever-changing world.

"Where is 'me' then?" one may ask;
Some say, "Nowhere."
Others say, "Somewhere,"
Or even "Everywhere."

But, does it really matter,
Once one realizes that
The translucent Light
Of One exhilarating Energy,
Ever flows unhindered,
Through all life forms,
And one *is*
This amazing Life Energy.

Vinod D Deshmukh
June 2, 2011

Chapter 5

INITIAL UNDERSTANDING AND INTEGRATION

असतो मा सद्गमय । तमसो मा ज्योतिर्गमय ॥ मृत्योर्मा अमृतंगमय ॥।

Lead me from the false to Truth; from the darkness of ignorance to Light of Self-understanding and from the fear of death to the Bliss of an enlightened, and fearless Life.

CONTENTS CHANGE; CONTAINING PROCESS DOES NOT

In 1982, I had presented an abstract at the annual meeting of the Society for Neuroscience. It was titled: "Presence as a new mode of human attention." (For the full abstract, please see Appendix 4). I had proposed that human attention had two fundamentally different modes. The commonly recognized human attention was called "Mnemic" as it is memory-guided, and the new mode was called "Presence" which is free from intrusive memories and verbal thinking.

The mnemic mode of attention is characterized by limited and distracted attention, in which habitual cognitive and emotional responses are based on personal memories and intentions. This creates the observer-observed duality and the experience of personal time, duration and transience. It creates, sustains, and adds to our egocentric self-image and images of others. It limits our perceptivity, attentional energy, intelligence, and the feeling of natural, unconditional happiness.

The presence mode of attention, on the other hand, is not dominated by personal memories. It is a complete, participant attention to the present - here-and-now. It is free of habitual, cognitive and emotional responses. It is free of past ego-image (and duality). It implies tremendous, frictionless, conflictless and holistic conscious energy, intelligence, Self-freedom, and a feeling of natural Being-in-Reality. Since it is completely one with the present – what is, it was called the "state of Presence."

Interestingly, on May 4, 2010, I wrote in my journal: "Presence is being fully present in the moment. Presence is freedom from the memory of my body, mind and ego. It is the freedom from I-Me-Mine. Presence is Self-qualia or a primal feeling of Self-existence, an intrinsic subjective awareness, the holistic Energy, and bliss. The Present is sacred."

Such a state of Presence is a holistic conscious state. Historically, such Superconsciousness was called Turīya तुरीय the fourth state of consciousness, as described in

Māṇ ḍ ūkyopaniṣ ad माण्डूक्योपनिषद्. It is called the "Fourth" as it is different from the other three conscious states namely, deep non-REM[1] sleep, dream REM sleep, and the dualistic, interactive wakefulness. Turīya or Brāhmī Sthitiḥ ब्राह्मी स्थिति: is an extraordinarily inspired state of calm, alert, and spontaneous consciousness, with completely integrated Being-in-Reality. It is proposed that such an extraordinary, superconscious state can be understood within the framework of modern Neuroscience and the Vedānta philosophy of human existence.

The author proposed in 2004, [30], that Turīya तुरीय is a unique holistic conscious state of Non-REM-Wakefulness (NREM-W) characterized by a) an optimal attentiveness, with freedom from daydreaming, irrelevant distractions and intrusive thoughts, b) an effortless or spontaneous behavioral quiescence, mental stillness and silence, with no random internal speech or thoughts, c) heightened perceptivity, intellectual clarity, and cognitive excellence, and d) an enhanced feeling of well-being, an unconditional bliss, serenity, Śāntiḥ शान्ति:, compassion, Karuṇ ā करुणा, love for Life, and spontaneous creativity, Srujatā सृजता. Figure 2.

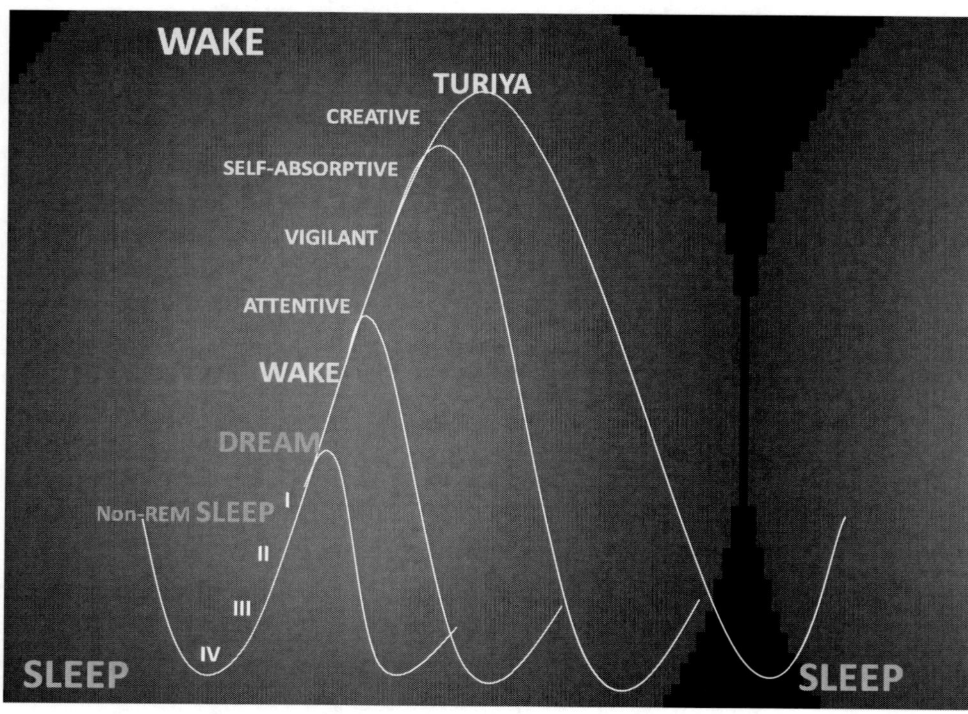

Figure 2. Four states of consciousness, i) Non-REM - Deep Sleep with I-IV sub-states depending on the depth of sleep, ii) REM - Dream sleep, iii) REM - Wakefulness with daydreaming and intrusive thoughts and distractions, iv) Non-REM - Wakefulness, or Turīya, with mental stillness, silence, self-healing serenity, profound insight and creativity.

In the current neuroscience, only three states of consciousness are recognized. The three states being i) slow wave or non-REM sleep, ii) dream or REM sleep, and iii) the daily,

[1] REM: Rapid Eye Movement

interactive wakefulness. The fourth state of Turīya is not formally recognized, but it is acknowledged as an advanced, meditative state, with altered unitive consciousness. Some new research is being performed on meditative states, especially using the functional magnetic resonance imaging (fMRI), electroencephalography (EEG), and magneto-encephalography (MEG).

Here is a brief summary of some of the current research on meditation. In Tibetan Buddhist meditation practices [31], three different types of meditative states are described, i) Focused attention, ii) Open Presence or Mindfulness, and iii) Non-referential compassion. During non-referential compassion meditation, EEG gamma activity (25-42 Hz) and gamma synchrony increased. Functional MRI[2] showed activation in the striatum, anterior insula, somatosensory cortex, anterior cingulate cortex and the left prefrontal cortex and a deactivation in the right inferior parietal region. Following 8 weeks of mindfulness based stress reduction (MBSR) program [32], participants reported reduced perceived stress significantly. Reductions in perceived stress correlated positively with decreases in the right basolateral amygdala gray matter density.

A conscious resting state questionnaire [33] has been developed to record the ongoing mental contents during the so called "resting conscious state." Five types of mental contents were found, namely, i) visual images, ii) inner speech, iii) somatosensory experience, iv) musical repetitions and v) numerical images. A ''neural switch'' [34] is most likely to be involved, when a cortico–striato–thalamo–cortical loop executes a set-shift of attention from external matters to the subject's own state of mind (and body) according to a previously established rule kept in working memory. Zen meditation, [35], in particular, is traditionally associated with a mental state of full awareness but reduced conceptual content, to be attained via a disciplined regulation of attention and bodily posture. Zen practitioners displayed a reduced duration of the neural response linked to conceptual processing in regions of the default network, suggesting that meditative training may foster the ability to control the automatic cascade of semantic associations triggered by a stimulus and, by extension, to voluntarily regulate the flow of spontaneous mentation.

Happy voices [36] elicited significantly more activation than angry voices in right anterior and posterior middle temporal gyrus (MTG), left posterior MTG and right inferior frontal gyrus. Furthermore, for the left MTG region, happy voices were related to higher activation only when paired with happy faces. Activation in the left insula, left amygdala and hippocampus, and rostral anterior cingulate cortex showed an effect of selectively attending to the vocal stimuli. A few general articles on meditation are listed [37-41].

An important difference between the Western and Eastern perspectives regarding the conscious mind is that in the Western perspective, the mind is considered as the totality of mental and psychic activity, including the psyche or the self. Whereas, in the Eastern philosophical traditions, the mind has a more limited definition and function. In Vedānta, for instance, mind is called the inner instrument of knowing and experience, Antaḥ karaṇ a अन्तःकरण, [42]. The mind is considered to be an observable phenomenon, which becomes an 'internal environment' for the essential conscious being. During meditation, one has a feeling of conviction, that this entire observable phenomenon is not me; "(this is) not me, not me,"

[2] Magnetic Resonance Imaging.

Neti, Neti नेति, नेति. I am the intrinsic, spontaneous, self-existent, self-content, and self-aware psychic Being, the true, primal Self, *Ātman* आत्मन् or Ādipuruṣ a आदिपुरुष.

Some of the modern neuroscientists have described such an essential conscious being as "the last sense of self, the intrinsic or subjective self." William James [43] called it the self-as-subject vs. self-as-object. He also described it as the spiritual or transcendent self: "By the spiritual self, so far as it belongs to the empirical me, I mean a man's inner or subjective being, his psychic faculties or dispositions, taken concretely; not the bare principle of personal unity, or 'pure' ego…For this central part of the self is *felt*...It is something with which we also have direct sensible acquaintance, and which is, as fully present at any moment of consciousness, in which it *is* present, as in a whole lifetime of such moments."

In Alternative Medicine and Nursing Disciplines [44], spirituality is accepted as an overall philosophy of one's life. "Spirituality, the search for meaning and purpose in life, through a connection with others, Nature, and/or the belief in a higher power, is at the core of each person's existence. In ancient times, spirit meant breath – as essential to life as air. Spirituality is that part of every person that yearns to share the beauty, love and joyfulness of the universe…We take our spirituality from many sources; Nature, God, Buddha, Higher Power, Goddess, Śri Krishna, B'ahaullah, Mohammed, Yahweh, Zoroaster and others. But sprituality is not religion, nor is religion spirituality. Spirtuality is the reflection of one's "spirit" and its relationship to the rest of the universe. Spirituality may be developed through self-reflection, prayer, and meditation."

J. Krishnamurti [45] defined religion as "the investigation, with all one's attention, with the summation of all one's energy, to find that which is sacred, to come upon that which is holy. That can only take place when there is freedom from the noise of thought, the ending of thought and time, psychologically, inwardly - but not the ending of knowledge in the world where you have to function with knowledge. That which is holy, that which is sacred, which is truth, can only be when there is complete silence, when the brain itself has put thought in its right place. Out of that immense silence, there is that which is sacred."

Meditation is an art of efficient and adaptive management of behavioral energy, with full self-regulation over attentional engagement and disengagement. In both of these conscious states, there is an experience of spontaneous, unitive being without a sense of ego, memory or personal time. There is a natural sense of well-being with self-understanding, spontaneous joy, serenity, freedom from the ego, and self-fulfillment. It is where the ultimate pursuit of happiness and search for meaning or purpose in life come to fruition. One realizes the truth of one's being in harmony with Nature and the Nature in oneself. Then each conscious moment becomes a dynamic process of self-discovery and learning of the ever-new Being-in-Reality. One's daily life becomes joyful Ānandīta आनन्दित and ever-enlightening beyond all measure and description.

Attention can be voluntarily or involuntarily engaged or disengaged. An attentional act creates the duality of the attended-attendee, resulting in a specific conscious experience with mental contents. Disengaging directed attention to the limit, results in a serene holistic alertness with nonspecific intrinsic awareness, Nirguṇ a निर्गुण. It may be expressed as the great nothingness or emptiness, Buddha's Śūnyatā शून्यता, verbal silence and essential awareness. Engaging attention to the limit, with a total participation in the present actuality, without any effort, sense of personal time, or autobiographical memories, results in Conscious totality, Pūrṇ atā पूर्णता. Between two consecutive attentional acts, there is an intrinsic awareness, with no attended-attendee duality. This results in a refreshing "experience of no experience," which is analogous to waking up from wakefulness or from a dreamless sleep with no recall of dreams. This intrinsic awareness can lead to a state of holistic, thought-free Awareness, Superconsciousness or Turīya.

Intrinsic awareness is like the preattentive gist-consciousness, which can occur within 30 msec, whereas conscious attention takes about 300-500 msec. So, the gist-awareness is 10-15 times faster than the conscious attentional process. My hypothetical proposal is that both of these pre-attentive and attentive processes are initiated simultaneously and they run in parallel. However, they are completed at different times, namely 30 msec and 300-500 msec, due to shorter and longer neural pathways and the specific neural networks involved.

The pre-attentive processing occurs subcortically, in the reticulo-limbic networks, whereas attentive processing needs complex and slow neo-cortical networks. Whereas conscious attentive processing is intermittent and 'particulate or impulsive,' the pre-attentive awareness has a 'continuum' like quality of the continuous self-aware, non-impulsive Being Sūtrātmā सूत्रात्मा. That is why the preattentive awareness feels spontaneous, indivisible, all-pervasive and enduring. The preattentive and attentive consciousness together make the Superconsciousness holistic Pūrṇ a पूर्ण, and indivisible Akhaṇ ḍ a अखण्ड.

A living organism's neurobiological energy can manifest in many forms: i) the neuromuscular energy for physical, biomechanical work, ii) the vocal energy for speech cognition and verbal communication, iii) the neuro-physiological energy for visceral processes, like respiration, digestion, metabolism, Prāṇ aśaktiḥ प्राणशक्तिः, iv) the conscious and preconscious mental energy, Citśaktiḥ चित्शक्तिः, iv) the spontaneous energy of essential being and self-awareness, Swayaṁ Jyotiḥ स्वयंज्योति, and v) the incomprehensible existential energy of the universe that ever supports all Life, Acintyaśaktiḥ अचिन्त्यशक्तिः. These energies can be in a potential or kinetic form. They are in kinetic form during common, interactive wakefulness and dream sleep, whereas, during non-REM sleep and non-REM wakefulness, turīya, they are in a potential form. During non-REM sleep, the conscious arousal-energy is low, whereas during non-REM wakefulness, the conscious arousal-energy is high. That is why the turīya state has been described to have a feeling of boundless holistic energy, unlimited capacity, creativity, and an intense sense of well-being and unconditional bliss.

The moment one resumes directed attention, the subject-object duality returns, the "potential" behavioral energy becomes "kinetic," and an egoistic mind suffers from various dualistic, interactive experiences. The ego continuously struggles to change itself or its situation, resulting in a wider gap between personal expectations and the reality. Therefore, it suffers from perpetual disappointments, stress, pain and transient pleasures.

There is a reciprocal relationship between two crucial neural networks: i) the goal-directed, task-specific, dorsal prefrontal - temporo-occipital-parietal network and ii) the resting, self-relational, midline prefrontal – medial posterior cortical, precuneus, posterior cingulate gyrus, and retrosplenial cortex "Default" network. When one network is active the other one becomes quiet, and vice a versa [46 - 48].

Meditation, on the other hand, is the art of being alert and serene in the midst of any situation. It is the ultimate, adaptive reality-consciousness, continuously learning and renewing itself. Then, the first and the third-person perspectives merge. It is a combined, holistic subject-object Awareness, Ubhaya Sākshī उभयसाक्षी, which becomes self-content, Ātmatuṣ ta आत्मतुष्ट. Such holistic consciousness remains cheerful and blissful, at-ease with itself, and at-home in the world. It is the art of self-mastering both skills of parallel and sequential mental processing as expressed in my poem below, "a River and a Lake." [49].

Ongoing meditation is the most essential state of one's being. One discovers and appreciates the wonder of presence, this ever-fresh mode of living. The spontaneous "essence" of our being remains the same. The conscious contents change; the container remains the same. It is the invariant aspect of our subjective experience. All conscious moments are essentially the same! "Sāre kshaṇ a sārakheca सारे क्षण सारखेच!" What remain are the infinite, ineffable essence, the Actuality, the Truth, and the wonder of living from the very source of one's Being. Learning goes on with appreciation and blessedness. Life remains good, when wisely lived. It is a precious gift, a Nature's blessing to all.

RIVER AND LAKE

Like a river, meditate in action.
Like a lake, reflect on the present.

A river meditates while running.
A lake meditates while standing.

A river is a sequence of actions.
A lake is present awareness.

A river is the sequential mind.
A lake is parallel awareness.

Listen to the river.
Look at the lake.
Learn from both.

A river is a lake that is in a hurry
To reach the ocean.

A lake is a river that pauses
To look at the blue sky.

A river carves out of time.

A lake reflects eternity.
A river knows the time.
A lake knows the timeless.

Speak like a river.
Listen like a lake.

A skillful mind
Can flow like a river and
Standstill like a lake.
It depends upon the terrain it faces
From moment-to-moment.
It lives freely and spontaneously.

Vinod D Deshmukh
November 7, 1992

Chapter 6

HOLISTIC CONSCIOUS STATE, TURĪYA तुरीय

अपाणि पादोः अहं अचिन्त्यशक्तिः | पश्यामि अचक्षुः स शृणोम्यकर्णः||
अहं विजानामि विविक्त रूपो ||| न च अस्ति वेत्ता मम चित्सदाहं ||२१||

I am that incomprehensible holistic energy that acts without hands or feet that can see without eyes and hear without ears. I can comprehend various forms, but, no one knows me as the timeless subjective awareness.

Kaivalyopaniṣ ad 21

Historically, holistic consciousness has been described as the unique, fourth state of consciousness, Turīya तुरीय, Sthitaprajñā स्थितप्रज्ञा, Ātmaprasāda आत्मप्रसाद, or Brāhmī Sthiti ब्राह्मी स्थिति. The four Vedās (Ṛg Veda, Yajur Veda, Atharva Veda, and Sāma Veda), which are supposed to be anonymous, apouruṣ eya अपौरुषेय, are probably more than 5000 years old. They have eloquently described a unique human state of blissful conscious being, Sat~Cit~Ānanda सच्चिदानन्द, serene, sacred, nondual Self, Śāntaṁ, Śivaṁ, Advaitaṁ *Ātman* शान्तं शिवं अद्वैतं आत्मन्, and the truth, goodness and beauty of nature, Satyaṁ, Śivaṁ, Sundaraṁ सत्यं शिवं सुन्दरम् and the Real, Conscious, Infinite *Brahman*, Satyaṁ Jñānaṁ, Anantaṁ, *Brahma* सत्यं ज्ञानं अनन्तं ब्रह्म |

The Māṇ dūkyopaniṣ ad माण्डूक्योपनिषद् clearly described four states of human consciousness, namely a) Suṣ upti सुषुप्ति the dreamless sleep with Prājña प्राज्ञ as the experiencing self, b) Swapna स्वप्न the dream sleep with Taijasa तैजस as the experiencing self, c) Jāgrat जाग्रत् the wakeful state with Vaiśwānara वैश्वानर as the experiencing self, and d) Turīya तुरीय the fourth, holistic conscious state, which is a highly awakened, self-integrated Source-state. The primal Source-Being with essential Self-awareness in such a state is called *Ātman* आत्मन्.

Māṇ ḍ ūkyopaniṣ ad माण्डूक्योपनिषद् contains twelve original Sanskrit verses, followed by a commentary, Kārikā कारिका by Gaudapāda, who was a Sanskrit scholar and a pioneer of a non-dualistic philosophy called Advaita Vedānta अद्वैत वेदान्त. Ādi Śaṅ karāchārya, who was a brilliant, eighth-century, Sanskrit scholar, philosopher, and a poet of India (788–820), has translated and commented on the Māṇ ḍ ūkyopaniṣ ad, as well as on Gaudapāda's Kārikā. The Māṇ ḍ ūkyopaniṣ ad, after describing the three commonly known states of human consciousness, goes on to describing Turīya in the seventh and the twelfth verses. S. Rādhākrishnan who was the President of India and a modern scholar of Vedānta, translated the seventh and the twelfth verses as follows:

नान्तः प्रज्ञं न बहिष्प्रज्ञं नोभयतःप्रज्ञं न प्रज्ञानघनं न प्रज्ञं नाप्रज्ञं |
अदृष्टमव्यवहार्यमग्राह्यमलक्षणमचिन्त्यमव्यपदेश्यमेकात्मप्रत्ययसारं
प्रपञ्चोपशमं शान्तं शिवमद्वैतं चतुर्थं मन्यन्ते स आत्मा स विज्ञेयः ||७||

अमात्रश्चतुर्थोऽव्यवहार्यः प्रपञ्चोपशमः शिवोऽद्वैत एवमोंकार
आत्मैव संविशत्यात्मनाऽऽत्मानं य एवं वेद ||१२||

"(Turīya is) not that which cognizes the internal (objects or events), not that which cognizes the external (objects or events), not that which cognizes both of them, not a mass of cognition, not cognitive, not non-cognitive. (It is) unseen, incapable of being spoken of, ungraspable, without any distinctive marks, unthinkable, unnamable, the essence of knowledge of the one self, that into which the world is resolved, the peaceful, the benign, the non-dual, such, they think, is the fourth state. He is the self; He is to be known…The syllable, AUM ॐ is the very Self. He who knows it thus, enters the (essential) Self with his (own) self." [50].

In differentiating the first state of dreamless sleep, from the fully awakened fourth state of Turīya, Gaudapāda comments, "in the dreamless sleep, Prājña, the experiencing self, is neither aware of himself nor of others. He neither knows the truth nor the untruth. He is truly not cognizant of anything. But in the state of Turīya, the essential self, Ātman, is always aware of all that is present in the Reality, in essence."

Pātañjali in his Yoga sūtras precisely expressed the reality of the state of Turīya: "The essential Self reveals itself when all mental activity such as thought, emotion and egocentric motives subsides. At all other times, one identifies oneself with the ongoing mental activity. When the mind stays undirected and settles in its original, unmodified state, the essential Self reveals itself." [51].

J. Krishnamurti [52] described beautifully such an advanced meditative brain state: "Meditation is to find out whether the brain, with all its activities, all its experiences, can be absolutely quiet. Not forced, because the moment you force, there is duality. The entity that says, "I would like to have marvellous experiences, therefore I must force my brain to be quiet" will never do it. But if you begin to inquire, observe, listen to all movements of thought, its conditioning, its pursuits, its fears, its pleasures, watch how the brain operates, then you will see that the brain becomes extraordinarily quiet; that quietness is not sleep but it is tremendously active and therefore quiet. A big dynamo, that is working perfectly, hardly makes a sound; it is only when there is friction that there is noise."

In explaining the fourth conscious state of Turīya in Śiva Sūtra, Jaideva Singh[1] eloquently stated, "The fourth state of consciousness is the everpresent witnessing consciousness of all the three. Even the three states of waking, dreaming and profound sleep could not be experienced as three different states without a consciousness, a knower that knows all the three. That fourth state is, then, our real Self. It is the everpresent, immortal *ātman,* the deathless, ceaseless consciousness that witnesses all that we feel, think, and do. It is the changeless permanent I that witnesses all of our changing I's."

(*Personal note*: Being a neurobiologist, I would use adjectives like 'immortal' and 'deathless.' I personally accept human vulnerability and mortality. However, the fourth conscious state is still a great wonder that remains to be appreciated by many!).

Fountain of Silent Peace

On waking up,
It just dawned spontaneously.
It was intense, all pervasive.
In it, there were no
Sounds, words or thoughts.
It was a sheer peaceful Silence.

At that time, speaking or thinking was
Like an avalanche of boulders,
That tended to disrupt the flow of
That pristine Awareness.

Nothing needed to be done,
But to stay rapped up,
In the ongoing wonder,
Otherwise, each word broke the Silence,
Each image obscured the clear sky,
And each action interrupted its flow.

So, do nothing, speak nothing,
Think nothing, see nothing.
But, listen with all your Heart and
Be one with the astonishing Wonder.

At that time,
One can't carry or take away anything.

1 Singh J. Translator-Commentor. Śiva Sūtras: the Yoga of Supreme Identity. Motilal Banarasidass Publishers, Delhi, India. 1979. Reprint 2008:39.

No true description of its presence.
One has to let go of everything,
Including one's ego
And its endless stories,
And one's own perception
Of the "me."
What continues is
The ever-present Reality,
The amazing truth of this Energy-Being.

The fountain of silent peace roars
In the infinite emptiness of no-thing.
Like the legendary
"Fountain of Youth,"
The "Fountain of Silent Peace" is
The greatest healer of human mind,
And a beginningless Source of
Self-understanding,
Serenity and Intuition.

It is a welcome return
Of our narrative self,
To the ever-fresh wellspring of
Serene and Silent Being.

Vinod D Deshmukh
December 2, 2005

Chapter 7

SELF-CONSCIOUS MIND IN NEUROSCIENCE

तदेजति तन्नैजति तद्दूरे तद्वन्तिके | तदन्तरस्य सर्वस्य तदु सर्वस्यास्य बाह्यतः ||

It, the *Brahman*, moves. It moves not. It is far. It is close. It is within all. It is beyond all.

Īśavāsyopaniṣ ad, 5

Lately, there has been a considerable interest in the scientific study of consciousness. Several new review articles and books have been published in an effort to understand and address scientifically this complex topic of human consciousness [53 - 58].

Mind means mental activity. Mind is the result of brain activity, which depends on brain's self-organization and self-integration. Brain and mental activities occur concurrently like two parallel streams. Mental activity includes three classical domains of conation, cognition, and emotion or affect.

Conation involves intention and volition with self-activation toward a goal. Conation is defined as the proactive activation or inhibition as opposed to habitual part of motivation. Intention implies a conscious decision to perform a behavior. Volition is the mental faculty by which an individual decides upon and commits to a particular course of action. Volition involves a sense of ego and an active control over the decision making process, and its veto power.

Cognition means information processing and thinking. It is the flow of information through an organism's brain and mind. Information is a reduction in uncertainty provided by the message or a stimulus. A biophysical stimulus has both energy and information. Stimulus energy can be both sequential and parallel in space-time. Information is knowledge about facts and ideas gained through experience and learning. Cognition includes subprocesses of perception, comprehension, memory, reasoning, judgement, imagination, and problem solving.

The executive, cognitive control is a set of processes that organize, plan, and schedule other mental operations. Cognition also means thinking or a thought process, which may be verbal, visual or tactile. Such a process is usually silent and has to be inferred from observable behavior or verbal report. It is also symbolic in the sense that it involves experience and manipulation of recalled mental representations stored in the brain.

Affect is any experience of feeling or emotion, ranging from suffering to elation. Affect can be irreflexive meaning experienced directly or reflexive when the person makes the emotion an object of his or her conscious perception. Emotion is an experience with physiological and behavioral responses to a personally significant event. Emotional control implies self regulation of emotions and their influence on thoughts and behavior. Emotional insight is an awareness of one's own and others' emotions. Emotional intelligence is the ability to process emotional information and to use it in reasoning and cognition.

Feeling is a self-contained phenomenal experience. Feelings can vary along three dimensions: pleasant-unpleasant, exciting-calming, and arousing-relaxing. Approach, avoid, and witness or wait-and-watch are the three fundamental emotional responses, that an organism can have, when facing a new situation. The witness mode involves momentary pausing, waiting, and learning about the evolving situation. Humans can experience a variety of feeligs including, happiness, sadness, anger, fear, surprise, boredom, and disgust. They may also have an intuitive feeling of knowing something without any sensation or focal attention. This may happen in certain meditative states. It has been variously described as the creative matrix or background Awareness-Being [59].

The concept of human consciousness is currently under intense investigation and debate in the neurosciences. One clear definition of consciousness is that it is a set of neuro-biological processes that allow an individual to perceive, comprehend, and act on the internal and external environments [60]. Consciousness defines the present experience, and the present experience defines current consciousness. Mental activity can be conscious, preconscious, or subconscious. Figure 3.

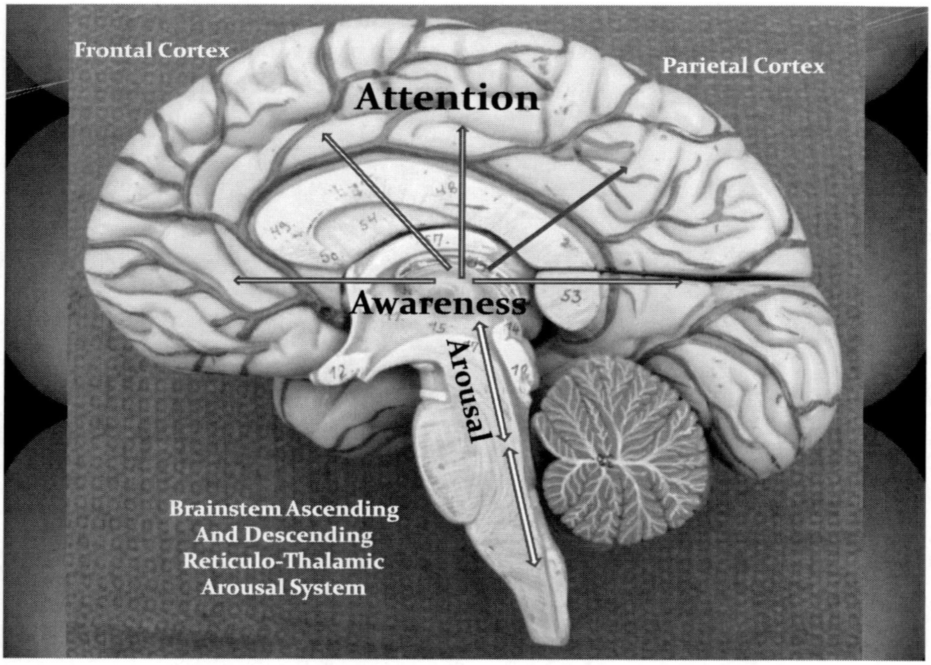

Figure 3. Brainstem-Diencephalic arousal system, ascending and descending reticulo-thalamo-cortical networks, with three components of consciousness: Arousal, Awareness and Attention. Each component has an independent, but inter-related, neural network. Conscious arousal~energy depends on the ascending reticulo-limbic-cortical and reticulo-thalamo-cortical networks. Conscious awareness depends upon the central thalamic nuclei and their related cortical network, and the conscious attention depends upon the fronto-parietal networks including frontal, supplementary and parietal eye-fields.

Consciousness has three main functional components: arousal, awareness, and attention. Conscious arousal describes the degree to which an individual is able to interact with the environments. General arousal is higher in a person who is more alert to sensory stimuli, more physically active, and emotionally more reactive [61]. Conscious arousal requires the interplay between the brainstem reticular activating system and the cerebral hemispheres. Like a pilot flame, the central brain or the reticulo-limbic system is continuously active in all living organisms. Without it conscious life is not possible.

The reticulo-limbic-cortical system subserves basic survival functions that include feeding behavior, "fight-or-flight" response, aggression and the expression of emotion, and the sexual response with the autonomic, behavioral, and endocrine aspects. The limbic system receives input from many parts of the cortex and contains multimodal association areas where various aspects of sensory experience come together to form a single experience. [62].

Conscious awareness implies that the individual is not only alert but also cognizant of self and its surroundings. Awareness is global and multimodal, but it is nonspecific in terms of any a particular sensory, motor, or cognitive modality. Awareness depends on arousal. The key neural structues required for conscious awareness are the central thalamic nuclei with their brainstem and cortical connections [63].

Conscious attention is the ability to respond and process modality-specific information at a specific time-place and person. Different sensory-motor-cognitive modalities include visual, auditory, tactile, olfactory, gustatory, locomotion, limb movements, speech, memories, thoughts, and images. Attention directed to a specific aspect of the experienced world or the self, requires both an intact general awareness and a well functioning, modality-specific thalamo-cortical network.

Neuroscience is a scientific study of the brain and mind. A lot of progress has been made in the understanding of how the brain mediates mental processes. The brain is the organ of mental activity. It forms an interface between the internal and external environments of a living organism. In general, the internal environment is monitored and managed by the brainstem-limbic-cortical system, whereas the external environment and situations are handled by the brainstem-thalamo-cortico-striate system.

The major conscious mental functions such as conation, cognition, and emotion are experienced and responded to by the multimodal associative cortex. The back part of the associative cortex, the temporal-occipital-parietal (TOP) region mediates perception, cognition, attention, memory, comprehension, self-situational monitoring, and self-awareness. It has been called the semantic-conceptual field. The front part of the multimodal associative cortex - the cingulate-prefrontal-premotor cortex, is involved in sensory-motor-cognitive and emotional integration, decision making, working memory, intention, voluntary action, and the executive control of behavior and mentation. Figures 4 and 5.

Most complex mental functions are mediated by cortical networks with multiple, reciprocal connections between different functional areas of both cerebral hemispheres. Some areas of the brain are specialized. For instance, Wernicke's area specializes in processing language comprehension and semantic integration. Broca's area specializes in language expression including semantic, phonological, and grammatical processing.

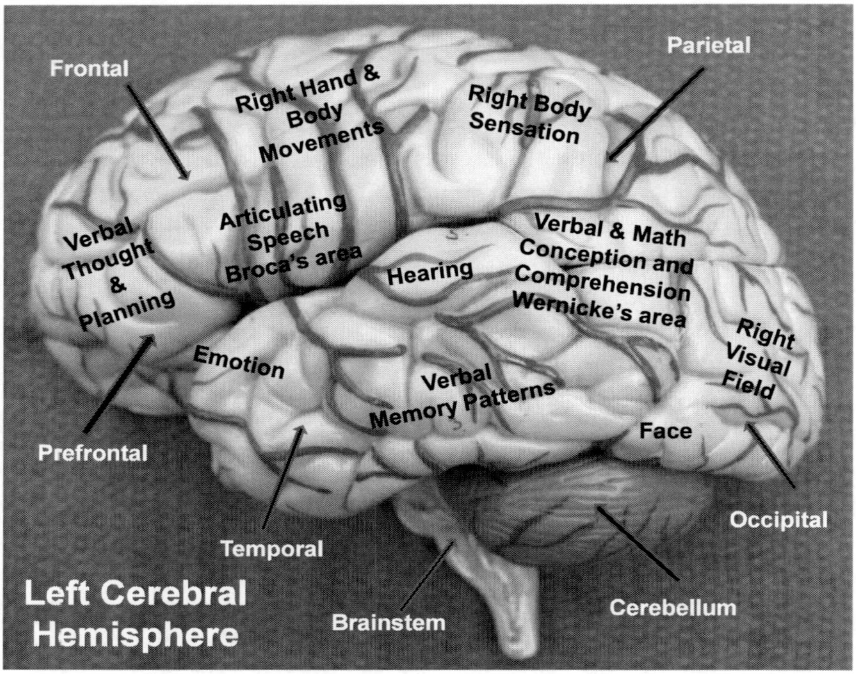

Figure 4. Left cerebral hemispheric functional areas, showing various modality-specific functional areas of the left cerebral cortex.

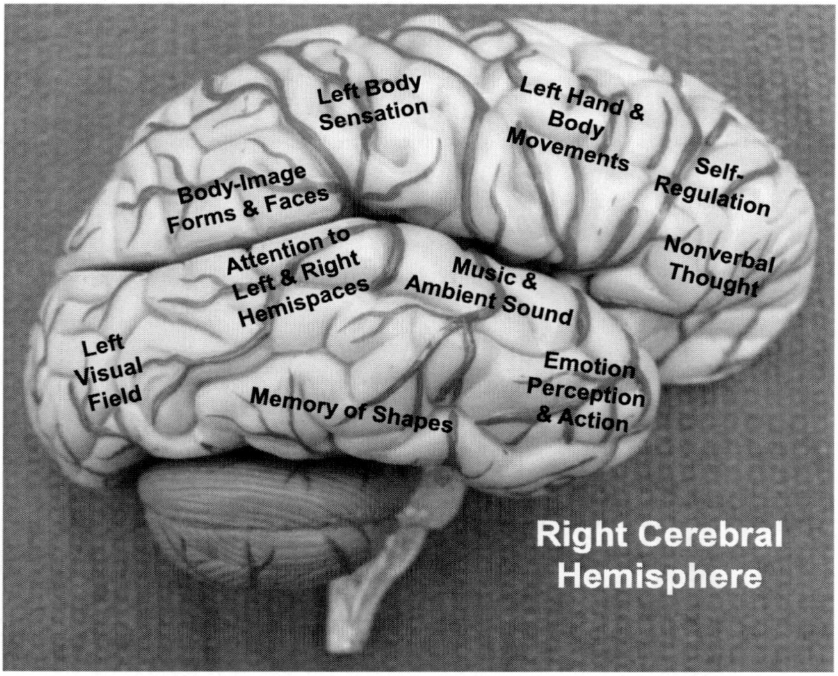

Figure 5. Right cerebral hemispheric functional areas, showing various modality-specific functional areas of the right cerebral cortex.

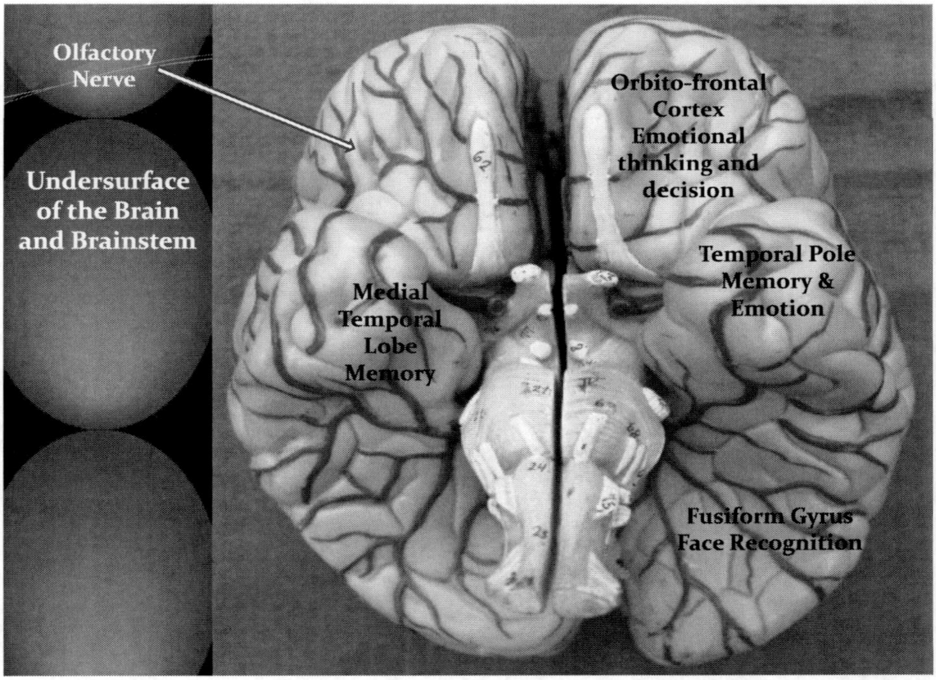

Figure 6.Undersurface of the brain and brainstem showing areas specializing in emotion, memory and face processing.

Hippocampus and the medial temporal lobe specialize in episodic memory including autobiographical memories. Right hemispheric, parietal association area specializes in attention to both right and left halves of the body and the sensory-perceptual fields. Fusiform gyrus specializes in face recognition. Prefrontal cortex with its "frontal intelligence" is crucial for working memory, decision-making, and executive functioning, which includes initiation, continuation, pausing, and stopping of attention, cognition and voluntary action [64]. Figures 6 and 7.

There are four different types memories represented in the brain: i) long term semantic memories, serving as the basis of general knowledge, are stored in the temporal-occipito-parietal (TOP) association cortex, ii) episodic memories of specific events, including individual life events, are represented in the hippocampus and medial temporal lobe, iii) procedural memory of skills and performance of learned actions is represented in frontal, premotor cortex, basal ganglia, and cerebellum, iv) working memory, by which one can hold and manipulate information, for a brief period of time, like remembering a telephone number for 20-30 seconds, is dependent on the dorso-lateral, prefrontal cortex.

Cognitive information is held in the field of awareness as working memory, by rehearsing it intentionally, as inner speech and thought. [65]. If the information is not rehearsed, it quickly dissipates out of awareness, like the cliché, "out of sight, out of mind." A new dictum could be: "Out of memory, out of mind." This is also true of all emotions, thoughts and intentions, which dissipate over time, unless they are voluntarily or habitually maintained in the present awareness. Like many functions of the body, the mind also follows the general principle of "dissipative homeostasis." Thus mind or mentation may be called "homeostatic or homeokinetic." More about this in a later chapter.

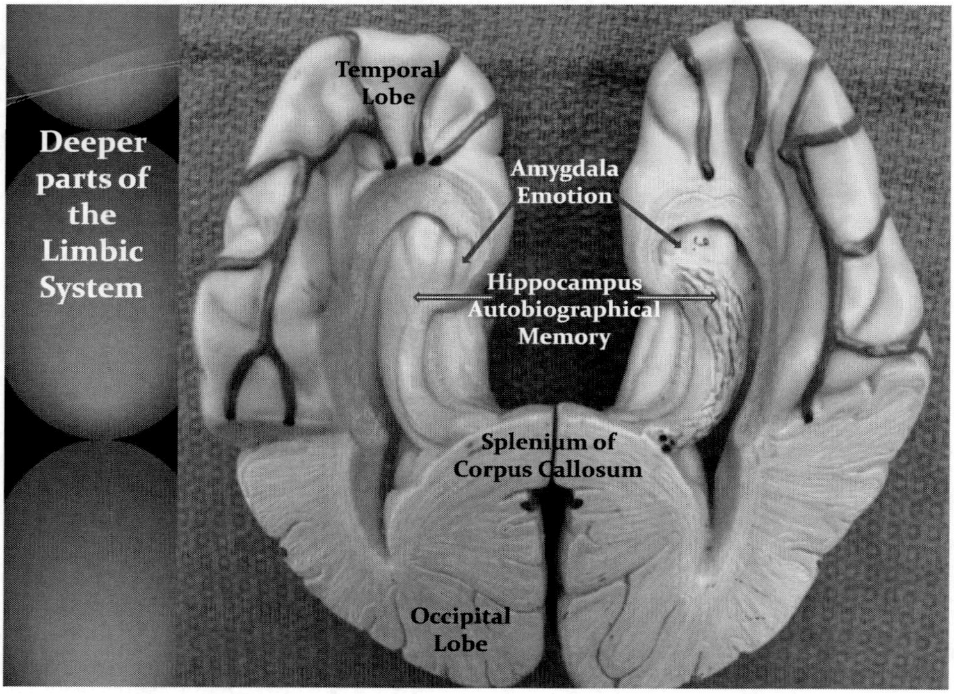

Figure 7. Temporal lobe including Hippocampus, which specializes in episodic, autobiographical memory and Amygdala, which specializes in emotional and threat processing. Splenium is the back part of Corpus callosum, which is a "bridge" between the two cerebral hemispheres for transfer of electrochemical energy, patterns of neural activation and behavioral information.

Human consciousness has three interdependent components: conscious arousal, awareness and attention. i) Conscious arousal depends upon a well functioning brainstem-diencephalic reticular activating system. Any damage or disease in this area could result in loss of consciousness, coma, or death. ii) Conscious awareness depends upon multimodal, nonspecific thalamo-cortical system, which includes central thalamic nuclei and their cortical and subcortical connections. Optimal arousal is essential for awareness. iii) Conscious attention directs and specifies arousal-awareness and behavior to a specific modality, time, place, and person. A lateral fronto-parietal network includes areas for directed eye movements, namely, frontal, parietal and supplementary-motor eye fields.

Attentional activity has two modes: i) a nonspecific, global matrix attention, eye-on-the-field or flood-light mode and ii) a specific vector attention, eye-on-the-ball or spot light mode [66]. The global matrix attention depends upon modality-nonspecific thalamo-cortical circuit. The specific vector attention depends upon specific thalamo-cortico-striate circuits. It creates a subject-object duality with a specific conscious experience and unique mental contents. Selective spatial attention is conceived as a mental spotlight, which improves perception of any or all objects within the attended ("illuminated") region. Attention can be conscious or subconscious, and voluntary or automatic.

Alert attentiveness depends upon a well-functioning, neuromodulatory system of central neurotransmitters, such as acetyl choline, norepinephrine, dopamine, serotonin, and orexin. The level of consciousness spectrum varies from deep sleep to hyperarousal. It is correlated with the activity level of these central neurotransmitters. Good correlation has been shown between level of consciousness and the activity level of Locus Coeruleus nuclei on both sides of the brainstem. These nuclei release norepinephrine in the whole of neuraxis in response to any change in the organism and its environment.

Preattentive 'gist' processing can be very fast. A fearful face flashed only for 30 milliseconds (msec) can influence subsequent cognitive processing, whereas conscious attentional processing takes 300-500 msec. Preattentive processing is very valuable for survival in sudden threatening situations. [67].

There are three specific cortical pathways that mediate "What," "Where" and "When" aspects of any experienced object or event. These aspects of perception and the organism's response to it are integrated. For instance, the ventral occipito-temporal pathway, which is also known as the ventral attentional system, identifies what the object is; the dorsal occipito-parietal pathway, which is known as the dorsal attentional system and is involved in processing where the object is, and the prefrontal-cingulate-parietal cortex network processes when to respond, not to respond, or to wait-and-watch.

Prefrontal cortex mediates executive-cognitive control. Cognitive control is multimodal, and it depends on working memory. It has limited capacity and flexibility. Prefrontal cortex has been called the great integrator. It synthesizes information from both the internal and external worlds and helps the organism to deal with them effectively and adaptively. Prefrontal cortex is connected with sensory, motor and limbic cortical and subcortical systems.

From moment to moment, each organism has to make a decision either to approach, to avoid, or to wait-and-watch, in response to a new event, an object or a situation. Frontal lobes specialize in the avoidance response, whereas, parietal lobes are involved in the approach response. Prefrontal inhibitory network is probably involved in wait-and-watch mode. Ideally, every organism has to be ever-prepared or ready, mentally clear and composed, and in full self-control with the ability to allow, pause, or stop one's actions, when necessary. Conscious preparedness depends on emotional arousal, conscious clarity and open working memory; a full cognitive-control depends on intelligent activational and inhibitory capacities. These are the skills that we have to learn and master in order to live a good and purposeful life.

INSIGHT

I know that I exist.
Knowing my self-existence is blissful.
I feel fulfilled and appreciate
The wonder of being alive and well.

Lasting peace is
In accepting oneself,

As one is in the present moment,
Effortlessly and spontaneously.

It is
Life's victory over death,
Mind's victory over fear.
One is Life till death.
One is Life itself.
Life is one.

Life is spontaneous and self-created.
Our breathing is spontaneous.
So is our being-energy,
And consciousness.

From the very first breath of life,
To the last,
The brainstem reticular formation
Fires spontaneously and continuously,
Organizing all vital functions
Of an individual,
Optimally and efficiently.

Let's appreciate
The wonderful holistic energy
That arises with each breath,
And heart beat,
And enables us to live life consciously,
One breath at a time.

With constant Self-witnessing,
One may understand and appreciate,
The wonder of this Life!

Self-discovery or self-realization is
Discovering the ever-new Reality,
Within and around us.
The amazing holistic Reality
Inspires us all!
Appreciate the wonder,
That IS
Present at this moment!
The Present is Sacred.

Vinod D Deshmukh
May 6, 2007

Chapter 8

SELF-CONSCIOUS MIND IN VEDĀNTA

पूर्णमदः पूर्णमिदं पूर्णात्पूर्णमुदच्यते | पूर्णस्य पूर्णमादाय पूर्णमेवावशिष्यते ||

This (experience) is whole. That (Existence) is whole. From the whole emerges whole. Even after the emergence of whole, the original, (the Absolute), remains whole.

Brihadāraṇ yakopaniṣ ad 5:1:1

According to Vedānta, the mind, which is known as Antaḥ karaṇ a अन्तःकरण, has four internal components or Antarendriya अन्तरेन्द्रिय. They are i) Citta चित्त, the storehouse of memory, ii) Manas मनस्, the cognitive experience including perception, comprehension, thinking, synthesis, and analysis, iii) Buddhi बुद्धि, the intelligent discrimination of experience, situation, personal action and decision making, and iv) Ahamkāra अहंकार, the sense of I-me-mine with accompanying motivation, intentionality, self-regulation and the feeling of being the agent or the ego. All of these components are self-observable and potentially resolvable in the superconscious, holistic matrix of Turīya. In such a meditative state, the mental activity Cittavṛ itti चित्तवृत्ति does not automatically or habitually intrude into the present conscious awareness or presence.

The self-as-subject or the essential source-being, *Ātman* आत्मन् is considered fundamental, foundational, spontaneous, intrinsic, and unobservable as a separate entity, object, event or a process. However, it is intrinsically aware of itself, by its noetic nature and its natural Self-acquaintance. It knows itself effortlessly, all the time. Such intrinsic, integrated information is the very property of a conscious human being. At one's core, there is a feeling of blissful conscious Self-existence, Swatvaṁ स्वत्वं. It is a matter of self-recognition or Pratyabhijñānam[1]. Figure 8.

The feeling of primal, existential being-in-the-world, Ātmabhāva आत्मभाव manifests as basic, foundational, affective consciousness of the blissful conscious being Sat~Cit~Ānanda

[1] Singh, J. Pratyabhijñāhṛ dayam: The Secret of Self-Recognition. Motilal Banarasidass Publishers, Delhi, India. 1979. Reprint 2008.

सच्चिदानन्द. On further differentiation, the commonly recognized three mental activities, namely, conation, cognition, and affection, become manifest as the observable mental phenomena. Our sense of self is considered as an integrated, multistream reality [68]. Its four component-streams, namely, biophysical, mental, social and existential, always act-in-synchrony-synergy to constitute our unitive self-in-the-world experience, from moment to moment.

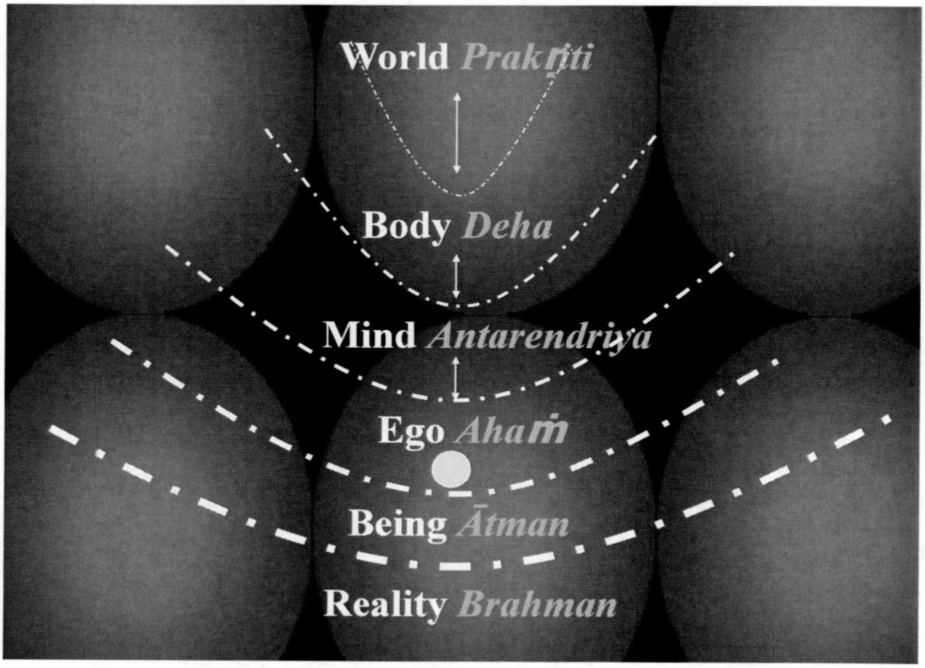

Figure 8. Vedāntic view of being-in Reality with nested levels of self-in-the-world experience. The yellow dot in the middle is the variable vantage point of mind-set and the current perspective of ego, Jīvabhāva जीवभाव. As the vantage point and the self-perspective shifts from ego to the essential source~being *Ātman* with Ātmabhāva आत्मभाव, the mindset as well as the self-in-world experience changes. Brāhmībhāva ब्राह्मीभाव is the spontaneous, intuitive feeling of being the Supreme Being, *Brahman* ब्रह्मन् itself.

The Sāṅ khya साङ्ख्य system of Vedānta philosophy looks at the observable reality as an ever-changing, but, holistic phenomenon called Prakṛ iti प्रकृति, and the ultimate, superconscious, holistic Being as the spontaneous, invariant subject or the experiencing person, called Puruṣ a पुरुष, [69]. The experienced world including one's body and mind are parts of Prakṛ iti. Puruṣ a is the ultimate subjectivity or the intrinsic witness, sākshī साक्षी or Upadraṣ taḥ उपद्रष्टः of the mind and everything that can be experienced. Puruṣ a, the holistic being can never be observed as an object or an event. Puruṣ a is the intrinsic, primal consciousness as such, Ādicaitanya आदिचैतन्य. It is self-sufficient Swārtha स्वार्थ. It is the living, conscious Being-in-itself. There is nothing beyond it for introspection. The direct and convincing knowledge of the holistic reality of Puruṣ a~Prakṛ iti is the enlightening culmination of Self-knowledge, Ātmajñāna आत्मज्ञान. Then, one is a light of insight, wisdom and compassion, to oneself.

Vedānta considers the natural environment, the body, as well as the mind, as the objectifiable and observable reality known as the experiential field, Kshetra क्षेत्र. The knower of this experiential field is Kshetrajña क्षेत्रज्ञ, as described in the 13th chapter of the Bhagvad Gītā. Please see Appendix 1 for the details of the twenty four elements of this experiential field, Kshetra. Despite our common belief, the mind is not our true nature. Mind is our observable, internal 'environment.' Mind is a momentary, mental activity. It becomes conscious when illuminated by spontaneous, intrinsic awareness.

The brain functions as an interface between the internal, Antar अन्तर and the external, Bāhya बाह्य environments. In order to survive and thrive within their natural environments, all organisms have developed effective sensory, motor, and cognitive organs for interaction. Vedānta names energy and information-processing organs of the body as a) sensory-perceptual organs, Jñānendriya ज्ञानेन्द्रिय, b) motor and vocal activity organs, Karmendriya कर्मेन्द्रिय and c) mental-cognitive-conceptual organs, Antarendriya अन्तरेन्द्रिय. Even our sense of self is divided into the external, Bāhyātmā बाह्यात्मा, internal, Antarātmā अन्तरात्मा and transcendent Self or Being, Paramātmā परमात्मा [70].

For each organism, the observed environment is continuously changing in a quantum way by the instantaneous combination of three primary modes of being, Guṇ aḥ गुण: namely, inertia Tamas तमस्, activity Rajas रजस् and homeokinetic equilibrium, Satwa सत्व. Such quantum transformation is the basis of experiential events in reality. A well known quotation in Vedanta is that the body is an instrument for achieving all of life's goals Śariraṁ ādyaṁ khalu dharma sādhanaṁ शरीरं आद्यं खलु धर्म साधनम्.

There are five Jñānendriyas namely, i) eyes for vision, ii) ears for audition, iii) nose for smell or olfaction, iv) skin for touch, and v) tongue for taste or gustatory experience. The five Karmendriyas are i) tongue, mouth, and nose for breathing, swallowing, tasting, eating, and speech, ii) hands for skillful manual and creative work and arts, iii) feet for standing, walking, running, and playing, iv) excretory organs for elimination of bodily waste, and v) genital organs for fulfilling sexual desires and reproductive activity. The four Antarendriyas, which make up Antaḥ karaṇ a अन्तःकरण are: i) Citta, a storehouse of memory, ii) Manas, perception, comprehension, thinking, synthesis, and analysis of cognitive experience, iii) Buddhi, the intelligent discrimination of experience, action, and decision making, and iv) Ahamkāra, a sense of I-me-mine with accompanying motivation, intentionality and emotion. Please see Appendix 1 for details. Figure 9.

Citta चित्त is the storehouse of genetic and epigenetic endowment and all past memories and experiences Samskāraḥ संस्कार: [71]. These Samskārās set the stage and context, for all of our experiences and actions. These long-term semantic and autobiographical memories are stored mostly in the Hippocampal network and the semantic-conceptual field of the posterior temporo-occipito-parietal, multimodal cortex. Ordinarily, we are heavily conditioned and limited by these memories of the past and expectations of the future. We feel as if we are imprisoned in this self-made "cage," as if we are ever committed to this life of bondage, limited understanding, and endless suffering.

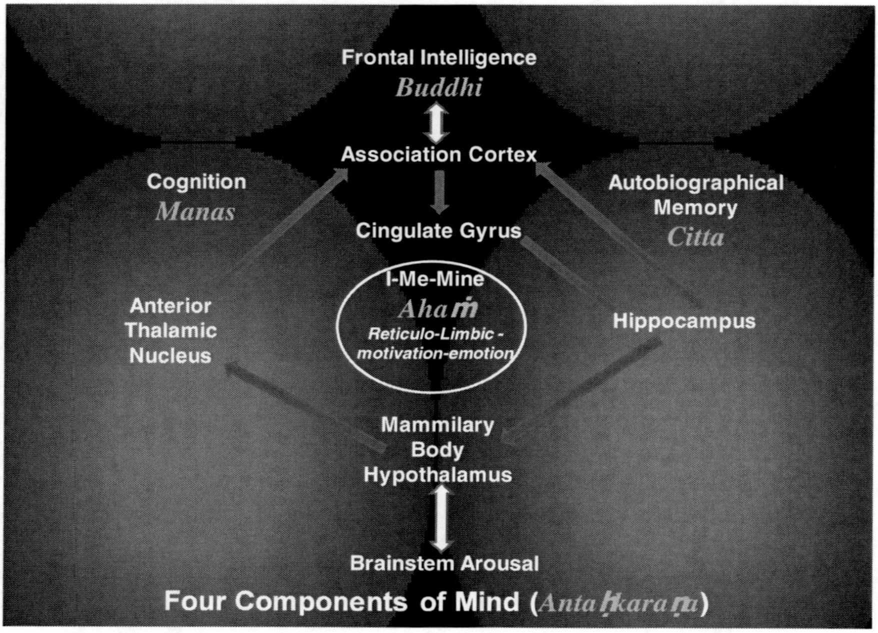

Figure 9. Mind with four components, Antaḥ karaṇ a are: Citta, Manas, Buddhi, and Ahamkāra. Reticulo-limbic-allocortical system and the associate neocortex form the crucial neural network underlying these mental functions. The components of this neural network include Hypothalmus, Anterior Thalamic nucleus, Orbito-Frontal associative cortex, Cingulate gyrus, Hippocampus and Amygdala.

But in all of us there is a natural instinct for self-freedom, Ātma Swātantrya आत्मस्वातंत्र्य, and curiosity. This natural desire for freedom and curiosity helps us rescue ourselves from this bondage, by intense self-awareness and self-understanding. We can realize the final goal of complete self-freedom, with an unshakable understanding, awareness, energy, wellness, and tranquility. This is the purpose of the Vedāntic philosophy of Life.

Manas मनस् is the internal faculty of perception, comprehension, thinking, analysis, and synthesis of cognitive experience. It also includes faculties of thinking, reflection, imagination, and invention. Most of such cognitive activity occurs in the multimodal, fronto-parietal associative cortex. Manas presents the cognized information to intelligence, Buddhi.

Buddhi बुद्धि is involved in discrimination of sensory and recalled experience, voluntary action and decision making. Therefore it is required for knowledge, understanding and action. Such intelligent activity predominantly depends upon the functioning of the prefrontal executive network, with activated working memory.

Ahamkāra अहंकार is a sense of agency, motivation and doer-ship, that arises as a result of repeated motivated actions, voluntary efforts and decision making. When one realizes that most events are controlled by multiple variables, including a chance factor or Providence

Daivaṁ दैवं, one's Ahamkāra or doer-ship diminishes [72]. One realizes the natural spontaneity of one's body, mind and being.

अधिष्ठानं तथा कर्ता करणं च पृथग्विधम् |
विविधाष्च पृथक्चेष्टा दैवं चैवात्र पञ्चमम् ||१४||
Bhagvad Gītā XVIII: 14

(As stated in the Saṅ khya doctrine, the five factors for the outcome of all human actions are): the seat or the situational field of action, the qualifications and readiness of the agent, the quality of instruments used, the amount and intensity of efforts made, and finally, the Providence or the chance factor (for success or failure).

The sense of self depends upon the midline, medial frontal-parietal and subcortical structures, forming the midline, self-relational neural network. As shown in figure 10, this network includes medial prefrontal cortex, medial posterior cortex, retrosplenial cortex, precuneus, the posterior cingulate gyrus and the crucial midbrain structures like tegmentum and tectum. The midline self-relational cortex, also called "the Default mode network" seems to be always active metabolically, even during resting states, and its activity decreases during goal-directed task performance. The self-relational cortex relates to itself with inward orientation to its spontaneous, intrinsic activities, whereas, the lateral fronto-parietal networks engage in outward orientation and interactions. These networks seem to have a reciprocal relationship.

The concept of the subconscious or unconscious mind, Citta has been elaborated in the Vedāntic literature. The repository of unresolved conflicts and memories form the contents of the subconscious mind. It is the arena of unfinished personal business and repressed conflicting impulses, emotions, desires, thoughts, and ideas. There are five primary instincts: i) self-preservation ii) socialization iii) sexuality and reproduction, iv) self-expression and creativity, and v) the desire to know everything including self, others, and the world. Vedānta recommends learning and developing personal skills of Self-awareness, ego-analysis, and ego-discipline. Such paths of growth and development of personality form the basis of Yoga and meditative practices.

The preconscious and subconscious or unconscious in current psychology and psychiatry include i) overlearned or automatic procedural memories, like walking, swimming, riding a bicycle, or tying shoe laces, reading, writing and speech ii) residual unresolved conflicts, painful, resentful, or lustful memories, and iii) the recent or remote contextual background for the current ego and its situation. [73]. Figures 10 & 11.

The spontaneous, meta-conscious being, Puruṣ a पुरुष, is beyond the scope of these instruments, Indriya, of indirect knowing, Paroksha Jñāna परोक्षज्ञान. The organs of perception, cognition and action transform the nonspecific awareness, into a specific conscious mental event. self-transcendence Apawarga अपवर्ग is the conviction of the experiencer that his/her true energy-being is distinct from all experienced phenomena. It is the ultimate Truth within each one of us and our ultimate subjective-objective Reality. It is one and the only Truth, not two, which is Ekaṁevādvitiyaṁ Satyaṁ एकमेवाद्वितीयं सत्यम्.

Pātañjali's Yoga Sūtra पातञ्जलि योगसूत्र continues to be the key reference for the study of mind in Vedānta. When the mind becomes calm due to the practice of Yoga, Yogaḥ cittavṛ itti nirodhāḥ योगः चित्तवृत्ति निरोधः, then, one realizes one's true nature spontaneously, Tadā dṛ aṣ tuḥ swarūpe avasthānam तदा द्रष्टुः स्वरूपेऽवस्थानम्. At other times, one identifies oneself with the ever-changing mental activities, Vṛ ittisārupyaṁitaratra वृत्ति सारूप्यमितरत्र. Five characteristic human mind-sets have been described: i) Muḍ ha मूढ, unenergetic, bored, disinterested, ii) Kshipta क्षिप्त, impulsive, unruly, chaotic, iii) Vikshipta विक्षिप्त, Distracted, wandering, iv) Ekāgra एकाग्र, focused, concentrated, one-pointed and v) Niruddha निरुद्ध, calm, composed, self-organized, integrated, effortless, spontaneous, ego-transcendent and selfless.

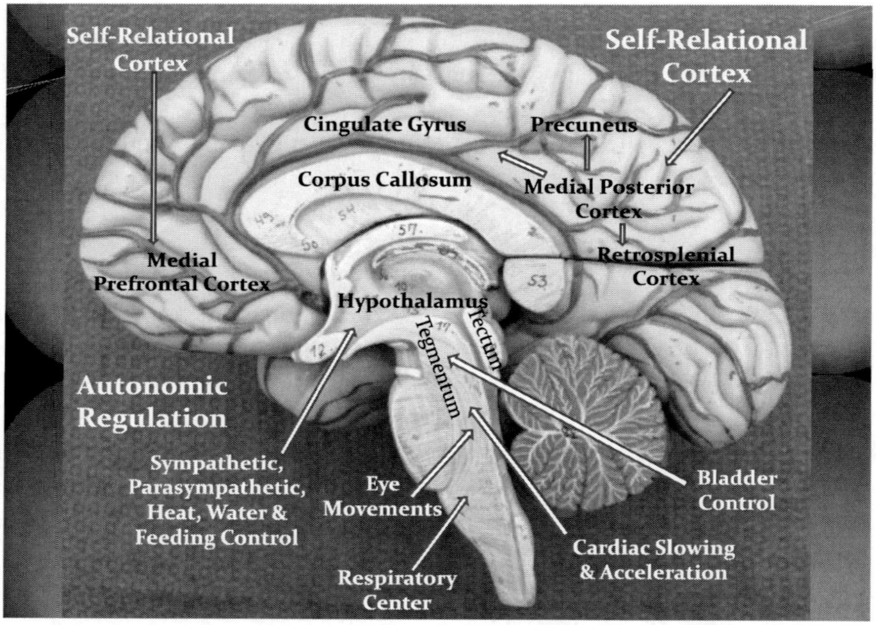

Figure 10. Autonomic and Self-Relational processes. The midline self-relational cortex, also called "the Default mode network" seems to be always active metabolically, even during resting states, and its activity decreases during goal-directed task performance. See Raichle and Snyder. The self-relational cortex relates to itself with inward orientation to its spontaneous, intrinsic activities, whereas, the lateral fronto-parietal networks engage in outward orientation and interactions. These networks seem to have a reciprocal relationship. The right fronto-limbic-insular cortex may be involved in the switching between these two networks.

Pātañjali's Yoga Sūtrās clearly define the stages of self-transformation, Samādhiḥ समाधिः or Ātmasākshātkāra आत्मसाक्षात्कार. Samādhiḥ समाधिः or enlightenment is the actualization of one's transcendent, superconscious and holistic Energy-Being, free of all specific, objective phenomena. The successive stages of Samādhi include freedom from four different types of mental contents, obstacles or opacities: i) Vitarka वितर्क is a deliberate, intentional, and self-reflective thought or choice, ii) Vichāra विचार is a mode of acting, judging, commenting, thinking, inner speech and deciding, iii) Ānanda आनन्द is a personal joy, pleasure and transient, conditional happiness and iv) Asmitā अस्मिता is the sense of I-me-mine or the transient, limited, executive ego or an agent.

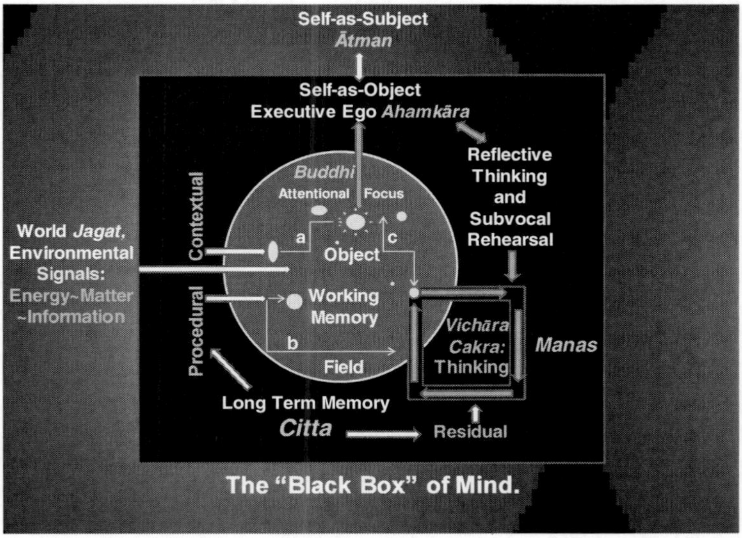

Figure 11. The "Black Box" of Mind. A functional model of mental activity with four main components of long-term memory Citta, with contextual, procedural and residual memories. Frontal Intelligence or Buddhi as the selective attentional and manipulative processes in the activated working memory field. Mentation or Manas as the verbal-visual-tactual cognition, reflective, ruminative thinking and subvocal rehearsal with the wheel of mentation Manaṣ cakra मनष्चक्र or Vichāracakra विचारचक्र. The ego or Ahamkāra as the central executive, the self-as-object, interacting with multidimensional environments and the field of experience, world, Jagat जगत्. Selective attention focuses on any one of the objects or events of interest, in the field of awareness and working memory. The working memory can hold and work on or manipulate up to seven +/- two objects at any given conscious moment. Objects in the field are shown as yellow ovals. Three pathways of information-flow and possible conscious cognition are shown: a) Direct sensory-perceptual-cognition from the phenomenal world, b) Indirect, slow, reflective, ruminative memory-dependent cognition due to mentation or thinking, and c) Spontaneous emergence of insightful, encouraging or disturbing information from the quiet preconscious or unconscious, implicit memories to the conscious level. Holistic conscious presence, Ubhaya Sākshī उभयसाक्षी includes both a) the direct sensory-perceptual objective reality inputs, as well as c) the spontaneous, inspired, intuitive, intrinsic sources, as holistic consciousness.

The word, Prajñā प्रज्ञा means to know wisely and to understand clearly and fully. The word Bīja बीज means a seed, with the potential to grow into a living being, like a plant or an animal. It can also mean a seed of a mental state, which can grow into a full-blown mental experience. With these meanings in mind, the states of Samādhi can be further classified into i) Samprajñāta सम्प्रज्ञात and Asamprajñāta असम्प्रज्ञात, meaning with or without awareness and ii) Sabīja सबीज or Nirbīja निर्बीज, meaning with or without a mental, experiential seed or mental content. The mental, experiential seed always indicates some content in the field of consciousness. Kaivalya कैवल्य or Mukti मुक्ति is the complete, unconditional freedom from all dualistic, phenomenal experience. Virām-Pratyaya विरामप्रत्यय is a freedom from personal thoughts and mental experience. It may lead to Asamprajñāta samadhi असम्प्रज्ञात with conscious clarity or Śūnyatā शून्यता, an unshakable serenity Śamatā शमता and profound self-understanding and equanimity, Sthita-Prajñā स्थितप्रज्ञा. It is the timeless, enlightened life with full Self-realization of the holistic Energy-Being-in-Reality.

FREEDOM AND LOVE

Freedom from
Pain,
Hatred,
Loneliness,
Dependence,
And the fear of aging,
And death.

Love for
Living,
Learning,
Discovering,
Creating,
And caring for family, friends,
Humanity and Nature.

Welcoming
Whole-heartedly,
The present moment,
And the next,
As it surges freshly,
By itself.

Appreciating
The great wonder of
Reality!

Vinod D Deshmukh
November 7, 2007

Chapter 9

IPSEITY *ĀTMAN* AND PRESENCE

"The self is the archetype of the ego; it is the innate potential for wholeness, and unconscious ordering principle, directing the overall psychic life that gives rise to the ego, which compromises with and is partly shaped by the external reality."

Jung CG

This archetypal self is similar to the *Ātman* in Vedānta. In a long tradition, Vedic scholars have contemplated on Being, the Self, *Ātman* आत्मन् and understood its true nature. They expressed their understanding in an amazingly precise way. The Vedic literature is ripe with great insights into our true nature, the Ātman and the nature of the ultimate cosmic Reality, the *Brahman* ब्रह्मन्. These visionaries concluded that Ātman and Brahman are the same, in essence. This great Vedāntic philosophy of Life has been an enduring source of inspiration, understanding, joy, courage, and altruism for many generations in India and also the rest of the world. Hopefully, it will continue to be so, for many generations of humanity to come.

In modern neuroscience and psychiatry, a new model of consciousness and self-consciousness has been proposed [74]. In this model, consciousness is divided into phenomenal and introspective consciousness. The phenomenal consciousness is a first-person-perspective, whereas, introspective, reflective consciousness is a third-person-perspective. The contents of phenomenal consciousness are pre-reflexive, raw feelings or qualia. The contents of introspective consciousness may be cognitive, emotional, sensory, or memory-related. These experiences may be conscious, preconscious, subconscious, or unconscious, depending upon the level of attentional awareness directed to them.

The phenomenal, self-consciousness is divided into two components, ipseity and self-qualia. Ipseity (Ipse: I or Self) is the unifying basic tone of the first-person's experience. It is the center of all conscious experience and is dependent upon a continuous, internally generated, interoceptive brain input. It gives us a sense of a single unitive being. Ipseity or I, in every experience, is implicitly and pre-reflexively present, in the holistic field of awareness, through which all conscious experiences pass. It is an intrinsic property of the self-relational, essential, holistic consciousness.

Ipseity is a spontaneous neurobiological phenomenon, which depends upon brain arousal and awareness. Ipseity itself is non-interactive and not a pole until one starts interacting with the 'other' by reflective consciousness. Self-qualia are responsible for the feelings of self-agency, self-unity, self-affectability, and implicit self-history. Ipseity is an unreflected presence, with self-luminosity and the self-conscious arousal-energy Swayaṁ jyotiḥ स्वयंज्योतिः.

From our common experience, we know that i) Self is distinct from the situation and the broader environment, ii) it is the source or author of our feelings, actions and thoughts, and iii) it is the same person across our life time. The contents of self-qualia, when reflected upon, become the contents of reflective consciousness. With reflective consciousness, we can communicate verbally and non-verbally with others and ourselves.

The concept of presence refers to a pre-reflective first-person experience, i.e. ipseity and a sense of immersion, absorption, or self-mergence, in the present moment. Subject and object are two abstract poles of a unique process, which is presence. The concept of presence was discussed in greater detail by the author [75]. Presence is the fact or state of being present. It means being present-minded as opposed to being absent-minded, which is 'absence.' Presence is being attentive to what is happening now and here. Presence is being in existence now. Presence is functioning fully or optimally at the present time. It implies freedom from the burden of the past and imaginary expectations of the future. It implies self-renewal from moment to moment. Presence is being well adapted to one's situation and self. Presence is the process of reducing uncertainty, a process of knowing and doing. Presence heightens awareness and may lead to an intuitive consciousness generating new ideas, new understanding, and creative solutions. Presence is a way to achieve mental clarity and serenity. It is the very essence of our Blissful Conscious Being, Sat~Chit~Ānanda.

PRESENCE

The Presence is
The process of existence.
It is being-in-existence,
Here-and-now and
Sometimes, then-and-there.

Presence is
The personal process,
That one is,
In the on-going Reality.
It is a nested process.

Presence is
a point
In the conscious space-time.
It is nested
In the existential cosmic process.

Presence is
A living wonder,
That some describe as

Eternal, infinite and sacred.
It is indescribable.

It is, what is;
Unfathomable and unknowable,
By our limited cognitive minds.

We just have to appreciate
Its wonder,
With our "Heart."
It is an all-inclusive
Natural process,
That is in-existence,
NOW!

Vinod D Deshmukh

January 7, 2007

Chapter 10

NEUROSCIENCE OF SELF-CONSCIOUSNESS

Somehow, the living brain self-organizes throughout life, and for a neuroscientist, the conscious brain~mind still remains a great mystery - a great puzzle to be solved.

The term consciousness is difficult to define, although all of us understand what it is from our first-person experience. There are many definitions and several reviews on the subject of human and animal consciousness [76 - 81]. In clinical neurology, consciousness is defined as a set of neural processes that allow an individual to perceive, comprehend and act on the internal and external environments. It has three functional aspects: arousal, awareness, and attention. Arousal describes the degree of wakefulness or alertness. It depends upon the adequate functioning of the ascending brainstem-diencephalic, reticular-limbic activating system. Awareness implies that the individual is not only alert but is also cognizant of self and surroundings. It reflects the depth and content of the aroused state. Awareness depends on arousal. For conscious awareness, proper functioning of the central thalamus and the cerebral cortex is essential. Only awareness, by itself, may not be directed and modality-specific. Attention is needed for directionality and modality-specificity. Attention depends both on awareness and arousal, and implies the ability to direct and respond to modality-specific stimuli. It implies directed awareness and response. It is modality-specific, e.g. tactile, auditory, or visual attention and a precisely directed perception, action or speech. The right cerebral hemisphere is dominant for attentive behavior. It is also dominant for visual-spatial and musical abilities. The left cerebral hemisphere is usually dominant for language and other symbolic processing, such as skills in pattern-recognition and mathematics. Figures 12, 13, and 14.

Consciousness is viewed as an organism's self-generating, self-organizing process, embedded in its ecological niche. This ecological perspective was described by Goerner and Combs [78] as follows: "The evolution of consciousness is seen in the context of energy-driven evolution in general, where energy and information are understood as two sides of the same coin. From this perspective, consciousness is viewed as an ecological system in which streams of cognitive, perceptual and emotional information form a rich complex of interactions, analogous to the interactive metabolism of a living cell. The result is an organic, self-generating or `autopoietic' system, continuously in the act of creating itself. Evidence suggests that this process is non-linear, chaotic, or at least chaotic-like and capable of assuming a number of distinct states best understood as chaotic attractors."

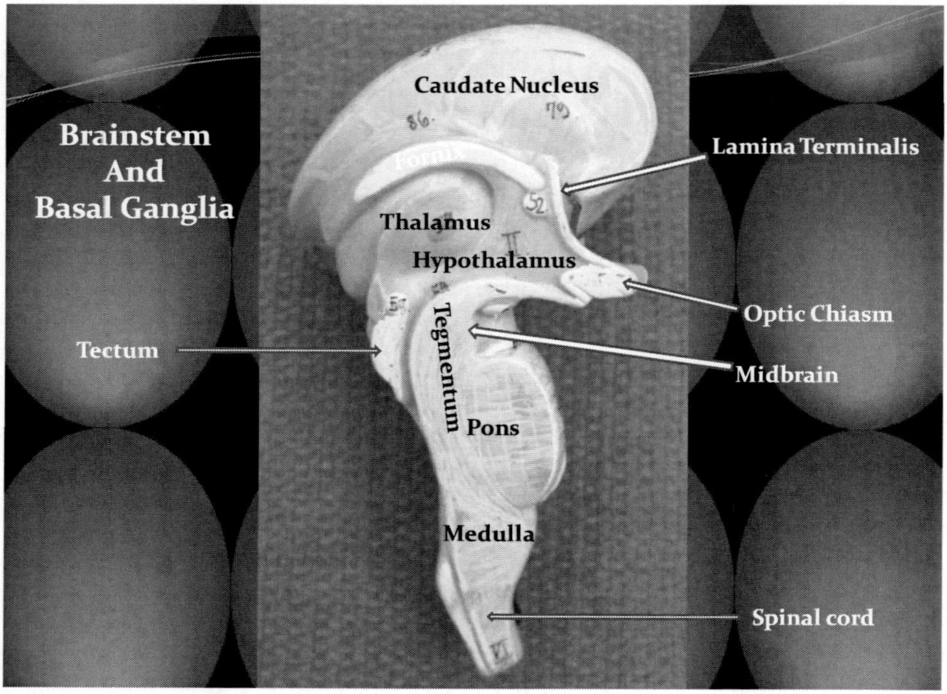

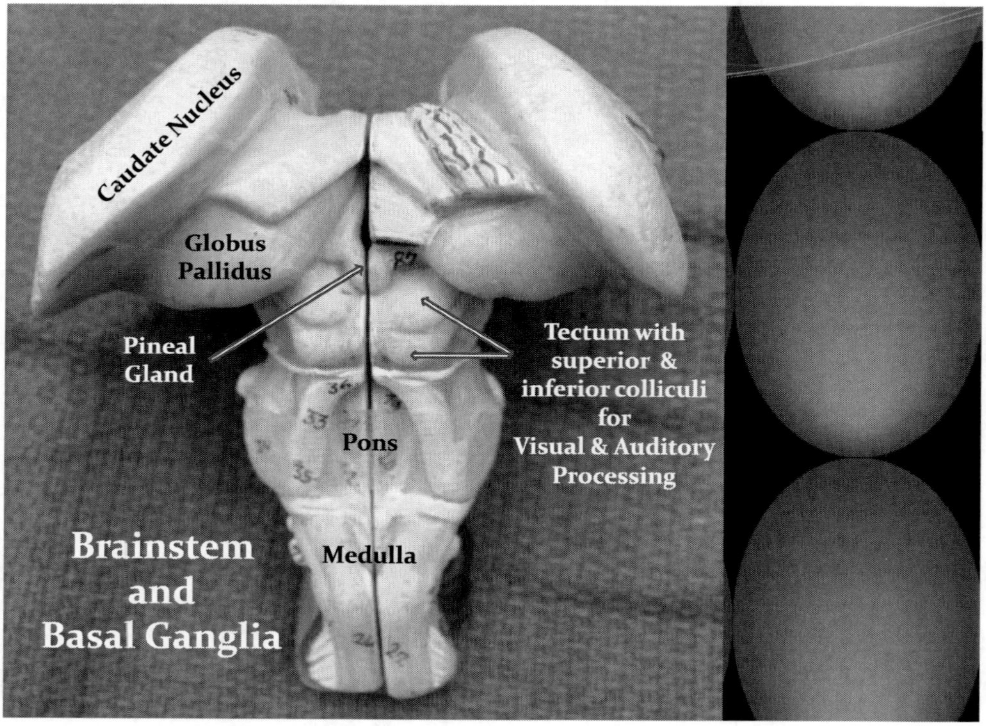

Figures 12 and 13. Brainstem and Basal Ganglia, inside and back views showing the key functional structures.

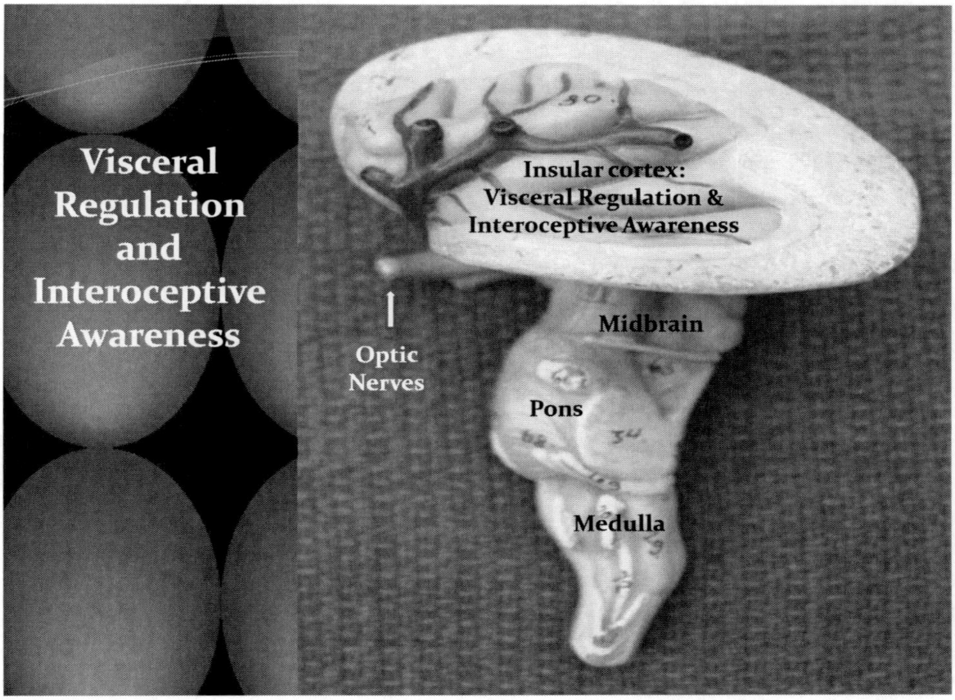

Figure 14. Left insular cortex and brainstem. Insular cortex processes interoceptive information and sub-serves body-awareness and visceral-affective regulation.

Tononi and Edelman [79] emphasized two properties of consciousness: i) conscious experience and ii) conscious state. "Conscious experience is integrated; each conscious scene is unified, and at the same time, it is highly differentiated; a huge number of different conscious states are possible at each conscious moment. They define integration or functional clustering as a property shared by every conscious experience, irrespective of its content. Each conscious state comprises of a single scene that is private and cannot be decomposed into independent components. We cannot be aware of two incongruent scenes simultaneously. So also, we cannot make more than a single conscious decision, within an interval of a few hundred milliseconds (300-500 ms), the so-called psychological refractory period. Conscious experience depends upon activation or deactivation of specific neocortical areas in response to external or internal stimulation and the activation by memory, intention, imagery or dreams."

Tononi [80] has recently proposed a theory of consciousness called "Integrated Information Theory," claiming that consciousness is integrated information. The quantity of consciousness is given by the amount of integrated information generated by a complex of elements namely neurons, and the quality of conscious experience or 'qualia' is given by the set of informational relationships within that neural complex.

The process of human waking from stage II sleep has been studied by using PET scanning. After waking from stage II sleep, brain blood flow is rapidly re-established in the centrencephalic regions, brainstem and thalamus, suggesting that the reactivation of these regions is essential for the re-establishment of basic wakefulness with conscious awareness. In the next 15 minutes, there is a further increase in the brain blood flow in the anterior cortical areas, prefrontal and anterior cingulate cortex, coinciding with the re-establishment of functional alertness and the dissipation of sleep inertia.

The word "Self" has multiple meanings. The dictionary defines self as i) the total, essential or particular being of one person, the individual, ii) personality, character, individuality, and iii) individual's consciousness of his own being, identity, subjectivity, ego. Self-consciousness implies conscious awareness of oneself, one's own being, one's actions, thoughts and emotions. In psychotherapy [82], it is acknowledged that self is a very personal matter and can never be known in its entirety. It is difficult to understand and to define it. However, self is tentatively defined as the totality of a complex, dynamic and organized system of learned beliefs that an individual holds to be true about his or her personal existence. It provides a consistency to the human personality.

The global Self is orchestrated and balanced like a spiral, and it is centered on the 'I', the Self-as-subject. This 'I' is the living connection with human experience. In addition to the I-as-the-Subject, the self also contains many observable self-images based on self-perception, as the self-as-object, the so-called "me." The self is modifiable in the sense that new perceptions are integrated into the self-image, throughout life, while old perceptions fade away. This continuous affective-cognitive flow of experience creates flexibility and modifiability of the self. A healthy self is highly flexible, well adjusted, creative and adaptive. It is continuously involved in creating new visions of personal growth and enhancement.

Antonio Damasio [83, 84] divided the sense of self into i) proto-self, ii) core self and iii) autobiographical self. Proto-self is defined as a coherent first-order collection of neural patterns, which map, moment-by-moment, the state of the physical structure of the organism in its many dimensions, at multiple neural levels, from brainstem to cerebral cortex. Proto-self does not perceive or hold knowledge. It has no language and we are not conscious of proto-self. It is a reference point in consciousness, but it is not an interpreter of anything.

The core self is a transient, second-order, non-verbal account that occurs whenever an object, a sensory, emotional, or memory input, modifies the protoself. Core consciousness is created in pulses, each pulse triggered by each objective input that we interact with or that we recall. We are conscious of the core self. The mechanism that produces the core self, undergoes minimal change across a lifetime. The core self requires the presence of the proto-self.

The autobiographical self requires the presence of the core self. It is based on the memory of multiple individual experiences of the past and the anticipated future. The autobiographical memory grows with life experiences and gets modified continuously by our new experiences. We are conscious of the autobiographical self.

The sense of self is also defined as a collection of schemata, a potential to act or to be in a certain way, regarding one's abilities, traits and attitudes that guide our behavior, choices, and social interactions. Self-awareness is our capacity to reflect on our sense of self. Such capacity depends on the proper functioning of medial prefrontal and posterior cingulate cortex. The frontal lobes, especially the prefrontal areas specialize in maintaining working-memory representations that integrate verbal and spatial information [85]. The non-dominant frontal lobe seems to be particularly important for accessing, integrating and maintaining self-knowledge as seen in patients with fronto-temporal dementia [86].

Frontal cortex, especially its prefrontal region is devoted to the organization of action in all neurobiological and cognitive domains: skeletal movement, eye movement, speech and logical reasoning [87]. Prefrontal cortex is in-charge of the temporal organization of behavior, speech and thinking. Three cognitive operations that are essential to serve these functions are i) preparatory set, ii) working memory, and iii) inhibitory control of interference. Prefrontal cortex, the great integrator, is able to sculpt behavior and perform diverse tasks through parallel excitatory and inhibitory regulation of neural activity in distributed neural networks [88].

Llinas considered 'Prediction' as the ultimate function of the brain. "Self is the centralization of prediction. "The self is not born out of consciousness, only the noticing of it (i.e., self-awareness). According to this view, the self can exist without awareness of its own existence. Even for us as self-aware individuals, self-awareness is not continuously present. […] "I" has always been a magnificent mystery; I believe, I say, I whatever. But one must understand that there is no such tangible thing. It is just a particular mental state, a generated abstract entity we refer to as "I" or "self." […] The "I" of the vortex, that which we work for and suffer for, is just a convenient word that stands for as global an event as does the concept of Uncle Sam vis-a-vis the reality of a complex, heterogenous United States." [89].

Chapter 11

SELF *ĀTMAN* आत्मन् IN VEDĀNTA

उत्पन्न शक्तीबोधस्य त्यक्तनिःशेषकर्मणः |
योगिनः सहजावस्था स्वयमेव प्रजायते ||४-११||

Samādhi dawns spontaneously on a yogi, whose holistic awareness-energy is awakened naturally, and who has let go of his ego-centered, selfish desires and actions.

Hatha-Yoga Pradipikā 4:11

In Vedānta, the essential, existential self or being is known as *Ātman* आत्मन्. There is a vast Vedic literature on *Ātman* and *Brahman*. Both terms are difficult to define, but in essence, both *Ātman* and *Brahman* point to the same absolute Reality, Sat~Chit~Ānand, expressed as the essential Being Sat सत्, intrinsic Consciousness Cit चित्, and unconditional Bliss Ānanda आनन्द.

Ātmopaniṣ ad आत्मोपनिषद् described the self, the person or Puruṣ a पुरुष, to be threefold, namely, the outer self Bāhyātmā बाह्यात्मा, the inner self Antarātmā अन्तरात्मा and the transcendental, holistic, source-being Paramātmā परमात्मा. The outer self Bāhyātmā is the physical body, which is composed of various body parts, organs, and biological processes. It is born and it dies. The inner self Antarātmā is the one that perceives various physical objects and also various mental states such as desire, aversion, pleasure and pain, lust, etc. He or she also comprehends languages, vocal and musical instruments, dancing, etc. He/she is the listener, smeller, taster, thinker, comprehender, doer, and a discriminating self, whose sign is memory. He/she is capable of studying, making decisions and taking selective actions. The transcendental holistic Self Paramātmā is to be realized according to the precepts of the Vedās. Such a self-realization dawns on someone who meditates on Adhyātmā अध्यात्मा, the proximate Self, who is the essential core of our being.

The self can be realized by mastering the paths of yogic self-integration including i) Prāṇ āyāma प्राणायाम, self-regulation and optimization of breathing ii) Pratyāhāra प्रत्याहार, the detached attitude of being a witness of all phenomena, iii) Dhāraṇ ā धारणा, focused attentiveness, iv) Dhyānaṁ ध्यानं, sustained, meditative awareness and v) Samādhiḥ समाधि: the ego-mergence in the absolute Reality. The transcendental, holistic Self-Consciousness is primal, like a banyan seed and it cannot be perceived or grasped by the limited mind. It is not born nor does it die. It is beyond all qualities, the witness, eternal and pure, of the essence of the indivisible, one-only subtle, without components, without taint, without egoism. It is beyond senses. It is all-pervading, unthinkable and indescribable. It purifies the defiled, the evil. It is spontaneous, without action, and without any residue. It is ever fresh and new.

In Ādi Śaṅ karāchāryā's Ātma-Jñānopadesh Vidhi [90], Ātman, the existential Energy-Being is described as follows: "*Ātman* is distinct from all things described before. It is the innermost (nothing else within it), all-pervading like space, subtle, eternal, without any parts, without qualities, spotless, having no activities like going and coming. It is devoid of ideas like me and mine and also of desire, aversion and effort. By nature, it is the Self-effulgent, Swayaṁ Jyotiḥ , like the radiant light and heat of fire or the light of the sun. It has no connections with the natural elements such as space, etc. It possesses no organs like the intellect, etc. It is free from the gunās like sattva, etc. and not having prāṇa and other vital airs. It is untouched by hunger, thirst, grief, delusion, bodily sense or body-image, old age and death. It is the self (the source) that resides in the "*heart*" of all beings and is the seer of all intellectual activities. It is the witness-consciousness of both the seer and the seen."

Śaṅ karāchārya elaborated on the ever-present reality of Ātman in his famous book, Ātmabodha [91] as follows: "*Ātman* alone illumines the senses, intellect and mind, like the light illumines various pots etc. *Ātman* however, is not illumined by these inert objects. Just as a light does not need another light to illumine itself, so too, Ātman needs no other knower to make it known, as its nature is awareness-as-such. On account of its being of the nature of awareness and bliss, there are no distinctions of the knower, knowledge and known in the supreme Self. It is the conscious energy, the knowing process itself. It verily shines by itself. *Ātman* indeed is an ever-present reality, yet because of our ignorance, it is not commonly known. When the self-ignorance is destroyed, the self is found like the lost necklace on one's own neck. Having relinquished the attachment to transitory pleasures, the enlightened one, content with the bliss of *Ātman*, shines alone inwardly like a flame, unperturbed by the wind."

INTUITIVE KNOWING

Intuitive knowing is
Realizing the knowing process.
It is the knowing of knowing!
The knowing process creates
The knower-known duality,
Like the two branches of the same tree.
The knowing process itself
Can be realized only intuitively.

All of us know this or that thing.
We think we are this or that person.
We know that we know something.

But, can we realize
The knowing process itself?

The intuitive realization of
The knowing process requires:
Stillness, unperturbed by movement,
Silence, unbroken by word,
Presence, not dragged by memory,
Spontaneity, un-driven by effort,
Serenity, not shattered by agitation,
Gentleness unspoiled by egoism,
Space, not shaped by face or form,
Clarity, un-obscured by thought,
Fearlessness, not touched
By the thought of death,
Joy, unsurpassed by any other,
Unaltered by all mental activity,
A conscious continuum,
Aware of its essence.

It is a knowing beyond
All words and descriptions.
It is neither crystallized nor grasped.
It is so fluid, yet so still,
Like a standing spiral.

It is primal, yet ever fresh.
It is the source,
As well as the sink, of cognition.
It is a knowing,
When the mind is empty of specifics,
Yet it is so full of boundless Energy.

It is a biophysical process.
It is a cognitive matrix,
Based on a dynamic brain network,
Where each experience arises and subsides,
Like a lone cloud in clear sky.

It is a meditation that continues on its own.
It requires no intentional action,
Since, any action would only be a needless intrusion.

It is a knowing
That dawns spontaneously.
It can't be willed or possessed.

Such knowing is a unique Awareness.
It has no name, nor face,
Yet, it is the source of all named faces.

I do not know what it feels like to be
A manatee, an osprey or any other being,
But probably, their essential awareness is
Similar to this great, primal feeling.

Such intuitive knowing is
The wonder of all wonders.
It is the wonder of
Our amazing existential Awareness.
It is the living Truth
Of our conscious Being,
Our self-aware Energy!

Vinod D Deshmukh

June 4, 2005

Chapter 12

MULTI-STREAM SELF

अत्र अयं पुरुषः स्वयंज्योतिः भवति।

In this superconscious, holistic state, the self becomes Self-luminous. It becomes a Self-effulgent light to itself.

The author had proposed to extend the standard bio-psycho-social model of mind and self to a more comprehensive concept of bio-psycho-social-existential or holistic self and mind. By adding the existential component to the self-concept and mind, the total human experience is better understood and explained. The word "existential" refers to the concrete lived experience of human beings, firmly rooted in the real world. Existential living is the capacity to live holistically in the present, and respond freely and flexibly to new experience without fear. Such an integrative living would create an experience of mindful presence, with an awareness and understanding of one's current, peaceful existence and a unique life of Self-actualization.

Well-being is defined as a state of happiness, contentment, lack of distress, overall good physical and mental health, a healthy outlook and a good quality of living. Maslow [92] defined self-actualization as "an episode in which powers of the person come together in an efficient and enjoyable way and in which he was more integrated and open to experience, more spontaneous and expressive, fully functioning, more creative, humorous, more ego-transcending, and more independent of his or her lower needs. He becomes more truly himself, more perfectly actualizing his potentialities, closer to the core of being, more fully human"

The self-actualized individual learns to overcome the four existential fears, the four 'I's, namely, Insecurity, Isolation, Insignificance, and Inexistence, or death. Yalom [93] wrote about the fears of one's nonexistence or death, lack of external support and being on oneself, with a need for free choice with responsibility, self-isolation from all creatures in the world, and a lack of meaning and hope in life. He suggested whole-hearted engagement in current life, creativity, self-actualization, and altruism, as possible solutions to these ultimate existential fears.

Vedic seers have beautifully expressed the value of self-freedom from all fears and development of friendliness with others and Nature.

अभयं मित्रादभयममित्रादभयं ज्ञातादभयं पुरो यः |
अभयं नक्तमभयं दिवा नः सर्वा आशा मम मित्रं भवन्तु ||

May we be fearless of friends as well as enemies, fearless of the known and the unknown, fearless during the day and at night. My hope is that all beings will be my friends.

Atharva Veda अथर्ववेद XIX XV ६.

The wisdom of self-integrity is beautifully expressed by Erikson [94]. It means acceptance of oneself and all aspects of one's life and integration of these elements into a stable pattern of living. It implies the experience of and adjustment to the trials and troubles of life as well as to its rewards and joys. Consequently, existence holds no fear; the ego has resigned itself to acceptance of life itself and to acceptance of the end of that life in death.

Integrity thus represents the fully developed personality, in its most mature self-realization. Integrity is acceptance of one's one and only life cycle, and of the people who have become significant to it, as something that had to be, and that by necessity, permitted of no substitutions. "The individual relinquishes the wish that important people in his or her life had been different and is able to love in a more meaningful way - one that reflects an acceptance of responsibility for one's own life."

The individual in possession of the virtue of wisdom and a sense of integrity has room to tolerate the proximity of death and achieve what Erikson termed a detached yet active concern[1]. "The style of integrity developed by his or her culture and civilization thus becomes the 'patrimony' of his or her soul...In such a final consolidation, death loses its sting."

Self is a complex, integrative process of a living organism. It self-organizes, coordinates, and integrates energy-information-matter, within and around itself, spontaneously, consciously as well as unconsciously. Self-process is understood in terms of synergetics, coordination dynamics, and energy-information–directed self-organization. It is dynamic, composite, ever renewing, and enduring. It can be convergent or divergent, and can function as the source or target of its own behavior-mentation.

The experience of self is continuously generated by spontaneous activation of neural networks in the cerebral neocortex by the brainstem-diencephalic arousal system. The multiple constitutive behavioral-mental streams develop concurrently, into a unique experience of self, specific for a person at his or her developmental stage. The chronological neuro-behavioral-mental development of self is described later in detail, from embryonic stage to old age. Self can be behaviorally and mentally oriented in three complimentary modes of being: egocentric, allocentric, and ecosystemic or holistic. The holistic mode of being can be both immanent and transcendent, and can be self-actualized, resulting in a healthy, conflict-free, creative, and meaningful life.

The human sense of self is hard to define since the word has so many connotations. The APA Dictionary of Psychology defines the word "self" as the totality of the individual, consisting of all characteristic attributes, conscious and unconscious, mental and physical. It refers to personal identity, being, and experience. A person can refer to self either as the

[1] This is similar to the attitude of being a loving, caring witness to the passing phenomena; also called Sākshi-bhāva.

source of its agency, the regulator of behavior, or as the target of perception-cognition-action. It is the essence of individuality – being, proprium, or ipseity.

The current or minimal self is the life-in-the-moment or the immediate experience of one's person, unextended in time. Narrative, autobiographical, or longitudinal self is based on autobiographical memories and projected future. According to the psychologist William James, nominative self is the Self-as-knower of the ego, whereas, empirical self is the self-so-known. The empirical self further consists of the material self, the social self, and the spiritual self, which is closest to one's core, subjective experience of oneself, [95].

I am also using the word "self" from the point of view of new biophysics, based on synergetics [96], dynamic patterns [97], coordination dynamics, energy-information–directed self-organization, and holistic-biological perspective of neuroscience [98]. "Synergetics is the cooperation of individual parts of a system that produces (new) macroscopic spatial, temporal and functional structures. It deals with deterministic as well as stochastic processes." Coordination dynamics is "a set of context-dependent laws or rules that describe, explain, and predict how patterns of coordination form, adapt, persist, and change in natural systems."

In a natural system, like a school of fish, or a flock of birds, there is an "upward causation" wherein an individual fish or bird interact and coordinate with others, and create a new, coordinative macrostructure, i.e., the school of fish or a flock of birds, which is a whole system, with its own new properties and rules of behavior. The school of fish – the whole, in turn, influences the behavior of all fish – a "downward causation." Two of these effects together constitute "circular causality" in the dynamic natural systems. The school of fish, or a flock of birds, is sometimes called a super-organism. These concepts are applicable to many complex, natural systems including living organisms and their societies, brain activity, animal behavior, cognition, human mentation and the Cosmos as a whole.

THREE STEPS TO INFINITY

The first step is
To make peace and be free of
The experience of the world,
With its valleys and mountains,
Rivers and oceans,
Trees, forests and deserts,
Animals and people,
With their war and peace.

The second step is
To make peace and be free of
The experience of the body
With all its agitations, lethargy,
Aches, pains and pleasures,
Its fight, fright and flight,
Hunger, sex and satiety,
Beauty and ugliness,

Aging and death.

The third step is
To make peace and be free of
The experience of the mind
With its thoughts and emotions,
Memory and imagination,
Success and failure,
Pride and prejudice,
Love and hate relationships,
Knowledge and ignorance of
Quarks to cosmos.

Like an impatient child, we may ask:
"Are we there yet? Close to Infinity?"

If we really took the first three steps,
And became free of all of
Our specific personal experiences,
Then, we would naturally be in
The ineffable, silent, serene,
Holistic, infinite awareness,
And blissful Being.

At such a timeless moment,
There is no need to climb any steps,
As there is no ladder to climb.
The Infinity is the Truth
Nearest to our *heart*.

Vinod D Deshmukh

October 6, 2007

Chapter 13

SYNERGIC ORGANIZATION OF SELF

In a holistic energy~being~awareness field, like a living organism or a school of fish, all elements are active, all over, at the same time. This is synergy-synchrony-integration of their matter~energy~information.

Self is a complex, integrative process of a living organism. The living organism is a functioning, behaving unit of Life. The living organism self-organizes, coordinates, and integrates information-energy-matter, within and around itself, spontaneously, subconsciously, and consciously. West [99] summarized the importance of neural integration: "How can diverse neuronal mechanisms provide coherent, subjective experience and volition? The answer is integration. Every living creature - beginning with the most primitive – is fully integrated; without integration, life is not possible." […] "What we are concerned with is not the search for a liaison between brain as a physical 'thing' and some other entity, which we call 'mind.' We need to understand brain as a functioning tissue that generates feelings, moods, and self-awareness that constitute the basic ingredients of mind."

Self-process is both convergent and divergent, it can function both as the source and target of its behavior and mentation. It is ever renewing itself since it is continuously generated as a result of spontaneous activation of cerebral cortex by the brainstem-diencephalic arousal system. The brainstem-cortical arousal system is crucial for the manifestation of a living, thinking and conscious self. Without such neurophysiologic arousal, consciousness, sense of self, attention, and volition are not possible.

The self is a dynamic, self-renewing process. Because of its dynamic nature, self is continuously changing, adjusting and adapting to its situational environment. The homeostatic and adaptive control of its behavioral arousal-energy is influenced by the sleep-wake cycle [100]. Differentiated self is a composite of many modalities, with concurrent, neuro-developmental streams. It plays many roles such as i) a biophysical consumer by breathing, swallowing, and sexual activity; ii) a mover-speaker-communicator by locomotion, gestures, and speech; iii) a sensor-perceiver-observer by all sensory modalities; iv) an image maker, a thinker by cognition, internal speech, imagination; v) an organizer-coordinator of experiential space-time, of personal, peripersonal, and extrapersonal fields, vi) a recaller and manipulator of working memory and information; vii) a simulator-imitator and modeler of perceived, imagined, and projected experiences; and viii) an adapter to an ever changing environment and to itself.

The current experience of an organism defines its present self, and the present self, in turn, shapes its current experience. Such a circular, multistream self is usually engaged in a relationship with someone or something, and is always embedded in a larger ecosystemic process. Such an interactive, experiential space or life-space is represented in the brain and can be understood as personal (body-mind and its activities), peripersonal (manually reachable space), and extrapersonal space beyond reach that can only be imagined and projected [101].

Life-space is defined as the totality of possible events for one person at a particular time, which is a person's possible options, together with the environment that contains them. It is like multiple streams being coordinated into a single, transient, convergent-divergent system with its complex, coordination dynamics. This is why we have to understand self in terms of new biophysics, synergetics, and coordination dynamics for complex, natural systems.

The existential being can be mentally-behaviorally oriented in three complimentary modes of existence, namely, i) an egocentric, dualistic, object-avoidant mode; ii) an allocentric, dualistic, object-approach and explore mode; and iii) an ecosystemic, holistic or field mode, which is self-existent, globally oriented, nondual and holistic. The latter holistic or existential mode can be self-actualized with a conflict-free sphere of ego, the intrinsic self-as-subject, or the invariant "I" the Ātman, which remains ever-the-same, throughout an individual's conscious life.

Pfaff [102] recently proposed a brain arousal and information theory. He described a model with an acronym "BBURP," which stands for a bilaterally symmetric, bipolar bidirectional (ascending and descending), universal (among vertebrates), response potentiating system. "Among all vertebrates, this system readies the animal or the human to respond to stimuli of all modalities, to initiate voluntary locomotion, (vocalization, speech) and to react with feeling to emotional challenges. [...] The totality of fundamental arousal is a function of generalized arousal plus an increasing function of specific arousal states (sex, hunger, thirst, pain, fear and so on)." He considers arousal as the most fundamental force of the nervous system and proposes an operational definition of arousal: "Generalized arousal is higher in an animal or a human being, who is more alert to stimuli of all sorts, and more motorically active, and more reactive emotionally."

At least six major neurotransmitter systems, using norepinephrine, dopamine, serotonin, acetylcholine, histamine, and orexin, work together to mediate brain's conscious arousal-energy. These independent, but coordinated, arousal systems originate in the brainstem-limbic regions and converge in the nonspecific thalamus, with dorsal and ventral paths to the associative and sensorimotor cortices.

Seeley and Sturm [103] described the ontogeny of self-representation: "From birth, humans iteratively construct the self, beginning with simple body state, 'building materials' and layering on new skills until we learn to think abstractly about ourselves, others, and the complex relations between them." The minimal self represents data available only to its owner including the current body state, and the conscious stream of internal dialogue and imagery. It is rooted in the ancient neural systems of the brainstem reticular formation and the limbic system.

These authors describe three processing streams of the minimal self: i) interoception maps the body states, into consciousness, probably mediated by a neural network connecting insula, amygdala, anterior cingulate cortex, and the orbitofrontal cortex; ii) exteroception maps the external reality, relying on bilateral, fronto-cingulo-parietal, spatial inputs, however, the attentional matrix is processed predominantly in the right parietal cortex and related subcortex; and iii) phrenoception or representations of spontaneous mental thoughts and acts, are probably mediated by a default mode network. Such undirected, spontaneous brain network includes dorsal and ventromedial prefrontal cortex, paracingulate region, posterior cingulate, precuneus, lateral posterior parietal cortex, and the hippocampi.

"If the minimal self describes self-representational acts that occur in the moment, the longitudinal self relates to elements of our extended individual life histories...The dorsomedial prefrontal cortex, which somehow participates in both semantic and episodic self-related memory, may be a node that helps bind the minimal and longitudinal selves together, marking elements of each, as originating from or relating to the self."

Embodiment, the sense of being localized within one's physical body, is a fundamental aspect of the self. The phenomenon of embodied self is processed in distinct cortical areas viz. temporo-parietal junction and the extrastriate body area [104]. The neural network that processes embodiment of self, its parts, and corporeal awareness include not only the posterior parietal-temporal cortex, but also premotor and motor cortices. Carruthers [105] proposes a model of the synchronous self, which includes the sense of control over one's body and mind, of being bounded in body and mind, of having perspective from within one's body and mind, and of being extended in time. Cavanna and Trimble [106] reviewed the role of the precuneus in self-processing. They suggest that the precuneus appears to play a crucial role in self-processing tasks, possibly through the involvement of mental imagery and the retrieval of self-related, episodic memories.

Damasio [107] proposed his solution to the conscious-mind problem with a movie metaphor: "The sense of self (ego), in the act of knowing, emerges within the movie. Self-awareness is actually part of the movie and thus creates, within the same frame, the 'seen' and the 'seer', the 'thought' and the 'thinker'. There is no separate spectator for the movie-in-the-brain. The idea of spectator is constructed within the movie, and no ghostly homunculus haunts the theater. Objective brain processes knit the subjectivity of the conscious mind out of the cloth of sensory (self) mapping. And because the most fundamental sensory mapping pertains to body states and is imaged as feelings, the sense of self, in the act of knowing, emerges as a special kind of feeling – the feeling of what happens in an organism caught in the act of interacting with an object."

The neural correlates of mental self were studied during yoga nidra relaxation meditation [108]. There was a relative decrease in blood flow in bilateral orbital and dorsolateral prefrontal, anterior cingulate, temporal, inferior parietal cortices, caudate nucleus, thalamus, pons, and cerebellar vermis, which are the structures associated with executive functions and working memory. Generally speaking, meditation shifted cortical activity from prefrontal to posterior regions. It was suggested that not only medial anterior, but also medial posterior cortical regions were essential for subjectivity. These regions seem to process a stable unified perspective of the organism relative to the environment, i.e., the "self".

Gazzaniga [109] suggested that a sense of self is constructed by the left hemispheric "interpreter" on the basis of input from a bi-hemispheric neural network. Zhu [110] concluded that human volition has at least three distinct aspects to its meaning as a mental act: i) decision making, ii) action initiation, and iii) executive control. These are complexly evolving, multistream, dynamic processes. Volition, of course, has a lot to do with our intentionality and sense of conscious self. Zimmer [111] described a "self network" located in the medial prefrontal cortex, which draws together perceptions and memories of self and combines them into an ongoing feeling of being oneself. Precuneus is involved in retrieving autobiographical memories and the anterior insula becomes active, when people look at pictures of their own faces.

In his recent book, “The Primacy of the Subjective,” Georgalis [112] proposed a new, non-phenomenal concept of minimal content, which is required to understand mind and language. He argues, “an agent constitutes minimal content and that this results in a unique intentional state: the ‘Fundamental Intentional State’.” He thinks that a strict third-person methodology is untenable; it must be supplemented with a first-person, subjective methodology. Another landmark publication on “Subjectivity and Selfhood” is by Zahavi [113]. He stated, “According to Sartre, consciousness has two different modes of existence, a pre-reflective and reflective. Whereas the former is an immersed, non-objectifying, self-acquaintance, the latter is a detached objectifying self-awareness that introduces a phenomenological distinction between the observer and the observed. The former has priority since it can prevail independently of the latter, whereas reflective consciousness always presupposes a pre-reflective self-consciousness.”

While describing Husserl’s concept of subjectivity, he quotes: “To be a subject is to be in the mode of being aware of oneself.[…] An absolute existent is existent in the form of an intentional life – which, no matter what else it may be intrinsically conscious of, is at the same time, consciousness itself.[…] For the latter [the life of consciousness] not only a lived experiencing, continually streaming along; at the same time, as it streams along, it is also immediately the consciousness of this streaming.”

Zahavi also addressed the relationship between consciousness and self. “An egological theory would claim that when I watch a movie, there is an object of experience (the movie), there is an experience (the watching), and there is a subject of experience, myself… In contrast, a non-egological theory would argue that experiences are egoless; they are anonymous mental events that simply occur, and minimal self-awareness should be understood as the acquaintance that consciousness has with itself and not as an awareness of an experiencing self.”

The non-egological perspective is consistent with the giveness of a lived, prereflective conscious being, proprium, or ipseity. It is only when we adopt a distancing and objectifying attitude toward the experience, i.e., when we reflect on it, that an ego appears. The act of reflection is similar to the act of directed attention. It is the attentional vector that creates the observer-observed duality.

Finally, there is a recent philosophical proposal of the “ultimate ground” of experience and existence. So called “physical” and “mental” are two aspects of the same unitive reality. Pred [114] alluded to it as “Onflow: organic monism of pure experience.” “The ultimate represents the underlying, energetic, creative ground for process, for concrescence, and for the ongoing flow or advance of events. The ground does not exist apart from its activity and has three basic inseparable aspects: creativity, diversity and unity.”

Huxley [115] described: “the divine ground of all existence is a spiritual absolute, ineffable in terms of discursive thought, but susceptible of being directly experienced and realized by the human being.” Similar holistic perspective of a unique, unitive, existential experience has been expressed by the author and others [116 - 118].

Pristine Being

Like the big Sky,
It contains clouds of many shapes,
But still remains ever so clear.

Like the giant Ocean,
It contains fish of many colors,
But still remains ever so transparent.

Like the Mother Earth,
It carries all trees, like little children,
But still remains ever so tireless.

Like a gentle Breeze,
It strokes all leaves tenderly,
But still remains ever so calm.

Like the glorious Sun,
It energizes every form of Life,
But still remains ever so inexhaustible.

Like the great Silence,
It absorbs all thoughts and songs,
But still remains ever so Serene.

Like a loving Heart,
It absorbs all feelings and emotions,
But still remains ever so Tranquil.

Like our face,
Mind has many expressions,
But its essence, its true being,
Remains ever so fresh and pristine.

Vinod D Deshmukh
May 10, 2005

Chapter 14

NEUROBEHAVIORAL DEVELOPMENT OF SELF

अन्तःपूर्णो बहिःपूर्णः पूर्णकुम्भ इवार्णवे |
अन्तःशून्यो बहिःशून्यः शून्यकुम्भ इवाम्बरे ||

Submerged in the ocean, a pot is full within and without. Being in the sky, a pot remains empty within and without.

Maitrayyupaniṣ ad मैत्रय्युपनिषद् 2:27

The concept of a neuro-developmental stream is now well established in neuro-embryology and pediatric neuroscience. For instance, in the Denver II assessment scale, for the neurodevelopment of a child, from the newborn to six year olds, four major streams of growth are described: i) gross motor, ii) fine motor adaptive, iii) language, and iv) personal-social. At each specific age, a child's growth can be assessed for normality, according to these four neuro-developmental streams. These streams evolve concurrently, from moment to moment, into a dynamic and holistic individual self, specific for that particular person and his or her developmental stage. The neurobehavioral development and the ontogeny of self are briefly described in a chronological order [119 - 133].

EMBRYONIC BEHAVIORAL DEVELOPMENT

1. 4th week: The human heart begins to beat at 65 beats/min.
2. 4–12 weeks: The circadian clock in suprachiasmatic nucleus begins to oscillate.
3. 6th week: The superficial musculature is developed. Cutaneous innervation and sensitivity begins around the mouth, extending to nose, and chin, eyelids, palms of hands, genitalia, and soles of feet.
4. 7th week: The cortical synapses begin, which continue to grow rapidly until 5 years, slowly until 18 years, and then continue to grow periodically throughout life.

Fetal Behavioral Development

1. 7–10 weeks: First muscle contractions, followed by lateral flexion movements of neck and trunk. Trigeminal nerve terminals are reactive to tactile stimuli. The **face** is recognizably human. Local stimuli may evoke squinting, opening of the mouth, incomplete finger closure, and flexion of toes. Swallowing begins.
2. 11–15 weeks: Fetal nose is well shaped and amniotic fluid circulates in the upper airways. Main olfactory system has mature neurons. Breathing motions appear and tactile stimulation elicits graceful movements.
3. 17–40 week: Appearance of grasp reflex. Fetal breathing movements induce displacement of fluids in the nasal airways so that the amniotic fluid in contact with chemoreceptors is continually renewed, marking the beginning of chemosensorium.
4. 24–30 weeks: Ability to suck develops. Eye opening occurs with sensitivity to light, but perception of form and color is not complete until long after birth.
5. 3–6 months: Spinal cord and brain stem reflexes are present. The fetus begins to swallow and absorb amniotic fluid.
6. 20–28 week: Fetus develops rest-activity cycles. Spontaneous and adaptive responses follow extensor-avoidance and flexor-approach behaviors. Neurosensory development with initially random, and then gradually synchronous, firing of retinal ganglion cells, auditory system, olfactory system, sensory-motor neurons in the spinal cord, brainstem and thalamus, associated with REM sleep in the third trimester. Gradually, sleep differentiates into REM and NREM type.
7. 24–36 weeks: Neural systems, including reticulothalamic, somatosensory (pain, touch), olfactory, auditory, limbic (comfort-emotion), and hippocampal (learning and memory), are functional. The auditory system is ready to learn and respond to meaningful sounds (language and music) by body movements and elevation of heart rate. These responses decrease after several repetitions, which is a sign of learning by habituation.
8. Before birth: From late gestation, the fetus has an ability to detect, selectively encode, memorize, and retrieve the odor information available in the womb.
9. 38 weeks prenatal to 6 months postnatal: Development of directional columns of primary visual cortex. These include columns for lines, patterns, movement, and direction. Visual system is functional and ready for visual experiences.

Neonate-Child-Adult Behavioral Development

1. Moment of birth: With the loss of placental connection with mother, there is an urgent need to begin breathing. This happens within seconds after a normal delivery and achieves a normal respiratory rhythm within 1 min after birth.
2. Newborn at birth: Alert and ready to respond and nurse. Neonates are nearsighted and have a fixed focal length of about 8–12 in. Visual preferences for a human face and preferential turning to a female voice. First social gazing lasts for about 40 min.
3. 0.5–8 h after birth: Ability to regulate arousal and organization of six discrete behavioral states — quiet sleep, active sleep, drowsy, alert, fussy, and crying. Term-

born infants show hedonic differentiation of odorants by displaying facial action indicative of acceptance or rejection.

4. Birth to 1 month: Sleep-wake cycles of about 90-min duration are distributed through 24 hours of day-night periods. Eyes follow to midline. Visual contact with faces and objects. Turns toward a novel sound. Can encode, store, and retrieve information about events experienced.
5. 2 months: Infants are more awake during the day. Responsive smile. Track with eyes past midline. Organize experiences by primitive reflexes like rooting and grasping. Actions relate to immediate environment experienced by the sensory-motor system. When over-stimulated, infants calm themselves by looking away, yawning, or sucking on their lips or hands.
6. 3–6 months: More awake during the day and more sleep at night. Coos and chuckles. Hand-mouth movements. Shows discrimination by interacting differently with each parent and strangers. Anticipates feeding. Begins to develop a mental model of how the world works.
7. 4 months: Reaches for objects. Tracks with eyes 180° horizontal and some vertical tracking. Rolls prone to supine. Bats at objects. Plays midline. Laughs. Orients to voice. Enjoys looking around. Associates experiences and related memories (sound of mother's voice with her face).
8. 5–6 months: Rolls supine to prone. Sits supported. Unilateral reach. Raking with all fingers. Babbles in one consonant syllables. Attached to primary caregiver. Follows object trajectory and its memory. Begin to control part of their world and realize their authorship.
9. 7–8 months: Transfers objects from one hand to the other. Imitates sounds. Anticipates object trajectory. Finger feeds. *Crawls* by dragging pelvis on floor. "Dada" nonspecific. Development of object permanence (peek-a-boo games) and primary caregiver permanence and stranger anxiety.
10. 9–12 months: Develops "joint attention", the ability to use gaze and gesture cues to share experiences with others, which matures by 18 months. Infants use these skills to develop theories of mind and to use others' affective cues to guide their behavioral choices. Waves "bye bye". Understands "no". Uncovers hidden objects. Picks up small objects with pincer movement. "Dada" and "Mama" specifically. Wernicke's temporal area for language comprehension myelinates before Broca's frontal area for language production. Primitive forms of explicit memory are thought to emerge late in the first year.
11. 11–12 months: Points with index finger. One-word, one-step command with gestures. Two words. Immature jargoning. Imitates. Develops reciprocal communication of asking and showing. Comes when called. Cooperates with dressing. Uses a cup.
12. 15–24 months: Runs, pivots, walks backwards. Scribbles. Removes shoes. Uses four to six words. Follows one-step command without gesture. Develops ability to pass mirror test and video self-recognition test. Piaget's sensorimotor development [104]. Erikson's basic trust vs. mistrust [105].
13. 18 months to 3 years: Walks upstairs with rail. Throws a ball. Imitates stroke on paper. Uses spoon with solids with little spilling. Takes off most clothes. Uses ten or more words. Combines two words. Understands two-part command. Names pictures.

Points to body parts. Realizes that they are truly separate from their parents and therefore vulnerable. Toddlers begin to use personal pronouns (e.g., "I", "me", "you") in reference to self and others. They come to realize that people are psychological beings with private, internal worlds; they distinguish behavior from thinking, desire from action, and reality from pretense. Memory systems develop including episodic and autobiographical memory, which provide the foundation for a longitudinal representation of self. In order to relieve stress, they develop self-consoling habits like thumb sucking, rocking, head banging, and using transitional objects ("lovies"). Preoperational symbolic-representational stage, (Piaget). Autonomy vs. shame (Erikson).

14. 24 months: Uses 50 words. Names body parts. Kicks ball. Walks downstairs. Imitates vertical line. Puts on some clothes. Vocabulary of 50–300 words. 25% of speech understandable. Follows commands with two actions on two objects. Increased locomotion and expansion of vocabulary and learning to change their environment and people through gestures and words. Practice independence by walking away. Demanding what they want. Doing anything without realizing consequences. Develop temper tantrums.
15. 2–4 years: Draws circle with perseverating lines. Can tricycle. Dresses with supervision. Vocabulary of 900 words. Knows first and last name, age, sex, colors. Three- to four-word sentences. Asks "why" incessantly. 75% understandable speech. Understands cold, tired, and hungry. Rapid language development provides concrete feedback and self-relevant information that enhances self-concept. By 2 years, begins to use mental state words, and by 3 years, routinely speaks of thoughts, beliefs, and feelings. Three-year olds know that thinking occurs internally and cannot be seen. By age 4, they reliably pass the tests of "theory of mind".
16. 3–6 years: Initiative and enjoyment of new locomotor and mental powers. Problem solving. "Magical" thinking. Self-centered with concrete, visual thinking. Lack logical explanation of events. They think they cause events. By 5 years, can print their first name. Can understand and verbalize the concepts of size, shape, and numbers. Combine sentences with conjunction. Follow three simple instructions. Read few letters and can tell the meaning of familiar words. Learn about the social world through interactive play with siblings and peers. Develop "pretend" play, which can ease anxiety. Act as superheroes to defeat evil villains. Perceive death as reversible. By 3 years, start becoming less "self-focused" and more social, being aware of other's needs. By 4 years, they become protective of younger children. By 5 years, they may show some leadership. Preoperational intuition (Piaget). Initiative vs. guilt (Erikson).
17. 6–12 years: Drive to be successful academically and socially. School-aged children enter "concrete operational stage" of thinking, meaning they can only operate on things present or experienced. Their representations are more connected and logical. They understand classification, seriation, and conservation. Seeing relationships and hierarchies. Develop symbol-associative learning, rule-governed play, and increased awareness of social expectations. Learn complex cognitive skills leading to their self-esteem. Learn to delay gratification by impulse control. Learn to control and sustain attention during 1st and 2nd grades. A 6-year old can focus attention on a task for 15 min. A 9-year old should be able to pay attention for an hour. A 6-year old should be

able to express feelings and thoughts. At 6 years, they learn to read and start understanding syntax and grammar. By 7 years, they can articulate all sounds of the language they are exposed to. Between 7 and 10 years, they learn irregular verbs, tenses, and expressive language. In the early grades, friendships are of the same sex, but as puberty approaches, friendships become heterosexual. Moral development and empathy continue to progress from the concrete level of rule following toward more independent thinking of right and wrong. As children learn to negotiate the rules of society, they may engage in behaviors of lying, cheating, and stealing to fulfill fantasies, save face, test limits, or fit into a peer group. Concrete, operational (Piaget). Industry vs. inferiority (Erikson).

18. 12–17 years: Establish self-identity and sexual orientation. Capacity for abstract thought, hypothetic-deductive reasoning. Can hypothesize about "what is possible" and develop strategies to solve problems. Increased ability to self-monitor and communicate thoughts and feelings. The adolescent develops an "armor of middle adolescence: the helmet of omniscience, the breastplate of omnipotence and the shield of invincibility." Formal operational, hypothetic-deductive logic (Piaget). Identity vs. role confusion. (Erickson).
19. 17–30 years: Intimacy vs. isolation (Erikson).
20. 30–60 years: Generativity vs. stagnation (Erikson).
21. After 60 years: Ego integration vs. despair (Erikson).

Chapter 15

TRIMODAL ORIENTATION OF THE MULTI-STREAM SELF

चित्तं न सुप्तं नो जाग्रत्स्मृतिविस्मृतिवर्जितम् ।
न चास्तमेति न उदेति यस्यासौ मुक्त एव सः ॥४:११०॥

One is truly free, whose mind is neither asleep nor awake, which is free of repetitive remembering and forgetting, and which neither arouses nor fades.

Hatha-Yoga Pradīpikā 4:110

The self process can be oriented in three complimentary modes of being-in-existence, namely (a) egocentric, object-avoidant mode; (b) allocentric, object-approach-and-explore mode; and (c) an ecosystemic, holistic, field mode, which may be non-interactive, globally oriented, conflict-free, and existential. The first two interactive modes of reflective consciousness create the subject-object duality, whereas, the non-interactive, prereflective, preattentive awareness is restful, spontaneous, nondual, and existential. Such a mode can be intuitive and creative. The existential, conflict-free sphere of self-awareness remains the same throughout an individual's conscious life.

The ego or "me" is viewed as the conscious sense of self-as-object, being the agent. According to the "Ego psychology" in psychoanalysis, the main function of ego is to control impulses and deal with the situational reality. Ego also contains a "conflict-free sphere" of functioning and has its own store of energy, with which to pursue goals that are independent of instinctual wishes. This is in contrast to "Id psychology," which focuses only on the primitive instincts of sex and hostility.

Kraft [134] described the process of creative revelations: "A little relaxation and distance change the mind's perspective on the problem – without us being aware of it. This change of perspective allows for alternative insights and creates the preconditions for a fresh, and perhaps more creative, approach. The respite seems to allow the brain to clear away thought barriers by itself. At some point, newly combined associations break into consciousness, and we experience sudden, intuitive enlightenment." Such exceptional, creative-intuitive moments have been described in meditative and artistic states.

Finally, Monnier [135] has well summarized the important concepts of psycho-neurobiology: He proposes "a scientific concept of the indissociability of the psyche (mind +

affectivity) and its brain (neuronal and neurochemical systems). This indissociability is revealed: (1) by the concurrent construction of the psyche and the brain during ontogenic development; (2) by the synergism of the psychic and cerebral activities; (3) by the isomorphism of mental-affective and cerebral-humoral structures; and (4) by the impossibility of detecting with scientific methods mental-affective and cerebral-humoral manifestations after death."

Mother's Face

A fetus cannot see its mother's face,
But, it is thrives well
In her womb, with her love.

Whether a fetus knows it or not,
Its life, mind and its very existence,
Depend on its mother.

She is the sole source of
Its nutrition, growth and activities.

Its very being is nested in her.
During an occasional period of quietness,
It may hear her loving song.

For the newborn, children and adults,
Motherhood is slowly transferred
From hman mother to Mother Nature.
We too cannot see Mother Nature's face.

Whether we are aware of it or not,
We too depend on
Her natural energies and nourishing elements.

We too are vulnerable, but protected,
In our little niche in Nature.

The earth we stand on, the air we breathe,
The water we drink, the food we eat,
The warmth of the Sun on our face,
On a lovely spring morning,
And the infinite universe that we thrive in;

All of these are constant reminders
Of our primal nurturing Source.

The Natural Reality
Is also the source of our mind -
All of our sensations, perceptions, emotions,
Knowledge, memories, language,
Inspirations and creativity.
She is the mother of all our experiences,
Conscious as well as subconscious.

We cannot see
The face of the infinite Cosmos.
We cannot palpate the whole galaxy.
But, if we stay still and listen
With our *heart*,
We may be able to hear
Her gentle whisper,
And realize
That our essential being is
Deeply rooted in her *heart*
And that we are ever guided by
Her love and great wisdom!

Vinod D Deshmukh

February 8, 2007

Chaptert 16

INTRODUCTION TO VEDĀNTA

ब्रह्मविद् ब्रह्मैव भवति ।

Knower of *Brahman* ब्रह्मन् becomes *Brahman* Itself.

Brahman is the ineffable, infinite, absolute, blissful, self-aware, existential, holistic Energy~Being~Awareness चित्ब्रह्मशक्तिः

DEFINITIONS

Vedānta means conclusion of intuitive knowledge, insight or wisdom. The origin of the Sanskrit word Vedānta वेदांत is Veda + anta वेद + अंत. The root verb Vid विद् means to know. Anta means end, conclusion, essence or a goal. So, Vedānta means the final conclusion as well as the goal of Vedās. There are four Vedās: Ṛgveda ऋग्वेद, Yajurveda यजुर्वेद, Sāmaveda सामवेद, and Atharvaveda अथर्ववेद, which are the timeless collection of inspired thoughts and intuitive wisdom. Vedāntic wisdom, philosophy and practice are based on three major sources of inspired writings namely, Upaniṣ ad उपनिषद्, Bhagvad-Gītā भगवद्गीता, and Brahma-Sūtra ब्रह्मसूत्र. These three together are known as the threefold foundation of ancient wisdom, Prasthāna-trayī प्रस्थानत्रयी.

PHILOSOPHY OF VEDĀNTA

It is a perennial philosophy of enlightened life, and a practical way of realizing it, by perrenial wisdom, Sanātana Dharma सनातन धर्म. The universe is an organic whole and has a Natural order called Ṛtam ऋतं. Every thoughtful individual is wonderstruck by its beauty, complexity, and infinite manifestations. One, who has understood the truth of being an integral part of this natural order, has an intuitive understanding of the Natural Reality within and without oneself, by the spontaneously inspired mind or Ṛtambharā prajñā ऋतंभरा प्रज्ञा. The search is for the fundamental Truth, which underlies the flux of all changing phenomena.

The author of Kenopaniṣad asked some fundamental questions about our conscious mind: "By whom willed and directed does the mind light on its objects? By who commanded does life make the first move? At whose will, do (people) utter this speech? And what god is it that prompts the eye and the ear?"

There are two forms of knowledge, a direct aparoksha अपरोक्ष, and an indirect paroksha परोक्ष. The direct knowledge is first-person, immediate and without any reflective thoughts or memories. The indirect knowledge involves slow, deliberate cognition with reflective thoughts, associations and reactive memories. Direct knowledge is like eating an ice-cream and personally enjoying its taste, flavor, and coolness etc. Indirect knowledge is like reading a description of a good ice-cream, or seeing some one else taste it.

The direct intuitive knowledge, Prajñānaṁ प्रज्ञानं, is based on a direct first-person experience. There is no subject-object duality in the direct experience, aparokshānubhūtiḥ अपरोक्षानुभूतिः. It is a pre-reflective, preattentive process. Such a direct, self-inquiry leads one on an inward journey to self, Antargaman अन्तर्गमन, self-knowledge, Ātma-jñāna आत्मज्ञान, and self-realization of energy~being, Ātmasākshātkāra आत्मसाक्षात्कार. The essential truth of our energy~being, Satyasya Satyaṁ सत्यस्य सत्यम्, can be realized only from within one self. It is the pathless path to the self~energy~being.

We have to learn to watch the drama of life dispassionately. This includes frequent changes in our environment or surroundings, parisara परिसर, our physical body, deha देह, our physiological activities like breathing, ṣwasana श्वसन, as well as the mind, manas मनस्, and its activities like thinking, vichāra विचार, intending, saṅkalpa संकल्प, recalling, smṛiti स्मृति. We need to learn to stay still, silent and serene in the present moment, until we realize the truth of our spontaneous, sahaja सहज, tranquil, śānta शान्त and exhilarating ānanda आनन्द Energy~Being.

Self-realization springs from within, because the fundamental truth of our existential being is within. It is not outside in the changing phenomena. There is something amazingly beautiful within each one of us – a primal feeling ādibhāva आदिभाव, of an endless, ananta अनन्त, and spontaneous wonder, vismayaḥ विस्मय. It is the whole-in-itself, pūrṇa पूर्ण. It lacks nothing. It is the greatest wonder within, which needs to be discovered by our own watchful self-enquiry. We are an integral part of this incredible Natural order, Ṛtam. We are in Nature and Nature is within us, at every level of our biophysical, mental and spiritual being. We have to realize this amazing integration in our own Heart. This is what Vedānta is all about.

The main thesis of Vedanta is that the ultimate reality of the universe, Brahman, and the ultimate reality of a conscious human being, Ātman, are two aspects of the same essential, existential Truth. Our task is to discover this Truth in our own being and appreciate the wonder of this amazing existence, Jagat जगत्.

BRAHMAN:
THE ULTIMATE ENERGY~BEING~AWARENESS चित्ब्रह्मशक्तिः
THE REALITY OF THE UNIVERSE

The word *Brahman* is derived from the root verb Bruh, which means to surge, grow, to expand or to mushroom. It is a ceaseless, spontaneous, bursting forth or emerging. It is the primal Reality as well as the organizing principle of the universe. Brahman is the real of real, the Truth of truths, Satyasya Satyaṁ, the source of all experience and existence. This absolute reality of *Brahman* is truth Satyaṁ, consciousness Jñānam, and infinity Ananta. It is also described as Blissful, Conscious Being, Sat~Cit~Ānanda. It is not merely a featureless absolute, but the whole universe as is with its infinite expressions.

सर्वं खल्विदं ब्रह्म तज्जलानिति शान्त उपासीत ||३:१४:१||

Chāndogyopaniṣ ad (3:14:1) described *Brahman* as Tajjalāna (tat-ja-li-an). "All this is *Brahman*. That (tat) from which the phenomenal existence-experience emerges (ja); that in which it merges (li); and that in which it breathes (an) and has its being. One should meditate on it with serenity."

It is the creative matrix of this dynamic universe. Universe is truly a uni-verse, a single verse, a holistic process. Like a spring-fed lake, it has circular causality – the process creates a product and the product influences the process. It is a single holistic system. Similar circular causality is evident between conscious contents and the conscious process itself. We are an integral part of this natural universe.

Brahman is not an object of thought or reflection. It is not the result of any human action or creation. It is beyond all possible descriptions. It can only be known intuitively in the core of one's energy-being. It is the unfathomable ground of the universe, which encompasses every thing in it. Brahman is both transcendent as well as imminent in the universe. It is both the real as well as the realized. The essence of the individual, *Ātman*, and the existential totality, *Brahman*, are two aspects of the same Truth.

ĀTMAN:
THE ULTIMATE ENERGY~BEING~AWARENESS चिदात्मशक्तिः
REALITY OF A CONSCIOUS HUMAN BEING

The word *Ātman* is derived from the verb an अन्, which means 'to breathe.' It is the breath of life. It is the essential energy~being of the individual, the self or the soul. *Ātman* persists when the not-self, Anātman अनात्मन्, or the observable field of experience, Kshetra क्षेत्र, is spontaneously eliminated from the essential, conscious awareness. *Ātman* and *Anātman* are two aspects of the same energy~being~awareness. Like an hourglass, they are two cyclical phases, a mental inhalation and exhalation. There is a complimentarity between them. It is a matter of one's perspective, as the phrase goes: "Glass, half full or half empty."

The not-self includes all observable phenomena like the world, body, mind, intellect and ego. Please refer to Appendix 1 for details. The *Ātman* is the ultimate conscious witness, sākshi साक्षी. Some Vedāntins think that Ātman is an unborn, aja अज, and immortal, amar अमर, element, bhāga भाग, of a person. *Ātman* is the essential, existential, self-conscious being. It is the foundational reality of an individual energy~awareness~being.

ĀTMAN IS *BRAHMAN*

The unity of Ātman and Brahman can only be realized directly and intuitively, within the calm and clear stillness of one's own energy-being. One can realize the self-renewing, spontaneity of one's own being. It is the nondual, advaita, experience of the existential singularity, ekatvam एकत्वं. That is why this philosophy of Vedānta is also known as Advaita Vedānta.

INDIVIDUAL SELF

The individual self is called jīva जीव, the one who breathes. It is the biophysical aspect of human individuality. The individual jīva is the agent or doer, kartā कर्ता, as well as the enjoyer or sufferer, bhoktā भोक्ता , of various life experiences. It has the biophysical body, deha, the subconscious organizing energy prāṇ a प्राण and the conscious mentation manas.

The manas is composed of five sensory faculties (hearing, sight, touch, smell and taste), five executive or motor faculties (speech, hands, feet, excretory and generative organs), and an overall executive intelligence, buddhi. In addition, mind also includes the matrix of memory, citta, and a sense of I or ego, ahamkāra. The four mental elements namely, manas, citta, buddhi and ahamkāra, together form an inner organ of conscious experience, antaḥ karaṇ a अन्तःकरण. Please refer to Appendix 2 and 7 for details.

Chapter 17

SKILLFUL PRACTICE OF VEDĀNTA

योगः कर्मसु कौशलम् ।

Yogaḥ karmasu kauśalam.

Yoga is the art of living.

To realize the Truth within, we have to become alert and aware of all that is happening from moment to moment, both within and around us. Such a mode of being fully and wholeheartedly present in the current moment is called presence, mindfulness or vipaśyanā. It is a unique orientation or perspective of being. It is a unique process of self-absorbing, renewing and staying undistracted. It is like bird-watching, when one is quiet, non-intrusive, passive, but totally engrossed in the very act of watching. One's whole heart and being are still, but fully attentive and silent in the moment. It is just being aware, watching, listening and eventually just "Being Present" in the timeless moment.

There is no world-teacher; the World IS the Teacher! The world includes all that is happening both within and without us. Each living moment can teach us something new, because no two moments are identical. The whole world is a process-product complex, which is continuously changing and evolving. One can learn continuously and directly from every change. An awareness of any change is cognition or knowledge. Human body and mind are both the means as well as the receptacle of personal experience, knowledge, and self-understanding.

In order to notice a change fully, one must be keenly attentive, free, still, silent, nonjudgemental, and present-minded. One has to wake up, not only from the day-dreams, but also from our busy wakefulness. Such an awakened awareness with direct, primal experience, aparokshānubhūti has been called the fourth state of consciousness, Turīya. According to Vedānta philosophy that is the goal of life. When, one is continuously in harmony with the primal, existential being, Ādipuruṣ a आदि पुरुष, one's life can be spontaneous sahaja सहज, effortless ayatna अयत्न, selfless nirahamkāra निरहंकार, all-caring sarvātmaka सर्वात्मक and direct, ever-inspiring, intuitive and creative, Prajñānaṁ Brahma प्रज्ञानं ब्रह्म.

THE INWARD PATH TO SELF-REALIZATION

An inward, pathless path has been described in many of the Vedāntic texts including Prasthāna Trayī, Pātañjali's Yoga Sūtra, Ādi Śaṅ karāchāryā's Ātmānusandhāna, Ātmabodha, Prabhodha Sudhākara, Aparokshānubhūti, and Vedānta Sāra.

Pātañjali's eightfold path, Aṣ tāṅ ga Yoga, has been expanded by Ādi Śaṅ karāchārya in his Vedānta Sāra and Aparokshānubhūti. He described fifteen specific skills to be learnt for Self-understanding and Self-realization.

1. Self-restraint, Yama यम is the development of one's ability to voluntarily quiet one's sensory-motor activities to reach a level of profound stillness, peace, bliss, and spontaneous content, silence-within - ṣ ānta or tuṣ ni bhāva. One should also remind oneself that the whole existence is a single holistic reality, *Brahman*.
2. Undistracted attentiveness, Niyama नियम is continuous, whole-hearted dwelling on what is happening at the moment, and to stay undistracted from any event of the past and any expectation of the future. This is also called presence or mindfulness.
3. Letting it happen, Tyāga त्याग of all phenomena that can be objectively experienced and reminding oneself that one's true nature, one's essence is Ātman, the ultimate reality within each one of us. Any of these objects is not 'me or mine', Idam na mama.
4. Verbal quiescence, Mounaṁ मौनं is being verbally still and mentally silent. Such mental silence can become spontaneous awareness, sahaja samjñā and verbally indescribable, shabda-vivarjit. One should let it happen within oneself. Let it blossom. It is the matrix of all verbal conversational activity.
5. Solitude, Vijanaḥ विजनः is a quiet personal place, in which there is no intrusion by distracting activities, sounds or other people.
6. Time-moment, Kālaḥ काल: can create an arousing mental phenomenon or it can take one to a blissful, nondual state in the blink of an eye, nimeshatah.
7. Steady posture, Āsana आसन is the effortless position of the body, in which one can dwell easily on the essential reality, Brahman. This can occur spontaneously, effortlessly, sukhena, and unceasingly, ajastra.
8. Mental quiescence, Chittabandhaḥ चित्तबन्धः is letting the mind come to a natural pause, a holistic state.
9. Body-mind equilibrium, Dehasāmya देहसाम्य is the collective quietness of the body and mind for realizing the Truth within.
10. Global intrinsic awareness, Jñānamayī Drishtī ज्ञानमयी दृष्टी is an expanded, limitless, nondual intrinsic awareness, when the totality of the experienced world is seen as a quantum Reality, *Brahman*. There is no subject-object differentiation in such an eco-systemic, expanded, global, intrinsic, holistic conscious space-time-field.
11. Conscious breathing, Prāṇ āyama प्राणायाम is awareness of every breath. During inhalation, pūraka, one should contemplate, "I am Brahman, the truth within." During exhalation, rechaka, one should think, "This objectively experienced world is not my true energy-being. The true Self is "not this, not this, neti, neti." During the internal/external pause, kumbhaka, one should let the mind heal by itself.

12. Inward self-withdrawal, Pratyāhāra प्रत्याहार is withdrawing the wandering mind from all experiential objects, events, activities and to let it get absorbed in the Truth within, *Brahman*.
13. Sustained attentiveness, Dhāraṇ ā धारणा is uninterrupted, conscious awareness of the Truth-within, like a continuous stream of oil, akhanda taila-dhāravat.
14. Meditation, Dhyānaṁ ध्यानं is a blissful state, contemplating on the feeling that "I am free, svatantra, and independent, nirālamba. I am Brahman, the Truth."
15. Self-absorptive Integration, Samādhiḥ समाधिः is an invariant, unchanging nitya, uninterrupted, indescribable, spontaneous anāhata, intrinsic awareness of the Truth. One forgets oneself as an isolated person, jīva or an ego. This actualizes the ultimate Reality. In this state, the person becomes Brahman, the Truth, itself. Brahmavid Brahmaiva bhavati. He or she lives an enlightened, inspired, blissful and selfless life naturally, effortlessly.

DIRECT INTUITIVE EXPERIENCE: APAROKSHĀNUBHUTI अपरोक्षानुभूति

The following are four, great statements of wisdom, Mahāvākya महावाक्य, from the Self-realized, Vedic sages, Ṛshi ऋषि. These are profoundly meaningful expressions about the fundamental nature of our conscious being, living in an incredible world:

सर्वं खल्विदं ब्रह्म तज्जलानिति शान्त उपासीत ||३:१४:१||

Sarvaṁ khalvidaṁ Brahma Tajjalāniti śanta upāsīta.

All this is *Brahman*. *Brahman* is Tajjalāna (tat-ja-li-an) "That (tat) from which the phenomenal existence (experience) emerges (ja); That in which it merges (li); and That in which it breathes (an). One should meditate on it with Serenity.

Chāndogyopaniṣ ad 3:14:1

अयं आत्मा ब्रह्म| Ayaṁ Ātmā Brahma.

The Self is *Brahman*. (Māṇ ḍ ukyopaniṣ ad 2).

अहं ब्रह्मास्मि | Ahaṁ Brahmāsmi.

I am *Brahman*. (Brihadāraṇ yakopaniṣ ad 1:4:10).

तत्त्वमसि | Tattvamasi.

You are That (*Brahman*). (Chāndogyopaniṣ ad 6:8:7).

Please see additional references on Vedānta and Meditation in Appendix 7.

Live Universe

This morning, after taking shower,
I went for a walk on the St. Johns River.
At the river's edge, all of a sudden,
I heard a sharp call of an Osprey,
From its perch, on a Cypress Tree.

I paused and just listened
With all my heart.
It was incredible.
It gave me the feeling and conviction,
That this universe is not only filled with
Energy-matter, the cosmic twin,
But, also with informative signals.

There is potential information,
At each point of space-time.
It only has to be deciphered by
A keen and intelligent observer.

Like energy, the information
In the universe, is limitless.
The only limit to human knowledge is
Our own perceptivity and intelligence.
The potential pattern becomes the actual,
When clearly observed and understood.

On my way back from the walk,
I noticed another Osprey,
Flying freely in the clear blue sky.
It correctly deciphered the call,
Of the first osprey.

Finally, both of them flew together,
In the freedom of the great, blue sky,
Leaving me with a blissful conviction,
That the Universe is truly ALIVE.

Vinod D Deshmukh

December 28, 2008

Chapter 18

MEDITATIVE BRAIN~MIND~REALITY

स्वल्पापि दीप कणिका बहुलं नाशयेत्तमः||२:२८||
स्वल्पापि बोधो निबिडं बहुलंनाशयेत्तथा ||२:२९||

Even a brief spark of light can eliminate dense darkness. Similarly, even a brief moment of insight can eliminate deep ignorance and misunderstanding.

Ātmabodhopaniṣ ad आत्मबोधोपनिषद्

Dhyāna Yoga ध्यान योग is a Sanskrit word for meditation derived from the verb Dhyāyati ध्यायति, which means to meditate, ponder, or be Self-aware. By practice of dhyāna, one can achieve a state of intuitive, self-absorptive consciousness, with stillness, silence, serenity and blissful presence of mind, which may lead to Samādhi or enlightenment. Such a mental state is conducive to Self-integration and understanding of the Truth of one's Being-in-Reality and the Reality-in-Oneself. The word Dhyāna was transformed into Jhāna in Pali, Ch'ān in Chinese, and Zenna or Zen in the Japanese language.

The word Yoga योग is derived from the verb Yuj युज्, which means to integrate or unify. Yoga is a way of integration through self-understanding and self-realization. It is a system of practices that facilitates the ultimate goal of an adaptive, creative and enlightened life.

Neuroscience has advanced considerably in understanding the mental phenomena of attention, memory, cognition, consciousness, social-emotional intelligence and the sense of self. These different domains of information processing can be understood in terms of activation or inhibition of specific brain regions and their connections.

BRAIN~MIND~REALITY

The following are some of the most interesting and well-established facts of neuroscience, which shed light on the brain and mind relationship:

1) A well-functioning brain is absolutely essential for human mental activity and behavior. Mind and consciousness are functions of a living brain. They cease to exist

when the brain fails to function. There is no bio-psycho-physical after-life. An individual survives only through one's progeny and personal legacy.

2) Human sleep, dream, and wakefulness are dependent on a well-functioning centrencephalic, reticular-limbic activating system. This system consists of chemically specific clusters of neurons that generate specific neurotransmitters like acetyl choline, norepinephrine, dopamine, serotonin, histamine, glutamate, GABA, and orexin. These neurotransmitters activate or inhibit the cerebral cortex and spinal cord. The sleep-wake cycle is regulated by a circadian clock in the suprachiasmatic nucleus of the hypothalamus. It is reset daily at dawn and dusk by the environmental and internal stimuli from the milieu.
3) The brainstem regulates most of the vital functions of the body including heart rhythm, circulation, breathing, swallowing, eye and head movements, phonation, and automatic movements, like walking, running, singing, speaking etc.
4) The cerebral cortex is essential for higher mental and cognitive functions. It consists of two cerebral hemispheres with specialized areas devoted to specific functions. In general, the left hemisphere, in a right handed person, specializes in language processing and mathematics, whereas the right hemisphere specializes in visuo-spacial and auditory processing, attentiveness, and inhibition of mental activities and behaviors.
5) The frontal lobes, at the front of the brain, modulate voluntary movement, speech, working memory, planning of complex, sequential actions, emotions, self-reflection and personality traits. The temporal lobes, along with the limbic system (hypothalamus, amygdala, hippocampus, cingulate gyrus and orbito-frontal cortex) are involved in emotion, motivation and memory processing. The temporal-occipital-parietal (TOP) lobes at the back part of the brain have specialized areas dedicated to the integration of perceptions, like vision, audition and touch, speech comprehension, object and face recognition, space perception, and processing of colors, numbers, mathematics, and music. These cortical areas have two streams of information processing: a ventral pathway of vision for the "what" processing, which is memory dependent, slow, and sequential; and a dorsal pathway for action in real time, the "where" processing, which is perception dependent, quick, and simultaneous [136,137].

The brain is an interface that mediates interactions between the internal milieu (environment) of the organism and its outer environment. In a broad sense, mental activity goes on within the organism's brain, with episodic interactions, with what is happening outside or inside. Most of the current neuroscientists disagree with a spiritual view, that mind is a supernatural entity, independent of the human brain. The current neurobiological perspective suggests a unified view of the brain-mind-reality. One of the strong proponents of such a neurobiological view was Young [138]. He stated: "The point for us is that all intellectual and emotional powers require activity in the brain and we are utterly dependent on it. No brain – no mind, no intellect, no nothing. The clinical evidence does not support the idea that there is some entity or spirit that can exist apart from the brain."

In reference to "sublime feeling", Churchland [139] made a valid point: "Real, the feelings certainly are. Worthy, in and of themselves, they also are – the more so if they inspire kindness and virtue, the less so if they inspire cruelty and terror. Do we trivialize a sublime feeling if we appreciate its dependence on the brain? Not in the least. Its significance does not depend on its being a soul-state rather than a brain-state. Indeed, self-deception is no virtue, and upon reflection, we may find it unworthy to give our experiences, wonderful though they may be, an inflated cosmic significance."

Damasio suggested a two-part solution to the puzzle of brain-mind-reality: "The first is the problem of how we generate what I call a 'movie-in-the-brain', an integrated composite of images in diverse sensory modalities – visual, auditory, tactile, olfactory, and so on. The second is the problem of 'self', which pertains to how we generate automatically the sense that we own the 'movie-in-the-brain'." His hypothesis is: "The brain uses mapping structures informed by both maps of the organism and maps of objects, to create a fresh, second-order representation, which indicates that the organism as represented in the brain is involved in interacting with the object. The second-order representation occurs in neural structures such as thalamus and cingulate cortices."

Cariani [140] emphasized the regenerative aspect of this biophysical process. He drew a parallel between life and mind, stating: "Living organization entails continual regeneration of material parts and functional relations (self-production). Similarly, dynamic stability of informational states in brains may entail coherent self-regenerating patterns of neural signals. If mind is the functional organization of the nervous system, then mental states can be seen as switching between alternate sets of stable, self-regenerative, neural signal productions." It is also called autopoiesis.

The neuro-ecological perspective, considering organism and environment as a single, functional system, was emphasized by Jarvilehto, [141]: "In any functional sense, organism and environment are inseparable and form only one unitary system. The organism cannot exist without the environment, and the environment has descriptive properties, only if connected to the organism."

Arthem and Liljenstrom [142] argued that "adaptation and learning are widespread and old properties of living organisms, even as old as life itself. Cognition or knowledge-processing mediated by a centralized nervous system… The evolutionary perspective suggests that consciousness can be understood as a biological phenomenon."

Recently, Ventegodt and his colleagues published a holistic perspective of biology and medicine. In a series of four articles on human development, they proposed the application of an energetic-informational interpretation of reality or a holistic perspective of many natural sciences [143 - 146]. In discussing the structure and function of the human brain, they suggest: "The concept of information-directed self-organization, gives a special meaning to the function of the brain. The brain is basically connected to itself, to the outer world through the senses, to the body through the nerves, and to the wholeness through the coherence given, from the fundamental structure of the world."

Chapter 19

NEUROSCIENCE OF ATTENTION

बीजावधानम् ||१५||

One should (always) attend to the 'seed' or the source (of all conscious experience).

Śiva Sūtra 15

Human attention depends on three neural networks [147,148]: (a) a subcortical, alerting network that maintains an adequate level of conscious arousal for cognitive processing; (b) a posterior cortical orienting network, which directs the body, head, ears, and eyes towards an interesting or alarming object, activity, event, or experience, chosen to be attended to; and (c) an anterior cortical selective-executive network, which enhances the perception of the selected target and suppresses interference by distracters like other objects, events, images, and thoughts. Attention can be focused on a specific place, time, and modality like vision, audition, thought, etc. Focusing in space enhances the processing of that region of interest, whereas, focusing in time enhances the processing of events, at the present moment. It is the basis of presence or present-mindedness, which is also known as mindfulness in the Zen Buddhist literature.

Attention functions in two different modes. The mnemonic mode is dominated by associations, memories and self-reflective, ruminative thinking. The presence mode is the key to adaptive mental excellence. It requires total attention to the present reality, with freedom from the past memories, biases, preferences, expectations and projections. When we direct our attention to objects around us, the knowing process creates a sense of duality of the observer and the observed; the knower and the known. During meditation, when situational or emotional conflicts, desires, wants and needs are resolved, and when there is no need to attend to anything specific, one can return to a naturally serene state of a silent, nonspecific Nirguṇ a निर्गुण awareness, with no sense of ego or authorship. Such a spontaneous, ego-absorptive, nondual state of being is known as Turīya. It is the primal ground of all of our conscious experiences. It is nonverbal, ineffable, silent and indefinable, but it can be verified intuitively by one's own direct experience.

Manly et al. [149] described the characteristics of an absent mind. "To be absent-minded is to be inattentive to the ongoing activity, to lose track of current aims and to become distracted from intended thought or action by salient but (currently) irrelevant stimuli." Assmus et al. [150] made an important point that perception of space and time is integrated in the left inferior parietal cortex or the supramarginal gyrus. Robertson and Garavan [151] defined vigilant attention as a continuous inhibition of task irrelevances... (This is similar to the classical definition of Yoga by Pātanjali: Yoga is a voluntary inhibition of irrelevant, mental activity, Yogah chitta vritti nirodhah). "We conceive of the right parieto-prefrontal network and its interactions with the midbrain arousal system, as the circuitry by which vigilant attention is maintained. This circuitry can be 'tuned up' (or down) endogenously or with exogenous support. Within this system, we believe that the prefrontal cortex plays a central role in maintaining and monitoring optimal arousal levels to match current task demands." In their event-related functional MRI study, Garavan et al. [152] identified an activation of the right hemispheric fronto-parietal network, during voluntary inhibition like pausing or stopping of a behavior or speech.

Mendez and Gershfield [153] described an overall neuroanatomical model of human attention. "Normal attention requires both the ascending reticular activating system (ARAS) in the upper brainstem and the multimodal, association areas of the cortex. Stimulation of the ARAS elicits general, nonspecific arousal and primes the cortex for stimulus reception, whereas the multimodal association cortex controls and focuses this prespecific, pre-modal arousal-energy for attending. These cortical areas are the 'attentional gate' for sensory input through feedback to the reticular nucleus of the thalamus. [...] The important multimodal areas are the right prefrontal and the temporo-parietal cortex, although bi-hemispheric cooperation is needed for maintaining attention."

There are two phenomena at the limits of our attentional capacity: attentional blink when a second stimulus is missed if it is presented within 200 msec after the first stimulus and a psychological refractory period when one is unable to respond to a second stimulus that occurs within 200 msec after the first response. There is also a phenomenon of central bottleneck as a limit to human information processing [154].

Chapter 20

SOCIAL-EMOTIONAL INTELLIGENCE

अद्वेष्टा सर्व भूतानां मैत्रः करुण एव च |
निर्ममो निरहंकारः समदुःखसुखः क्षमी ||१३||

He or she hates no one. He is friendly and compassionate. He is not egocentric. He is even-minded in pain and pleasure and he is forgiving.

Bhagavad Gītā; 12:13

Emotional intelligence is defined as the competence to identify, understand, and express emotions; assimilate emotions in thought; and regulate both positive and negative emotions in oneself and others [155]. "Understanding the emotions of oneself and others is the key to a satisfying life. Those people who are self-aware and sensitive to others manage their affairs with wisdom and grace, even in adverse circumstances… Emotional intelligence is claimed to be positively related to academic achievement, occupational success, satisfaction, emotional health and adjustment."

Goleman [156] subdivided it into four domains: personal competence with self-awareness and self-management, and social competence with social awareness and relationship management. Bar-On [157] characterized it as an array of non-cognitive capabilities, competencies, and skills that influence one's ability to succeed in coping with environmental demands and pressures. This is similar to the well-known yogic aphorism: Yoga is skill in volitional action, Yogaḥ karmasu kouśalam योग कर्मसु कौशलम् |.

Panksepp [158] described the role of neocortex in emotion processing. "When the mushrooming of the cortex opened up the relatively closed circuits of our old mammalian and reptilian brains, we started to entertain alternatives of our own rather than nature's making. We can choose to enjoy fear. We can choose to make art of our loneliness. We can even exert some degree of control over our sexual orientations. Most other animals have no such options. Affectively, we can choose to be angels or devils, and we can construct or deconstruct ideas at will. We can choose to present ourselves in ways that are different from the ways we truly feel."

Pritchard and Alloway [159] described the neural regulation of emotional behavior. "A rich supply of afferent projections from the association cortex provides the amygdaloid complex with visual, somato-sensory, auditory and viscero-sensory information. In addition, the amygdaloid complex has dense, reciprocal connections with hypothalamus and several brainstem nuclei, which allow it to coordinate a wide range of autonomic responses. These anatomic pathways suggest that amygdala plays a role in mediating emotion, personality, and other psychological processes."

Rauch et al. [160] observed increased brain blood flow in anterior cingulate, anterior temporal, and ventral globus pallidus regions, in eight healthy men during competitive and sexual arousal. Beauregard et al. [161] observed that right amygdala, right anterior temporal, and hypothalamus were activated during sexual arousal, whereas, right superior frontal and right anterior cingulate areas were activated during attempted inhibition of arousal. They conclude that humans have the capacity to influence the electrochemical dynamics of their brains, by voluntarily changing the nature of their mental processes.

Baron-Cohen et al. [162] described a concept of "social brain", which mediates social intelligence. It consists of orbitofrontal cortex, superior temporal gyrus, and amygdala. Best et al. [163] provided evidence of dysfunction of the orbitomedial, prefrontal cortex in patients with impulsive aggressive behavior.

Wild et al. [164] define the "laughter neural network". They summarize: "The expression of laughter seems to depend on two partially independent neural pathways. The first, an 'involuntary' or 'emotionally driven' system involves the amygdala, thalamus, hypothalamus, subthalamic areas and the tegmental brainstem. The second 'voluntary' (or a self-driven) system that originates in the premotor/frontal areas and leads through the motor cortex and pyramidal tract to the ventral brainstem. These systems appear to be coordinated by a laughter-coordinating center in the dorsal, upper pons."

Heller et al. [165] have provided a synopsis of the relation between emotion and cognition and the skill of emotion regulation. "Human emotion can be conceptualized as a set of processes that include attention, appraisal, subjective feelings, and visceral and motor responses… The dorsolateral prefrontal cortex is implicated in executive control and working memory, whereas orbito-frontal cortex has been associated with emotional and affective processing. […] The right hemispheric system plays an executive role in modulating attention and vigilance in anxiety, especially in anxious arousal (i.e., panic and fear). This right hemisphere system promotes sympathetic nervous activity, spatial attention, visual scanning of the environment and sensitivity to meaningful nonverbal cues."

Chapter 21

FEELING OF SELF

The feeling of self implies an intuitive perception and understanding of one's being or selfness. According to the dictionary, the self is "the total, essential, or particular being of a person." Some of the recent publications in neuroscience on the subject of biophysical self are discussed below.

Llinas [166] argued that "prediction, which is a forecast of what is likely to occur, is the ultimate function of the brain. All moving animals use this predictive ability to efficiently guide their behavior in an ever-changing environment. Self is the centralization of prediction. Why this predictive ability arose is clear: it is critical to survival, guiding it at the level of both the single animal (moment-to-moment) and the species (in fact, of all actively moving species throughout evolution). 'I' has always been the magnificent mystery; I believe, I say, I whatever. But one must understand that there is no such tangible thing. It is just a particular mental state, a generated entity we refer to as 'I' or 'self'."

Wegner [167], in his book "Illusion of Conscious Will" stated: "Conscious will is something that is experienced when we perform an action – actions feel willed or not, and this feeling of voluntariness or doing a thing 'on purpose' is an indication of conscious will. [...] Intention is normally understood as an idea of what one is going to do that appears in consciousness just before one does it." Wegner and Sparrow [168] described "authorship processing supports the perception of events, actions and thoughts as issuing from the self as a causal agent. To discern whether a given item is authored by self or has arisen from some other source, this processing mechanism consults authorship indicators – sources of information about the likely origin of the item. The elemental indicators include body and direct bodily feedback, feed-forward, visual and other indirect sensory feedback, social cues, action consequences, action-relevant thoughts and environment orientation."

Deshmukh had proposed a model for self-consciousness as the "Situational, Transient, Executive Process or the STEP." It was elaborated as: "Self-consciousness is transient and it arises from conscious attention and decision-making, due to the executive activity in the prefrontal-parietal network in a given situation. The common experience of apparent continuous selfness results from a) the continuous self-orientation in person, place and time and b) the phenomenon of sensory-perceptual fusion of discrete experiences in time and space, which is analogous to the apparent continuity experienced while watching a movie. Prefrontal cortex and its related network mediate attention, self-consciousness, and self-organization of behavior, cognition and the self-regulation of various mental states. Prefrontal network play a crucial role in the STEP model."

In describing the neuroanatomy of the self, Miller et al.[169] suggested that selfness depends on three core cognitive domains: i) abstract or general information about personal attributes (semantic knowledge); ii) concrete, often affectively laden, experiences, on which self was formed (autobiographical memories); and iii) motivation to maintain self-schemas or self-images (will). They studied 72 patients with fronto-temporal dementia who had impaired sense of self and found correlated changes in the right frontal region.

Johnson et al.[170] described the neural correlates of self-reflection. "The capacity to consciously reflect on one's sense of self is an important aspect of self-awareness. A sense of self is a collection of schemata regarding one's abilities, traits and attitudes that guide our behaviors, choices and social interactions." They studied functional MRI in healthy volunteers, and found that the medial prefrontal cortex and posterior cingulate areas were involved in self-relational process.

LeDoux [171] suggested a synaptic view of the self. "Genes and experience or nature and nurture are, in the end, not different things, but different ways of doing the same thing – wiring the synapses of our brain. [...] Obviously, much of who we are is based on memories learned through personal experience, including either conscious or unconscious memories."

Ramachandran [172] explained: "Obviously self and qualia are two sides of the same coin. You can't have free-floating sensations or qualia with no one to experience them and you can't have a self completely devoid of sensory experiences, memories or emotions. The defining characteristics of the 'self' are fivefold. First of all, continuity: a sense of unbroken thread running through the whole fabric of our experience with the accompanying feeling of past, present and future. Second is the idea of unity or coherence of self. Third is the sense of embodiment or ownership. Fourth is a sense of agency, what we call free will, being in charge of our own actions and destinies. Fifth, and most elusive of all, the self, almost by its very nature, is capable of reflection – of being aware of itself."

Samson et al. [173] provide evidence that the inhibition of one's own point of view and the ability to infer someone else's point of view, rely on distinct neural processes. The right inferior frontal lobe is necessary for self-perspective inhibition, whereas, the left temporo-parietal junction is necessary for inferring someone else's perspective. Turk et al. [174] present their evidence for the left hemispheric "interpreter" module, which generates a unitary sense of consciousness even in the disconnected brain and gives rise to a unified sense of self.

Chapter 22

HEALTHY MIND AND MEDITATION

सत्यं ब्रूयात्प्रियं ब्रूयात्, न ब्रूयात्सत्यं अप्रियं।
प्रियं च न अनृतं ब्रूयात्, एष धर्मः सनातनः॥

Satyaṁ brūyāt, priyaṁ brūyāt, na brūyāt satyaṁ apriyaṁ |
Priyaṁ ca nānṛ utaṁ brūyāt, eṣ a Dharmaḥ Sanātanāḥ [1] ||

One should speak the truth. One should speak, what is pleasant to the listener. One should not speak, what is true, but hurtful. One should also not say, what is pleasant, but untrue. This is the eternal wisdom.

From ancient times, people have been fascinated by the wonder of their own mind and the experience of the surrounding universe. This pondering, about one's being-in-Reality, may have been the beginning of a meditative mind, and the origin of various philosophies and religions. Currently, there is a considerable interest among the medical and scientific community, in promoting mental health, subjective well-being, happiness, and spirituality.

Vaillant [175] reviewed different models of mental health. He considered mental health as i) normality, ii) positive psychology, iii) maturity, iv) social-emotional intelligence, v) subjective well-being, and vi) resilience. Mental normality implies healthy ability to work, love, and play; efficient problem solving; investment in life; and self-autonomy.

Klamut [176] defined happiness as a state of the spirit (mind), which consists of internal peace, satisfaction with one's life, the joy of life, benevolence, and cordiality towards oneself and others; sensitivity to the beauty of nature, culture, and art; harmonious coexistence with the surroundings. Achievement of such happiness depends on oneself and a rich, encouraging environment. McGrath [177] recently defined the term "spirituality" as a personal worldview (and self-view) that emphasizes the importance of discerning purpose in one's life.

Yoga is also about mental health and excellence. Yoga is a way of adaptive self-integration, being at-peace with oneself and at-home in the world. Self-integration results from constant self-awareness and letting go of irrelevant memories, imaginations, mental agitations, and distractions. Such a person functions with a truly undistracted, attentive and serene mind. When the mind is undirected and assumes its original, unmodified state, the Self

---

[1] Shrotriya VK. Sanskrit Subhāṣ ita Saritā. Part 2. Pune, India: Nitīna Prakāśana; 1989: 122.

experiences itself. Yoga is a skillful quieting of a distracted and ruminative mind with a natural resolution of emotional conflicts, culminating in a truly peaceful and intuitive, conscious state.

Three essential steps of Yoga Saṁyam संयम include i) Dhāraṇ ā धारणा, conscious focusing of attention on an object, an activity, a thought or an ongoing experience; (b) Dhyānaṁ ध्यानं, continued, sustained dwelling of attention on the same experience; and (c) Samādhiḥ समाधिः, effortless, self-absorptive, and intuitive state of understanding and realization of one's true nature or Energy-Being. Here are a few excerpts from Pātañjali's Yoga Sūtra पातञ्जलि योगसूत्र:

योगष्चित्तवृत्तिनिरोधः | तदा द्रष्टुः स्वरूपेऽवस्थानाम् || वृत्ति सारूप्यमितरत्र |||

"Yoga is calming the fluctuations of a (wandering, ruminative and agitated) mind (Verse 2). Then the self abides in his or her own (natural silent, serene) state (Verse 3). Other times, the self is associated with the ego (and ownership) of ongoing mental activity (Verse 4)."

"Mental calming can be achieved by disengagement or letting go (of a ruminating mind) and a constant self-awareness (presence, mindfulness or vigilant attentiveness) (Verse 12). [...] Impending pain and suffering can be prevented (by meditation and healthy life style) (Verse 67), [...] Self-regulatory activity and its continued experience as a controlling self are falsely associated. (Verse 74). The cause of selfishness or egoism is a lack of self-awareness (Verse 75). On becoming fully aware, the false association between self-regulatory activity and the essential self disappears, which leads to complete Self-freedom (Verse 76). The uninterrupted deployment of vigilant awareness on the reality (presence or present-mindedness, vigilant attention) is the means of dispersing self-centered thinking and self-ignorance (Verse 77). With vigilant attentiveness comes fitness of mind (Verse 104). [...] The capacity to change mental state manifests in three different ways: ability to stop ongoing mental activity, ability to focus attention on a specific event in space-time, and the ability to maintain attention on a given task or event leading to an enhanced cognitive capacity (Verse 122). Being free from any selfish motivation, instinctual pressure and mental conflict, one can live peacefully with spontaneity, presence, and natural wisdom (Verse 195)."

There is a vast literature on Buddhist and Zen meditation. James Austin's book, "Zen and the Brain" is a landmark publication, integrating two very complex fields of knowledge. There are many insights in this book with attempts to understand meditation and consciousness in terms of neuroscience. However, it is beyond the scope of this chapter to review several, interesting observations made in that book.

Here is an excerpt from the Ṣ wetaṣ watara Upaniṣ ad ष्वेताष्वतर उपनिषद्: "let the wise man restrain his mind vigilantly as (he would) a chariot with vicious horses. (Verse 9)... Even as a mirror stained by dust shines brightly when it has been cleaned, so the embodied one when he has seen the real nature of the Self becomes integrated, of fulfilled purpose, and freed from sorrow. (Verse 14)."

An excerpt from Maitri Upaniṣ ad मैत्री उपनिषद् "This is the rule for achieving this (spiritual oneness): control of breath, withdrawal of senses, meditation, concentration, contemplative inquiry, and absorption; (this is) said to be the six-fold yoga, (Verse 18). [...]

That which is non-thought, which stands in the midst of thought, the unthinkable, the hidden, the highest, let a man merge his thought there. Then will this living being be (free) without any support (or dependence). (Verse 19). […] For by the serenity of thought, one destroys deeds, good and evil, with the serene Self abiding in itself, he enjoys enduring happiness. (Verse 20)."

An excerpt from the sixth chapter of the Bhagavad Gītā भगवद् गीता on Dhyāna Yoga ध्यानयोग [178, 179]: "Let a man lift his self by his own self; Let him not lower himself; One's self alone is one's own friend or foe. (Verse 5). […] Unflickering, like a lamp in a sheltered place: So the man of disciplined thought practices yoga of the Self. (Verse 19)… That in which thought ceases, stopped by the practice of disciplined concentration, and in which, seeing himself through himself, one is content in oneself (Verse 20); The one whose self is disciplined by yoga, sees the Self abiding in every being, and sees every being in the Self. (Verse 29)."

An excerpt from Śiva Saṁhitā शिवसंहिता "Out of consciousness is born all the animate and inanimate objects (experiences) of this world. Hence, abandoning all these, one should abide in consciousness itself. (Verse 49). […] Indivisible by time and space, Ātman in its natural state is always truly complete or whole. (Verse 54)… In a world full of ignorance and with extreme paucity of knowledge, happiness comes only when sorrow is removed. The Ātman, however, is ever happy. (Verse 57). […] The Ātman alone is without duality and beyond words. (Verse 61). […] All desires disappear only through knowledge (Self-understanding). When the sense of plurality fades away, the light of Oneness, ekatvaṁ एकत्वं , dawns. (Verse 57)."

Gheraṇ ḍ a Samhitā घेरण्ड संहिता described an ancient, six-fold system of Yoga: postures, mudras or mystic hand gestures, control of senses, breath control, meditation, and superconsciousness. Here is an excerpt: "Getting into (an absorptive) mental trance, let the mind be united with the self *Ātman*. When both (mind and ego) merge into the supreme Self *Paramātman*, Samādhiḥ ensues, (Verse 16). […] All living creatures on land and in the sky, all trees, bushes, creepers, plants, grass, all rivers, and mountains – all are seen as the one supreme Brahman, and one's own Self is seen in all. (Verse 19)."

Chapter 23

ART OF MEDITATION

शान्तोऽयमात्मा ।

Śantoyamātmā.

This *Ātman* is blissfully silent!

"This moment has never been before. It is ever-new and sacred.
It will not repeat itself. It deserves our full attention and reverence.
Let us learn and appreciate its wonder."

Meditation[1] is a unique way of being~in~Reality. It is a set of skills to live consciously with full Awareness, Learning and Love for Life (ALLL). It is an art of presence, which implies being present in the current moment whole-heartedly, with all of one's arousal-energy-being, sensitivity, deep feeling, intelligence and creativity.

Meditation implies living with full awareness and understanding of oneself and the present moment. It is a skill of being at-ease with oneself and at-home in the world. It is being highly adaptive, peaceful, self-content, friendly and caring for oneself and others. It is an art of being a true friend to oneself and the world.

If we start observing ourselves, our behavior and mind, we come to realize that usually we are not present-minded. Our mind and heart are not in the here-and-now. Our mind, including our attention, thoughts and emotions, wanders constantly. Our mind seems to drift and dwell on something else, somewhere else, as if, at some other time. The mind commonly dwells on the past memories and future expectations. It is hard for most of us to be fully present and to really experience what is happening right at this moment.

"Mind matters the most. Let us watch and shape it, if we can.
Mind is like a flickering flame affected by many influences.
Let us help it burn and shine bright and beautiful."

It is uncommon for most of us to pause for a moment to smell a rose, to see the sunset, to listen to a bird or to just appreciate the present reality. It is because we are so preoccupied with our own thoughts, chores, plans, mistakes, reactions, memories and imaginations. Once,

1 Deshmukh VD. The Art of meditation. The South African journal of Natural Medicine, May 2008, 37:124-125.

we learn to pay attention to the present reality, we learn a lot from what is truly happening, right in front of us and within us.

There is always a lot to learn from the present reality, because the reality is infinite and it is continuously changing from moment to moment. Reality is the great teacher. No two moments are exactly alike. The present moment has never been before and will never repeat itself. Each moment is new, unique, and sacred. By sacred, I mean it deserves our full attention, understanding, appreciation, and reverence. The reality of the moment is sacred. That is why it is so important for us to learn the art of presence or present-mindedness. The key is Awareness, Learning and Love for Life (ALLL).

There are two ways to define human experiential reality. One is by the consensus of a group of people, for instance, the group may agree that "This is a round table." Then, that becomes the reality of the "round table" by mutual agreement. The other way to define reality is by direct, personal experience, for instance, realizing one's essential, Self-aware Being. Only an individual can have such a realization of Reality-by-experience.

The present is sacred, infinite, and indescribable. The present is the start as well as the finish of our momentary conscious journey to our Self. But all these are just words. Do we realize the truth in these words? A word is only a symbol. In order for us to really understand the truth behind the symbol, we need to see and read it clearly, understand its meaning and associations and then, actually realize the truth behind the symbol within ourselves.

During walking or moving meditation, we need to learn to be a silent witness of our bodily movements and mental activities, as they are occuring from moment to moment. We need to learn to listen to the silence within, which is an essential part of meditation. Words, inner speech, thoughts and memories keep us at the surface of the fountain of conscious mind. Language is important for communication and expression, but it is unnecessary or even a hindrance for a quiet, silent awareness. During meditation, it is more important to listen whole-heartedly to one's existential being than to continue to chat with one's ego, at the surface of consciousness.

When we listen whole-heartedly, and when our mind is really quiet, we may hear a unique, spontaneous sound of silence, Anāhat nāda. This can be a good cue of a silent and peaceful mind. One also has a great sense of wellbeing, boundless arousal-energy and an unconditional bliss. Such a unique meditative state, Turīya, the fourth state of consciousness, cannot be described fully and accurately, but it can be lived, felt and experienced directly during meditation and in our everyday life.

There are two modes of meditation, all-exclusive and all-inclusive. In the all-exclusive mode, there are no contents in the conscious mind. It has also been described as Śunyatā, the great emptiness or the unique, experience of no experience. This may happen during formal sitting meditation, Zāzen, with absolute stillness, silence, egolessness, and serenity. In the all-inclusive mode, there is a feeling of full participation or "Oneness" with all that is. Nothing is excluded. It has been described as Pūrṇ atā, a fullness of conscious being or a perfect mindful Presence. It may happen spontaneously during inspiring moments like peak experiences, dynamic meditation, artistic creations, sports, or even some everyday events.

How can we achieve such a wonderful, happy, inspired and intuitive frame of mind? There is no one specific path or technique, but there are some mental skills that all of us can learn to live a good, inspired life. The following are some of the suggestions for meditation with Self-awareness, Ātmapreksħā, which can be practiced at any time, for a few minutes, and every-now-and-then, ideally throughout the day:

1) Pause in what you are doing now and just watch attentively.
2) Finish the current train of thought and remain quiet at this moment.
3) Disengage from the past context and let go of any mental pursuits, searches, expectations, worries, plans and wishes.
4) Be aware of your posture, breathing, mood, emotions and thoughts, as they occur.
5) Witness the present reality as is, without any comments, corrections, descriptions, associations, or recollections.
6) Listen to the spontaneous, background sound of the Serene Silence within.
7) Expand your attention from a specific object to the global field of background or matrix Awareness.
8) Remain calm, and observant. Be a silent witness, Sākshī, to all that is happening.
9) Enjoy the natural wonder of Being in the present moment and especially, the Reality of Being present with Awareness, Learning and Love for Life (ALLL).
10) Appreciate this moment of inspiration, the wonder of the ever-new Reality, unfolding and one's being in it, open, receptive, cognizant and Self-content.
11) Let these skills become a part of one's daily life. Let your present experience be the teacher and healer.
12) This moment has never been before. It is new and sacred. It deserves our full attention, appreciation and reverence. The present reality is sacred, only if, we would realize its wonder from moment-to-moment.

"The present Reality is sacred. We are in it. We are it.
We can realize its truth spontaneously,
By our own full presence and blissful existence."

There is a vast literature on Yogic, Buddhist and Zen meditation. Briefly, there are two main modes of Buddhist meditations: Śamathā – Tranquility meditation and Vipassanā – Insight meditation. Śamathā includes development of i) concentration by breath awareness anapanasati, ii) friendliness or loving kindness, metta bhāvanā, iii) compassion, karuṇ ā, iv) spontaneous joy, muditā, and v) equanimity, upekkhā. Vipassanā or insight by direct perception or experience, Pratyak Jñāna, includes development of i) mental clarity regarding nature of Self, ii) inner peace and freedom, and iii) wisdom and compassion. Śamathā can calm the mind, but only Vipassanā or insight can reveal how the mind was disturbed to start with. Such Self-understanding, Prajñā, leads to wisdom by Self-learning, Ātma Jñāna.

In Jainism, meditation is called Sāmāyika, a Prākrit word, derived from Samaya meaning time. It means being in the moment of continuous real time. If the present moment is considered as a moving line between the past and the future, Sāmāyika happens by being fully aware, alert, and conscious, in that moving timeline, when one experiences one's true nature or Ātman. The aim of Sāmāyika is to transcend our constantly changing daily experience of being a vulnerable and suffering individual, Jīva, and to realize our changeless, blissful Being, the Ātman. This act of being a conscious witness, Sākshī, of the continually renewing universe, with the individual Jīva being in it, is the first step in realizing one's true nature.

Chapter 24

MEDITATIVE BRAIN

लोकानन्दः समधिसुखम् ||१८||

The delight that the yogi feels in abiding in his/her true nature as the knower with respect to both the ego and the object in the world, is his/her natural delight of samādhi.

Śiva Sutras 18

We do not exactly know, what happens in the human brain, during meditation. Obviously, it is difficult to bring together individuals accomplished in meditation, during their enlightened state of mind, in a high-tech laboratory with functional MRI[1], EEG[2], MEG[3], and PET[4] scanning. Lazar et al. [180] used functional fMRI to identify the brain regions that are active during a simple form of meditation and relaxation response. A significant increase in signal was observed in the dorsolateral prefrontal and parietal cortices, hippocampus, temporal lobe, anterior cingulate, striatum, and precentral and postcentral gyri during meditation. The results indicate that the practice of meditation activates neural structures involved in attention and control of the autonomic nervous system.

Newberg and Iversen [181] described two types of meditation: "The first type is one in which the subjects simply attempt to clear all thoughts from their sphere of attention and to reach a subjective state, characterized by a sense of no space, no time, and no thought. This state is also fully integrated and unified, such that there is no (dualistic) sense of a self and other. The second form of meditation involves focusing attention on a particular object, image, word, or phrase, which may lead to a subjective experience of self-absorption with the object of focus. […] In eight Tibetan Buddhist monks, voluntary meditation with sustained attention was initially accompanied by activation in bilateral, but right more than left, prefrontal cortex and cingulate gyrus. This was followed by activation of the inhibitory reticular nucleus of the thalamus, which in turn deaffarented the posterior temporo-occipital-parietal (TOP) areas, minimizing the (cortical) sensory input. The perception of one's bodily self, depends on the activation of posterior, superior parietal lobule. The hippocampus acts to modulate cortical arousal-energy and responsiveness via connections with the prefrontal

---

1 Magnetic Resonance Imaging
2 Electroencephalography
3 Magnetoencephalography
4 Positron Emission Tomography

cortex, amygdala, and hypothalamus. These structures are involved in generating attention, emotion, and imagery."

"Activation of right amygdala results in stimulation of the hypothalamus, with subsequent stimulation of the parasympathetic system. This is associated with a sense of relaxation and profound quiescence, reducing breathing and heart rates, which in turn, reduces the activity of Locus Coeruleus. Decreased NE[5] from Locus Coeruleus would decrease the stimulation of hypothalamus, thus, decreasing the stress-related production of CRH[6], ACTH[7], and cortisol. [...] Argenine vasopressin (AVP[8]) is known to be released during meditation and has been shown to contribute to the maintenance of positive affect, to decrease self-perceived fatigue and arousal, and to significantly improve the consolidation of new memories and learning. The activation of prefrontal cortex increases the levels of free glutamate[9] in the brain, which can stimulate the hypothalamus to release beta-endorphin. Beta-endorphin is known to reduce pain and fear, and to produce a sense of joy and euphoria. Moderately increased levels of serotonin[10] during meditation also appear to correlate with positive affect."

McCraty et al., [182], defined intuition as a process, by which information that is normally outside the range of conscious awareness, is perceived by the psycho-physiological systems. They conclude that the heart and brain, together, are involved in receiving, processing, and decoding intuitive information. The intuitive perception and human creativity are closely linked [183].

Creativity is defined as the ability to produce work that is both novel (i.e., original, unexpected) and appropriate (i.e., useful, adaptive). Dietrich [184] summarized by stating, "Creativity results from the factorial combination of four kinds of mechanisms. Neural computation that generates novelty can occur during two modes of thought, deliberate and spontaneous, and for two types of information, emotional and cognitive. Regardless of how novelty is generated initially, circuits in the prefrontal cortex perform the computation that transforms the novelty into creative behavior. To that end, prefrontal circuits are involved in making novelty fully conscious, evaluating its appropriateness, and ultimately implementing its creative expression."

EEG was recorded in long-term Vipassanā meditators and a control group with "rest" (usual wandering mind) state. Meditation was associated with a decrease in frontal delta (1-4 Hz) power, an increase in frontal theta (4-8 Hz) power, and a significantly increased, parieto-occipital gamma (35-45 Hz) power. [185].

A specific form of yoga can generate controlled high-frequency gamma waves. For the first time, paroxysmal gamma waves were observed in eight subjects practicing a yoga technique of breathing control called Bhrāmarī Prāṇ āyāma. EEG signals were analyzed using time-frequency representations, independent component analysis, and EEG tomography. [186].

An association between the endogenous neurotransmitter release and conscious experience was demonstrated for the first time in human subjects. Using 11C-raclopride PET,

5 Norepinephrine.
6 Corticotrophin Releasing Hormone.
7 Adrenocorticotrophic hormone.
8 Argenin Vasppressin Peptide.
9 Excitatory neurotransmitter.
10 5-Hydroxy Tryptamine.

an increased endogenous dopamine release in the ventral striatum, during yoga nidra meditation was demonstrated. Yoga nidra is characterized by a decreased level of desire for action, associated with decreased blood flow in prefrontal, cerebellar, and subcortical regions, structures thought to be involved in executive control. [...] During meditation, 11C-raclopride binding in ventral striatum decreased by 7.9%. This corresponds to a 65% increase in endogenous dopamine release, [187].

The subjective reports and physiological correlates of the experience of "consciousness itself," an existential self-awareness, or self-acquaintance, isolated from the processes and objects of experience were explored during transcendental meditation practice. Subjectively, this state is characterized by the absence of the framework (time-space, and body-sense) and contents (qualities of inner and outer perceptions) that usually define waking experience. Physiologically, this state is distinguished by the presence of apneustic breathing, autonomic orienting at the onset of breath changes, and increases in the frequency of peak EEG power. [188].

Meditation is an ancient spiritual practice, which aims to still the fluctuations of the mind. In 31 subjects, during the onset of meditation, activations were found bilaterally in the putamen and the supplementary motor cortex, while deactivations were found predominantly in the right hemisphere, the precuneus, the posterior cingulum, and the parieto-temporal area. During sustained meditation in 21 subjects, activation in the head of the caudate nucleus, and extensive deactivations were found in the white matter of the right hemisphere, mainly in the posterior occipital-parietal-temporal area and the frontal lobes. [189].

Activation of a default mode network including frontal and parietal midline structures varies with cognitive load. It is more active during low-load tasks and less active during high-load tasks, requiring executive control. Meditation practices entail activation in areas that overlap the default mode network during TM practice suggests that meditation practice may lead to a foundational or 'ground' state of cerebral functioning that may underlie eyes-closed rest and more focused cognitive processes. [190].

Meditators seem to have better attentional capacity and skills. This study found that meditators i) noticed more changes in flickering scenes and noticed them more quickly, ii) counted more accurately in a challenging concentration task, iii) identified a greater number of alternative perspectives in multiple perspective images, and iv) showed less interference from invalid cues in a visual selective attention task, but v) did not differ on a measure of sustained inattentional blindness. Together, results show that regular meditation is associated with more accurate, efficient, and flexible, visual attentional processing, across diverse tasks that have high face validity outside of the laboratory. Meditator's better visual attention is not just immediate, but extends to contexts separate from meditation practice. [191].

Failure to switch off emotion is due to the activation of mental representations of present, past, and future that are created independently of external contingencies. Mindfulness training can be seen as one way to teach people to discriminate such "simulations" from objects and contingencies as they actually are. [...] Participants can learn to uncouple the sensory, directly experienced self, from the "narrative" self. [192].

Significantly larger gray matter volumes in meditators, in the right orbito-frontal cortex as well as in the right thalamus and left inferior temporal gyrus, were detected. Meditators also showed significantly larger volumes of the right hippocampus. Both orbito-frontal and hippocampal regions have been implicated in emotional regulation and response control. Thus, larger volumes in these regions might account for meditator's singular abilities and habits to cultivate positive emotions, retain emotional stability, and engage in mindful behavior. [193].

Using MRI, higher gray matter density in lower brain stem regions of experienced meditators compared with age-matched non-meditators was observed. These changes may be related to cardio-respiratory control and parasympathetic effects and traits, as well as the cognitive, emotional, and immune-reactive impact reported in several studies of different meditation practices. [194].

Meditation involves attention-regulation and may lead to increased activity in brain regions associated with attention such as dorsal-lateral prefrontal cortex (dlPFC) and anterior cingulate cortex (ACC). The dlPFC and ACC regions were more active throughout meditation in comparison to the control task. The long-term practitioners had significantly more consistent and sustained activation in dlPFC and ACC during meditation versus control in comparison to short-term practitioners. This may correlate with better sustained attention and attentional error monitoring.

A set of brain regions are metabolically active during wakeful 'rest' and consistently deactivate during the performance of a variety of demanding tasks. This "default mode network" has been functionally linked to the stream of thoughts occurring automatically in the absence of goal-directed activity. Zen meditation is traditionally associated with a mental state of full awareness with reduced conceptual content. Zen practitioners displayed a reduced duration of the neural response linked to conceptual processing in regions of default network, suggesting that meditative training may foster the ability to control the automatic cascade of semantic associations triggered by a stimulus and, by extension, to voluntarily regulate the flow of spontaneous mentation. [195].

This study was designed to compare changes in brain gamma-amino-butyric acid (GABA) levels associated with an acute yoga session versus a reading session. Outcome measures: GABA-to-creatine ratios were measured in a 2 cm axial slab using MRI spectroscopic imaging, immediately prior to and immediately after interventions. Results: There was a 27% increase in GABA levels in the yoga practitioner group, but no change in the reading group. [196].

Chapter 25

INTEGRATION OF MEDITATION

मध्य विकासात् चिदानन्द लाभः ||१७||

By the self-development of the Madhya (in-between, center, interval or at the edge of phenomenal time) is there a spontaneous emergence the blissful Energy~Awareness~Being.

Pratyabhijñāhṛ dayam: The Secret of Self-Recognition: 17

Meditation is an art of efficient and adaptive management of neuro-behavioral arousal-energy with total engagement or disengagement. In both of these conscious states, there is an experience of spontaneous, unitive being without a sense of ego, memory or time. There is a natural sense of well-being, with self-understanding, spontaneous joy, serenity, freedom, and self-fulfillment. It is where the ultimate pursuit of happiness and search for meaning in life resolve. One realizes the truth of being in harmony with Nature and Nature in oneself. Then each conscious moment becomes a dynamic process of self-discovery and learning about the ever-new, spontaneous reality. One's daily life becomes full of joy, Ānanda आनन्द and inspired beyond description.

Attention can be voluntarily or involuntarily engaged or disengaged. An attentional act creates the duality of the attended-attendee, resulting in a specific conscious experience. Disengaging attention to the limit results in a bare resting awareness (Jñānamayī Drishtī ज्ञानमयी दृष्टि), with global, nonspecific nirguṇ a, meta-awareness or awareness of awareness. It may be expressed as the great Nothingness, Emptiness or Transparency, Śūnyatā शून्यता, Silence or the essential Awareness. Engaging attention to the limit, with a total participation in the present moment, without any effort, sense of time, or ego-awareness, results in a holistic consciousness, Pūrṇ atā पूर्णता . It has been also described as the "Flow" state [197] or "Meditative Presence" [198].

Between two consecutive attentional acts, there is an inter-attentional Awareness, with no attended-attendee duality. This results in a refreshing experience of no experience, which is analogous to waking up from a sound, non-REM sleep without any dreams. This inter-attentional awareness can lead to a state of non-REM alertness, Turīya तुरीय. During non-REM alertness, conscious mentation exists only in a potential, pre-form state. Neurobehavioral arousal-energy and mentation can be in potential or kinetic forms. They are in kinetic form during common, interactive consciousness and dream sleep, whereas, during non-REM sleep and non-REM alertness, they are in potential form. During non-REM sleep, the conscious arousal-energy is low, whereas, during non-REM alertness, the conscious arousal-energy is optimally high. That is why the turīya state has been described to have a feeling of boundless energy, Ananta Śaktiḥ अनन्तशक्तिः, unlimited capacity and intense well-being. This enlightening process is nonlinear and dynamic, whereas the common state of self-consciousness functions within a chaotic attractor basin [199].

The moment one resumes directed attention, the ego-object duality returns and the potential, neuro-behavioral energy becomes kinetic; the egoistic mind takes on the role of various, personal conscious experiences. The ego continuously struggles to change the situation or itself, and suffers from pain or pleasure, throughout its transitory life. Meditation, on the other hand, is the art of being alert and serene, in the midst of all situations. It is the ultimate, adaptive Reality-Consciousness, continuously learning and renewing itself. It is the art of mastering both skills of parallel as well as sequential processing, from moment to moment. It is the ideal state of one's being, at each moment, discovering and appreciating many wonders of this Infinite, ever-new reality.

Chapter 26

HOMEOKINETIC MIND AND EQUANIMITY STHITAPRAJÑĀ स्थितप्रज्ञा

निर्वात दीप इव ।

Nirvāta dīpa iva.

Serene energy~being~awareness is like an unperturbed flame of a lamp.

"The conscious awareness of self springs from the ground of spontaneous, self-organized (wakeful) activity."

From "The Complementary Nature" by Kelso and Engstrom

It is interesting to note that the modern homeokinetic physics is not only consistent with, but also provides a scientific explanation for the ancient, introspective observations of Vedic Ṛishis or seers. The ancient concept of mental equanimity, Sthitaprajñā स्थितप्रज्ञा, with ego-mergence, can now be better understood in the light of homeokinetic physics. Homeokinetics is a logical extension of the commonly used term 'Homeostasis' in Biology. This chapter will provide an introduction to homeostasis, homeokinetic physics, and its novel application to human mental activity and the concept of equanimity. The ideal state of mental equanimity Sthitaprajñā is well described in the Bhagavad Gītā, Upaniṣ ads, Brahma-Sūtra, and Yoga Sūtra.

HOMEOSTASIS

Homeostasis is a well established term in Biology. 'Homeo' means the same or similar and 'stasis' means a steady state. Homeostasis is defined as a tendency toward a relatively stable internal environment, in organisms through interactive, physiological processes. Homeostasis implies maintenance of an internal, steady state of an organism by means of visceral auto-regulation and behavioral self-regulation.

Claude Bernard, a nineteenth century French physiologist first recognized the tendency toward stabilization of the internal environment of the animal body. In 1932, Walter B. Cannon, [200], an American Physiologist at Harvard University, used the term 'Homeostasis' and published his well-known book, “The Wisdom of the Body.” Cannon described the fundamental adaptive process of homeostasis as the ceaseless balancing and rebalancing of physiological processes that maintain internal stability and restore a normal state, when it has been disturbed.

Homeostasis applies to many physiological variables at multiple levels of organization in both unicellular as well as multicellular organisms. For the optimal functioning of an organism, these physiological variables are maintained within a certain range of tolerance. Some of the examples of homeostatic regulation in humans and animals include the maintenance within a normal range of blood pressure, heart rate, blood oxygen, carbon dioxide, and hydrogen H+ ion concentration, water metabolism, osmotic pressure, body temperature, energy metabolism, neuro-endocrine regulation and behavioral self-regulation, including our conscious decision making. Homeostatic regulation applies to all levels of organization, including molecular, cellular, tissue, organ system, individual organism, and societies [201].

Antonio Damasio, [202], recently proposed an interesting hypothesis about the possible relationship between subconscious or automatic homeostatic mechanisms and the evolution of adaptive, conscious behavior. He states: “Homeostatic regulation, which includes emotion, requires periods of wakefulness (for arousal-energy gathering); periods of sleep (presumably for the restoration of depleted chemicals necessary for neuronal activity); attention (for proper interaction with the environment); and consciousness (so that high-level of planning of responses, concerned with individual organism and the group, can eventually take place).”

He went on to say that consciousness is valuable, because it introduces a new means of achieving homeostasis. The neural mechanisms in the brainstem and hypothalamus can coordinate non-consciously, with great efficiency, the visceral functions of the heart, lungs, kidneys, endocrine system, and immunological system, within an adequate range to make life possible, whereas the neural mechanisms of consciousness handle the problem of how an individual organism may cope with unpredictable, environmental challenges, which is essential for its survival and the survival of the species.

Damasio, [203]: “Creatures with consciousness have some advantages over those who do not have consciousness. They can establish a link between the world of automatic regulation and the world of imagination.” He recently summarized his position eloquently: “Consciousness permits an extension of these automatic, homeostatic mechanisms by allowing for flexibility and planning, important functions in complex and unpredictable environments. Conscious organisms know about their past and can make guesses about their future. They can implement this knowledge and manipulate it through planning, in an endeavor to approach that which is beneficial and avoid the harmful.”

HOMEOKINETICS

The term ‘Homeokinetics’ was coined by Soodak and Iberall in 1978, [204, 205]. They considered the origin of life as a self-organizing process and propose ten principles to describe the physics for complex living systems. “Self-organizing systems use cyclic processes to regulate their inner environments. These cyclic processes transport matter-energy (information) and therefore in effect, import and export entropy. We call this thermodynamic cyclic conception of the life phase of complex systems homeokinetics, by extension of Claude Bernard and Walter Cannon's concept of homeostasis. In the homeostatic view, internal mechanisms regulate the organism so as to return the organism to equilibrium. Homeokinetics emphasizes the role of kinetic processes, particularly in the form of ongoing, periodic, thermodynamic engine processes, in carrying out the regulatory functions of the organism."

"A river represents a typical homeokinetic system. A river is not a fixed form, but is a process cycle. It is not a hydraulic element in a fixed channel, but the effect of rainfall in a hydrological cycle. The rainfall causes, both water runoff and the appearance of a bed-load of transportable material that erodes and maintains the form of the river."

Another good example of a homeokinetic system is a school of fish swimming freely in an ocean. Each fish is an element or atomism of the system, but the school as whole, the continuum, behaves like a single holistic entity or an organism. Iberall and Soodak wrote a primer on Homeokinetics in 1998 [206] and on the biophysics of the origin of life on earth in 2001, [207].

Scott Kelso and David Engstrom's recent publication, "The Complementary Nature" in 2006, is another landmark publication in this field. They explain "Complementary Nature" as the name they have given to Nature itself, while at the same time voicing their belief that Nature itself entails complementarity in its manifold expression. They suggest that the Nature is experienced by humans as complementary pairs. The sense of self or agency of action emerges from the spontaneous self-organizing coordination tendencies. Meaningful information is the joint product of a coordinated system of parts and processes that span organism and environment. Coordination establishes meaning. The conscious awareness of self springs from the ground of spontaneous, self-organized activity.

They described the ontogeny of our sense of self. "As a fetus moves spontaneously within the womb, it eventually discovers arms and legs that flex~extend, a mouth that opens~closes, a body that bends~twists. In other words, the neonate begins to make sense of itself as a living thing (being). 'These movements belong to me! I am doing this!' From spontaneous self-organized behavior emerges the self - 'I am,' 'I do" – and from there a huge range of potentialities ('I can do'). 'I-ness' thus arises from spontaneity, and it is this 'I' that may be said to direct action."

THE UNBREAKABLE

A slip of hand breaks a wine glass.
A crack in the mirror breaks a face.
A child's giggle breaks silence.
The rejection of love breaks Heart.

A dripping paintbrush divides a canvas.
A scratchy violin destroys symphony.
An interruption wrecks a train of thought.
A knock on the door breaks meditation.

An earthquake breaks the ground.
A surf wave breaks the ocean's calm.
A ripple breaks the stillness of a pond.
A falling star breaks the night sky.

A drop of ink breaks the innocence of a page.
A point shatters the heart of infinite space.
A moment divides the continuity of time.
A perception breaks unawareness.

What is it that is never broken,
By any action, thought or emotion?

It is the reality of a pristine mind,
When Silence hums freely,
When Stillness moves creatively,
When eyes see the Transparent,
When Peace forgives and forgets,
When Life Loves itself and
The unbreakable
Energy~Being~Awareness
Endures!

Vinod D Deshmukh
April 14, 2007

Chapter 27

MIND IN INDIAN PSYCHOLOGY: ANTAḤKARAṆA अन्तःकरण

एकं ज्योतिर्मयं शुद्धं सर्वगं व्योमवद्दृढं ।
अव्यक्तं अचलं नित्यं आदिमध्यअंतवर्जितं ||५||

The holistic energy~being is one, self-effulgent, pure, steady, all-pervasive, space-like, unmanifest, unmoving, unchanging, without any beginning, middle or end.

Nirguṇ aṁ Dhyānaṁ निर्गुणं ध्यानं, in Yoga Yajñavalkya[1]

The concept of mind, Antaḥ karaṇ a अन्तःकरण as the internal organ of mentation is different in the Indian Psychology than the one in the Western Psychology. The APA[2] dictionary of psychology (2007) defined mind as: "i) all intellectual and psychological phenomena of an organism, encompassing motivational, affective, behavioral, perceptual, and cognitive systems; in other words, the organized totality of the mental and psychic processes of an organism and the structural and functional, cognitive components, on which they depend. The term, however, is often used more narrowly to denote only cognitive activities, such as perceiving, attending, thinking, problem-solving, language, learning and memory, ii) the substantive content of such mental and psychic processes, iii) consciousness or awareness, particularly as specific to an individual, iv) a set of emergent properties automatically derived from a brain that has achieved sufficient biological sophistication, v) human consciousness regarded as an immaterial entity distinct from the brain and vi) The brain itself and its activities."

The Handbook of Indian Psychology [208] on the other hand defined mind and consciousness differently: "In contrast to the bio-centric bias of Western psychology, Indian psychology has consciousness as its core concept. Centrality of consciousness is its defining characteristic. Consciousness is considered to be a primary principle irreducible to brain

---

1 Dinakar LG. Yoga Yajñavalkya. Pune, India; 2006:67.

2 American Psycholgical Association

states. The brain does not generate consciousness[3]; it simply reflects consciousness and often by filtering, limiting and embellishing it. […] Mind and consciousness are considered to be qualitatively different. Unlike consciousness, mind is assumed to be material but subtle. It is the interfacing instrumentality that is connected to consciousness at one end and with the body at the other end. Mind is seen as the gateway and one's connection to reality. It is the tool of awareness, but not awareness-as-such. When the mind connects us with the world outside through the sensory system, we have phenomenal awareness. When the connection is to consciousness-as-such, there is transcendental realization. […] Psychology cannot study consciousness-as-such because humans are cognitively "closed" from understanding it. Consciousness-as-such is not an object; it is considered undifferentiated subjectivity without any content. […] The 'person' is consciousness embodied. The person functions as a composite of consciousness, mind, and body. Mind and body have the effect of limiting, obscuring, veiling, and distorting consciousness."

The true Self, which is consciousness-as-such, is considered independent of and free from the incessant mental activity. In fact, for Self-realization to occur, all mental activity, Antaḥ karaṇ a vritti, has to merge spontaneously, in its ground matrix-state - the consciousness-as-such. This happens in the so called "the fourth state of consciousness, Turīya sthiti." The realization of one's essential subjectivity can neither be objectified by senses, imagined by a thinking mind, nor described in any human language. Such Self-realization is knowing by being. The knower of *Ātman* becomes *Ātman* itself, Ātmavid Ātmaiva bhavati आत्मविद् आत्मैव भवति |. Yoga is defined by Patanjali as a state of spontaneous, effortless, ego-mergence in the essential ground of our self-luminous, conscious Energy-Being-Awareness, which is our essential nature. At other times, we remain preoccupied with our limited, ongoing mental activity.

The concept of "Person" in Advaita Vedānta is that of a nested, multi-layered entity, like the multiple sheaths of an onion or the trunk of a banana plant. A person (Jīva) has at least five layers or sheaths, made up of matter-energy-information, varying from gross to subtle: a) Material or physical sheath, Annamaya kośa, b) Vital or physiological, Prāṇ amaya kośa, c) Sensory-Perceptual-Cognitive, Manomaya kośa, d) Intentional-Discriminating, Vijnānamaya Kośa and e) Joyous-Blissful, Ānandamaya kośa, which is the essence of all. [209].

The mind, Antaḥ karaṇ a in Vedānta is considered an internal organ or a tool of mental action or conation Karma, cognition Jñāna, and emotional experiences of pleasure, pain, fear, anger, etc, Bhogaḥ . It includes four component processes: i) Citta is all memories including the conscious working memory, long-term semantic memory, and the subconscious memories, both individual and collective, ii) Manas is mentation, thinking-imagining, dealing with the sensory-motor organs, iii) Buddhi is decision-making, choosing, discriminating intelligence, and iv) Ahamkāra is a sense and feeling of being an ego, self, interpreter, predictor, volition, intentionality, planning, organizing, central executive. There is a certain nested hierarchy in these regulatory capacities of the four mental subsystems. The hierarchy from below up would be memory Citta, mentation Manas, intellect Buddhi, and ego Ahamkāra. This nested hierarchy is manifested in both human and animal ontogeny as well as phylogeny.

---

3 Modern neuroscientists do not agree with this statement at all. For them, brain is the organ of consciousness. Without a living-functioning brain, there is no consciousness. The above perspective becomes speculative and purely spiritual.

According to the nondualistic Advaita Vedānta view of Ādi Śaṅ karāchārya, the essence of human personality is the self *Ātman*, which is beyond body, life, mind and intellect. Self is attributed to have consciousness, continuity in consciousness, and awareness of itself as the knower and the agent of activities. The self lives through all states of consciousness, which mind does not. The two are different. The self is the knower of the experiential field Kshetrajña, the seer Dṛ iṣ ṭ in, the witness Sākshī, the immutable Kuṭ astha, and pure consciousness Cit Śaktiḥ *Ātman*. [210].

Chapter 28

EQUANIMITY IN BHAGAVAD GĪTĀ AND BRAHMA SŪTRA

प्रजहाति यदा कामान्सर्वान्पार्थ मनोगतान् |
आत्मन्येवात्मना तुष्टः स्थितप्रज्ञस्तदोच्यते ||५५||

When a person grows out of all egoistic desires, ambitions and action-plans, and becomes content in his or her own essential self or being, then he deserves to be called a person of steady wisdom.

The Bhagavad Gītā II: 55

In the Bhagavad Gītā, a person of self-realization with perfected wisdom, Prajñā प्रज्ञा is described as Sthitaprajña स्थितप्रज्ञ. Such a person has outgrown egoistic desires and delusional ambitions and conflicting action-plans. He is self-content Ātmatuṣ ta आत्मतुष्ट, wise and at-peace with self, Sthitadhīḥ स्थितधिः. He is free of extreme negative or positive emotions, and resilient to changing circumstances. He has mastered the art of self-regulation, Saṁyama संयम and he is free of episodic feelings of I-me-mine, Ahamkāra अहंकार. He realizes the true nature of Self-in-Reality. He looks at everyone with an eye of equanimity. Unperturbed by changing circumstances, he enjoys spontaneous inner bliss Ātmaprasāda आत्मप्रसाद. He is compassionate Karuṇ ā and cares for all living beings and Nature. He is ever-free Mukta and a light to himself, Swayamjyotiḥ स्वयंज्योतिः. [211].

Brahma-Sutra described the process of ego-mergence Swāpyayāt स्वाप्ययात् of the momentary ego, Kshaṇ ika jīva क्षणिक जीव, into the self-aware, enduring self Śāśwata Jñaḥ शाश्वत ज्ञः. During activity, ego appears different from its inmost source, but both are the same just as the light and the source of light are the same, due to self-effulgence Prakāśa Āṣ rayatwāt Tejaswāt प्रकाश आश्र्यत्वात्तेजस्वात्. It described the state of equanimity and stillness acalatwaṁ अचलत्वं , after mergence of speech Vāk वाक् into mind Manas, mind into breath energy Prāṇ aśaktīḥ प्राणशक्तिः, breath awareness into Self-awareness Ātma Jñāna

आत्मज्ञान, and self into the self-witnessing conscious energy~being Citśaktīḥ चित्शक्ति Cidātman चिदात्मन्, which is its true nature Tat Ātmakatvaṁ. Such a person is truly free Mukta मुक्त and has no other ruler Ananya Adhipatiḥ अनन्य अधिपति: [212].

Chapter 29

DISCUSSION ON EQUANIMITY

यत्र यत्र मनस्तुष्टिर्मनस्तत्रैव धारयेत् ।
तत्र तत्र परानन्दस्वरुपमं सम्प्रवर्तते ॥७४॥

Wherever the mind of an individual finds deep satisfaction (without agitation), let it dwell on that. In every such case, the bliss of one's true nature will manifest by itself.

Vijñānabhairava or Divine consciousness, 74.

All of our mental processes, like conation, cognition, emotion, perception, attention, memory, intelligence, ego, and imagination, are self-organizing and homeokinetic. They go through periodic cycles of activity and rest. Whereas, rest is a state of relative equilibrium or homeostasis, homeokinetic activity include phases of emergence Udaya उदय, existence Vṛ itti वृत्ति and mergence Laya लय of arousal-energy-awareness and conscious as well as subconscious experiential processes. It is clearly important to appreciate precise definitions of the key terms such as "mind," "consciousness," and "self." Lot of misunderstanding has occurred, in both western and eastern literature, when these terms were used with imprecise definitions and context. These are summary terms and each has so many implied meanings and connotations. The differences in the use of these terms in the Western and Indian psychology have already been emphasized above.

The possibility of spontaneous mergence of transient, mental activity into the essential matrix-consciousness, which can still endure, without any mental specificity, was clearly considered and discussed in a very recent chapter by Giulio Tononi and Steven Laureys, [213]. The authors have successfully differentiated between consciousness-as-such and almost all other mental activities namely i) sensory input – motor output, ii) language, iii) reflection, introspection, iv) attention, v) memory, vi) sense of personal space, vii) sense of body and self (ego). They have convincingly argued that all of these mental activities can be dissociated in different circumstances, from the essential consciousness-as-such, with an existential feeling of a timeless, speechless being - the last sense of self or the intrinsic, subjective self, Antaryāmi अन्तर्यामि. Here is their quote: "Perhaps states achieved through transcendental meditation techniques, can approximate a loss of awareness of space, body, and self (ego): experts report a feeling of silence, no bodily feelings, unboundedness (no space, and possibly no self), and no time. Even in such cases, though, the experience would still be happening to one entity – it would be 'centered' if you wish, but not in the conventional spatial sense. This last sense of 'self', which we may call 'intrinsic' or 'subjective' self – would be one and the same as the (existential) experience, not further dissociable."

This final conclusion is remarkably similar to the Vedāntic concept of spontaneous sound of serene silence, Anāhata nāda अनाहत नाद, spontaneous serenity of being Śantoyaṁ Ātmā शान्तोयऽमात्मा, and the essential, witness consciousness Sākshī साक्षी. The concept of such existential, essential self-awareness and its possible realization through different meditative practices has been reviewed recently by this author. The concept of existential conscious being is also consistent with Damasio's concept of basic or core consciousness and Thomas Bleck's explanation of consciousness as an integrative function of three subsystems, namely, conscious arousal, awareness, and attention.

According to Damasio, core consciousness provides the organism with a sense of self about one moment, now, and about one place, here (like a stroboscopic action photo). It is a simple biological phenomenon and operates in a stable fashion through the lifetime of an organism. It is independent of working memory, long-term memory, language, and reasoning. It is a central resource and serves the entire compass of brain's neural patterns. This core sense of self is newly created for each moment in time; conscious individuals continuously generate 'pulses of consciousness.' (Strobe light, *Spanda*). According to Thomas Bleck, basic awareness, in an aroused individual, implies that the individual is not only alert, but also cognizant of self and surroundings. It does not imply any specificity for the modality of stimulation, which could be external or internal, [214].

The neurobiology of breathing and emotion has recently been reviewed. The basic spontaneous respiratory rhythm is generated in the lower brainstem. However, it is highly influenced by emotion and volition. Respiration is important in maintaining physiological homeostasis and it co-exists with emotions, speech and cognition. The emotional modulation of respiration is mediated by the reticulo-limbic network consisting of orbitofrontal cortex, amygdala, piriform cortex, entorhinal cortex, and the hippocampus [215]. The value of slow mindful breathing during meditation, as a means of achieving homeokinesis, has been emphasized in the Vedic and Yogic literature. Heightened emotions can lead to rapid shallow breathing, while intentional slow deep breathing can help to calm extreme emotions. This science of optimal breathing, Prāṇ āyāma has been practiced for thousands of years in India [216].

The neurobiology of human volition or free will has been recently reviewed. The consensus seems to be, that modern neuroscience rejects the traditional dualistic view of volition as a causal chain from the conscious mind or 'soul' to the brain and body [217 - 219]. Rather, volition involves brain networks making a series of complex, open decisions, between alternative actions. Such a neocortical network includes pre-supplementary motor area, anterior prefrontal cortex, and multi-modal parietal cortex. Free will is not a driving force for movement, but a conscious awareness concerning the nature of the movement. Movement is generated by subcortical networks subconsciously, and the conscious sense of volition comes later as a result of self-perception.

Some Vedāntists seem to have a dualistic, spiritual perspective of self and consciousness-as-such. They seem to reject the role of brain in the generation of consciousness-as-such. However, most of the neurobiologists are convinced that all of our conscious mental activities, including our sense of self (ego), are generated by the optimally functioning brain and its complex neural networks. Therefore, there is a wide gap between these two views. There have been many attempts to bridge this 'great divide' between the spiritual and the biophysical aspects without much success; although, some proposals are worth mentioning.

Ralph Pred, [220], talked about "organic or experiential monism," To quote Pred: "The physical and mental poles, like the perceptual and actional, are aspects of a unitary experience enjoyed in the ongoing flow. It is in this sense of unitarity and seamlessness, in contrast with mind-body dualisms, that I talk of an experiential monism."

Schafer, [221], proposed a transcendental, non-empirical Reality in the order of "One." Schafer proposed: "The reality appears to us in two domains: the open and well-known domain of empirical, material things – the realm of actuality – and a hidden and invisible domain of non-empirical, non-material forms – the realm of potentiality. [...] Reality is an indivisible wholeness that is aware of its processes, like a Cosmic Spirit, and it reveals its awareness in the mind-like properties of elementary processes, as well as in the human consciousness."

FACES FASCINATE ME

On a sunny afternoon in Lisbon,
I took a yellow tram, number 28E,
And sat by an open window,
With my camera in hand.
The tram went through the old parts of town,
With ancient buildings, small shops, and narrow streets.

Initially, I was fascinated by
The incredibly narrow paths for trams,
Old churches, historic houses and monuments.
I took many pictures of the winding streets,
The red and yellow trams, and some private cars,
Skillfully negotiating through places and people.

Then I started noticing people and their faces,
Patiently waiting at the tram stops.
I mentally paused and looked at each face,
With curiosity, interest and enthusiasm,
Without any bias or judgement.

Every new face fascinated me.
Each had a unique story of its own.
I started taking pictures of these anonymous faces.
I could relate to each person,
And could feel their being - their spirit.

I saw the wonder of happiness and love
Of a father leading his three well-dressed daughters,
Of a toddler, securely holding her grand father's hand,
Of a newly wed couple kissing each other passionately,
And two old ladies enjoying a leisurely conversation,
Unaware of the passing tram and rushing passengers.

I also saw sad loneliness and fear on the face,
Of an old lady
Walking with a stick and a grocery bag,
Of a young woman
Frantically smoking and cursing on the cell phone,

Of a middle aged man
With a vacant look, in front of a closed door,
Of three men
Drinking beer, smoking cigarettes and arguing,

Of an old man
Sitting probably hungry, at a street corner,
Of a dignified man
Singing Fado-like songs,
And petting his little dog every-now-and-then.
Of a lady
Posed as a marble statue,
And a lonely woman trying to sell flowers.

Every face fascinated me.
Each face had a unique story,
And an unspeakable dignity.
Each face was reflecting
Its humanity.

The human spirit was shining through
And expressing itself,
Through each and every pair of eyes.
I could feel their essential energy and liveness.
No face was imperfect or ordinary.
Each had its own living brilliance.

Every face fascinated me.
Every life-form taught me something new.
Every person was reminding me,
Of our commonality, of our basic dignity,
And the Great Spirit that smiles through us all,
Through all faces, all forms

And everything that exists.
All faces fascinate me, including my own!
I bow down to the great Spirit within us all.

Namaste! नमस्ते!

Vinod D Deshmukh

September 8th 2010

Chapter 30

HOLISTIC CONSCIOUSNESS, TURĪYA, AND THE STEP MODEL OF EGO

आत्मनि संविशति आत्मनात्मानम् |

Ātmani samviśati ātmanātmānam.

The ego-self spontaneously merges within itself, by itself, into the essential energy~being~awareness, the *Ātman*.

HISTORICAL BACKGROUND

The fourth, holistic conscious state, Turīya तुरीय was described in an ancient Sanskrit text called Māṇ ḍ ūkyopaniṣ ad माण्डूक्योपनिषद्. The Upaniṣ ads are short insightful texts in verse form, which were preserved by the ancient philosophers in India, by passing them, from generation to generation, in an oral tradition, before the advent of written language. Most scholars date the written form of Upaniṣ ads back to 3,500 to 5,000 years ago. One hundred and eight such Upaniṣ ads, including thirteen essential ones, have been translated in English [222 - 225]. Oral recitation of these meaningful Sanskrit verses still continues amongst the Sanskrit scholars all over the world. It is a living philosophy, practiced by many Hindus, in their daily lives.

At a symposium on consciousness, held in honor of Herbert H. Jasper, a pioneer neurophysiologist from the Montreal Neurological Institute, a panel of renowned neuroscientists made outstanding presentations on the complex subject of human consciousness [226]. Barbara E. Jones, [227], of McGill University, reviewed the current understanding of the neural basis of consciousness across the sleep-wake cycle. In her introduction and conclusion, she acknowledged that the currently established three states of consciousness, namely dreamless sleep, dream sleep and wakeful state had been described about 4000 years ago in an ancient Sanskrit text, called Upaniṣ ad, [228]. We know now that this referenced Upaniṣ ad was Māṇ ḍ ukyopaniṣ ad [229].

In this chapter, I wish to elaborate on this profoundly insightful, ancient source of knowledge, based on human experience. The Māṇ ḍ ukyopaniṣ ad has twelve verses. It clearly described four states of human consciousness, namely i) the dreamless sleep state, Suṣ upti सुषुप्ति, with Prājña प्राज्ञ as the experiencing self, ii) the dream sleep state, Swapna स्वप्न, with Taijasa तैजस as the experiencing self, iii) the preoccupied, dualistic, interactive, REM wake state, Jāgrat जाग्रत्, with Vaiṣ wānara वैश्वानर as the experiencing self, and iv) the fourth, Turīya तुरीय, holistic conscious state of nondual, intrinsic, field-awareness, which is an extraordinarily awakened, self-integrated state. The primal, existential Being with essential Awareness, in such a state is called *Ātman* आत्मन्, the essential, existential, self-aware energy~being.

The Sanskrit word Turīya literally means the fourth aspect [230]. The Encyclopedia of Eastern Philosophy and Religion defined Turīya as a super-conscious state of illumination, called the fourth because it transcends the three familiar states of deep sleep, dream and wakefulness [231]. This state of essential consciousness is beyond thought, causality, personal time and identification with the body. It is pure, unified awareness, of indescribable clarity and serenity. It is of the nature of essential existential Being, the Ātman.

This book of Māṇ ḍ ukyopaniṣ ad contains twelve original Sanskrit verses, followed by a commentary, Kārikā by Gaudapāda, who was a Sanskrit scholar and a pioneer of holism, a non-dualistic philosophy called Advaita Vedānta अद्वैत वेदांत. Ādi Śaṅ karāchārya, who was a brilliant, 8th century, Sanskrit scholar, philosopher and a great poet of India (788–820), has translated and commented on the Māṇ ḍ ukyopaniṣ ad as well as on Gauḍ apāda's Kārikā. The Māṇ ḍ ukyopaniṣ ad, after describing the three commonly known states of human consciousness, goes on to describing the fourth conscious state, Turīya, in the seventh and the twelfth verses. Both Eastern and Western interpretations of the possible, fourth state of holistic consciousness are described below.

EASTERN INTERPRETATION

S. Rādhākrishnan, who was a modern scholar of Upaniṣ ads, translated the seventh and the twelfth verses as follows: "(Turīya is) not that which cognizes the internal (objects), not that which cognizes the external (objects), not that which cognizes both of them, not a mass of cognition, not cognitive, nor non-cognitive. (It is) unseen, incapable of being spoken of, ungraspable, without any distinctive marks, unthinkable, unnamable, the essence of knowledge of the one Self, into which the world is resolved, the peaceful, the benign, the non-dual, such, they think, is the fourth quarter. He is the Self; He is to be known. [...]The syllable AUM, ॐ is the very Self. He who knows it thus enters the (essential) self with his (own) self."

In differentiating the state of dreamless sleep from the fully awakened fourth state of Turīya, Gaudapāda commented: "in the dreamless sleep, Prājña, the experiencing self, is neither aware of himself nor of others. He neither knows the truth nor the untruth. He is truly not cognizant of anything. But in the state of Turīya, the essential Self is essentially aware of all that is present in reality." Pātanjali in his Yoga sūtras precisely expressed the reality of the conscious state of Turīya: "The essential self reveals itself, when mental activity, such as thought, emotion and egocentric desires, subsides. At all other times, one identifies oneself with the ongoing mental activity. When the mind stays undirected and assumes its own original unmodified state, the essential Self experiences itself," [232, 233].

WESTERN INTERPRETATION

James H. Austin, a neurologist has accomplished a difficult task of understanding and expressing various states of consciousness, from the Zen Buddhist literature, in the light of modern Neuroscience and compiled them in his landmark book, Zen and the Brain [234]. He described six advanced, conscious states (IV–IX), which are beyond the commonly recognized states of (I) Slow-Wave or dreamless sleep, (II) Desynchronized, dream sleep and (III) wakefulness. "Conscious state (IV) is a level reached during concentration and receptive meditative modes. The conscious state (V) is a state of heightened emotionalized awareness without sensate loss. The conscious state (VI-A) is a state of absorption without sensate loss i.e. external absorption and conscious state (VI-B) is a state of absorption with sensate loss i.e. internal absorption. The three more advanced and extraordinary, conscious states are: (VII) a state of insight-wisdom, Kensho, or Satori, (VIII) a state of ultimate being, beyond expression and (IX) the stage of ongoing enlightened traits." The last three advanced states have many features in common with the holistic, superconscious state of Turīya.

In order to achieve extraordinary conscious mental state like Turīya, some of the meditative techniques are being studied in the field of mental health. Roger N. Walsh, [235], defined the term "Meditation" as "a family of practices that train attention, in order to heighten awareness and bring mental processes, under voluntary control. Their ultimate aim is the development of the deepest insight, into the nature of mental processes, consciousness, self-identity and reality, and the development of optimal states of psychological well-being and consciousness."

He further described these optimal conscious states as "without exclusive identification, (in which) the "me - not me" dichotomy is transcended and the individual thus perceives himself or herself as both no-thing and every-thing. Such people experience themselves both as pure Awareness or no-thing and also as the entire universe or every-thing. Defenses drop away, because when experiencing oneself as no-thing there is nothing to defend; when experiencing oneself as every-thing there is nothing to defend against. This experience of unconditioned or pure Awareness is apparently very blissful. It is described in the Hindu tradition as Sat~Cit~Ānand: Blissful~Conscious~Being."

In the Hindu-Buddhist literature, the "awareness of no-thing" is called Śunyatā, which means an emptiness or awareness, with no specific content or objects. The "awareness of every-thing" is called Pūrṇ atā, which means the total, holistic awareness of the present reality. In Śunyatā, the personal attitude is to let go of all that one is experiencing presently, whereas, in Pūrṇ atā the personal attitude is to embrace all that one is experiencing at the present moment. Both of these personal attitudes have been beautifully combined in a Zen saying, "To study the Self is to forget the self (ego). To forget the self (ego) is to be enlightened by all things." [236]. This concept is beautifully described in Śiva Sūtra: भूयः स्यात्प्रतिमिलनम् ||४५|| It means, "In the case of an enlightened person, there is an awareness of the Divine Reality both inwardly (Nimilanam) and outwardly (Unmilanam), again and again."

A team of psychiatrists and psychologists have recently used mindfulness meditation as a stress reduction intervention in the treatment of anxiety disorders [237]. They define mindfulness meditation as "an effort to intentionally pay attention non-judgmentally to the present moment experience and to sustain this attention over time. The aim is to cultivate a stable and nonreactive present awareness."

There is a remarkable similarity between mindfulness and Freud's characterization of the ideal state of mind, for a psychoanalyst during psychotherapy [238]. Freud [239] described the latter as one of "evenly suspended attention". He defined it operationally as to "suspend judgment and give impartial attention to everything there is to observe." This is very similar to meditative awareness like mindful presence, Turīya, the ideal state of calm, composed and clear holistic awareness.

Two concepts "global vs. local attentiveness" [240] and "spotlight" vs. "floodlight" or "strobe light" attentiveness [241], from the Behavioral and Cognitive Neurology fields, are useful for understanding these advanced states of consciousness. In such global or "strobe light" mode of attention, not only the external reality, but also the internal mental event, becomes perceptible as contents of the total attentional field. It may be a beginning stage, which can lead to the advanced mental state of Turīya.

Csikszentmihalyi in his book, "Flow: The Psychology of Optimal Experience," [242], described attention as "psychic energy, without it no work can be done, and in doing work it is dissipated. We create ourselves, by how we invest this (psychic) arousal-energy. Memories, thoughts, and feelings are all shaped by how we use it. And it is energy under our control, to do with as we please; hence, attention is our most important tool in the task of improving the quality of experience." He also remarked about the circular causality between attention and self: "the self directs attention and the attention determines the self. In fact both these statements are true: consciousness is not a strictly linear system, but one in which circular causality obtains. Attention shapes the self, and is in turn shaped by it."

Some of the recent reviews in Neuroscience point to the Prefrontal Cortex as an important region in the cortical networks, significant in mediating at least nine major higher cortical functions[1]: i) bodily regulation, ii) attuned communication, iii) emotional balance, iv) response flexibility, v) empathy, vi) insight or self-knowing awareness, vii) fear modulation, viii) intuition and ix) morality. Knight and colleagues, [243], concluded, "Prefrontal cortex provides both inhibitory and excitatory input to distributed neural circuits required to support performance in diverse tasks. [...] Prefrontal cortex is able to sculpt behavior through parallel inhibitory and excitatory regulation of neural activity in distributed neural networks."

Miller and Cohen [244] proposed: "The Prefrontal cortex has long been suspected to play an important role in cognitive control and ability to orchestrate thought and action in accordance with internal goals. [...] Here, we propose that cognitive control stems from the active maintenance of patterns of activity in the prefrontal cortex that represent goals and the means to achieve them." Bunge and colleagues report that the "Prefrontal region is involved in keeping information in and out of mind. [...] Goal-directed behavior depends on keeping relevant information in mind (working memory) and irrelevant information out of mind (behavioral inhibition or interference resolution). Prefrontal cortex is essential for working memory and for interference resolution." [245].

[1] Siegel DJ. The Mindful Brain: Reflection and Attunement in the cultivation of well-being. New York, NY: W. W. Norton & Company; 2007: 337-345.

In reviewing brain imaging of attentional networks, Fernandez-Duque and Posner [246] divided the attentional network into three subdivisions: i) Vigilance network involved in achieving and maintaining the alert state, b) Orienting network involved in orienting to sensory stimuli, particularly to locations in visual space, and c) Executive network orchestrating voluntary actions.

AUTHOR'S INTERPRETATION AND SUGGESTIONS

Mān ḍ ukyopaniṣ ad described a fourth state of consciousness called, Turīya, after defining the three well known states of consciousness namely, dreamless sleep, dream sleep and wakefulness. The fourth conscious state is a state of Self-integration and Self-liberation, which cannot be objectified or spoken of, and into which the world-experience and the ego-experience are resolved. Therefore, it is the nondual, serene and essential state of Energy-Being. In this state, the essential Being is always aware of all that is present in the reality of the moment. Such a liberated person exhibits many characteristics, like the ability for vigilance, optimal level of arousal-energy, optimism, equanimity, compassion, love and creativity. This unique state of consciousness can be explained in terms of modern neuroscience.

A model of conscious mind is proposed, where the working memory, which is a function of the prefrontal cortex, is at the center of the moment-to-moment consciousness. For the execution of different voluntary activities, prefrontal cortex interacts with the autobiographical memories in hippocampal network and the long-term memories stored in various regions of the multimodal association cortex. Prefrontal cortex through its thalamo-cortico-striate network interacts with the autobiographical memories in the hippocampal-limbic-cingulate network and the subconscious storehouse of long-term memories in the multimodal association cortex during the execution of voluntary activity. (See Figure 14).

The current consciousness with working memory is further polarized into conscious space-time. The current conscious space is polarized into autobiographical self and others, resulting in the common dualistic experience. The conscious time is polarized into past, present and future, based on the current working memory and the phenomenon of sensory-perceptual fusion, resulting in the common experience of conscious mental time. Polarization of conscious space occurs when the working memory gets polarized into an autobiographical self and its environment, which leads to the experiential duality. A sensory-perceptual fusion of sequential conscious states in working memory, results in a sense of mental time and an apparently continuous ego [247].

Self-consciousness during voluntary action, perception and emotion, is understood in terms of attention and its neural mechanisms. The executive function of the prefrontal cortex directs attentive behavior, which in turn defines the sense of ego, at the present moment. There is a circular causality between the two.

A new model for understanding of the executive process was proposed by the author. It was called, the Situational Transient Executive Process or the STEP model. According to this model, ego-consciousness is transient and it arises from intentional action, attention and executive activity, in the form of decision-making, in a given situation. The common experience of apparently continuous selfness results from i) continuous self-orientation in person, place and time and ii) the phenomenon of sensory-perceptual fusion of discrete experiences in personal time-space, which is analogous to the apparent continuity experienced, while watching a movie. Prefrontal cortex and its associated networks mediate attention, self-consciousness, and self-organization of behavior, cognition and the self-regulation of various mental states. Prefrontal cortex and its network play a crucial role in the STEP model. The STEP model is consistent with the overall consensus, expressed in a recent review article on consciousness by Zeman. [248].

In summary, the fourth state of consciousness, Turīya, as described in Māṇḍukyopaniṣad, is an extraordinarily inspired state of calm, alert and intuitive consciousness, with Self-integration. It can be understood within the framework of modern Neuroscience. The author had proposed that Turīya is a unique conscious state of Non-REM Wakefulness (NREM-W) characterized by i) an optimal attentiveness, with freedom from day-dreaming and irrelevant, intrusive thoughts, ii) behavioral quiescence, with no rapid eye movements and internal speech, iii) heightened perceptual clarity, from moment to moment, with cognitive excellence and iv) an enhanced sense of well-being, serenity, compassion and intuitive creativity. Many exceptionally gifted people throughout human history seem to have verified this truth of a holistic, super-conscious state. Just as we stand on the shoulders of past intellectual giants to understand and discover the new in science, so too, we may be guided by the genius and experience of the ancient seers and philosophers to discover and understand the new in the neuroscience of human subjective experience. Figure 15.

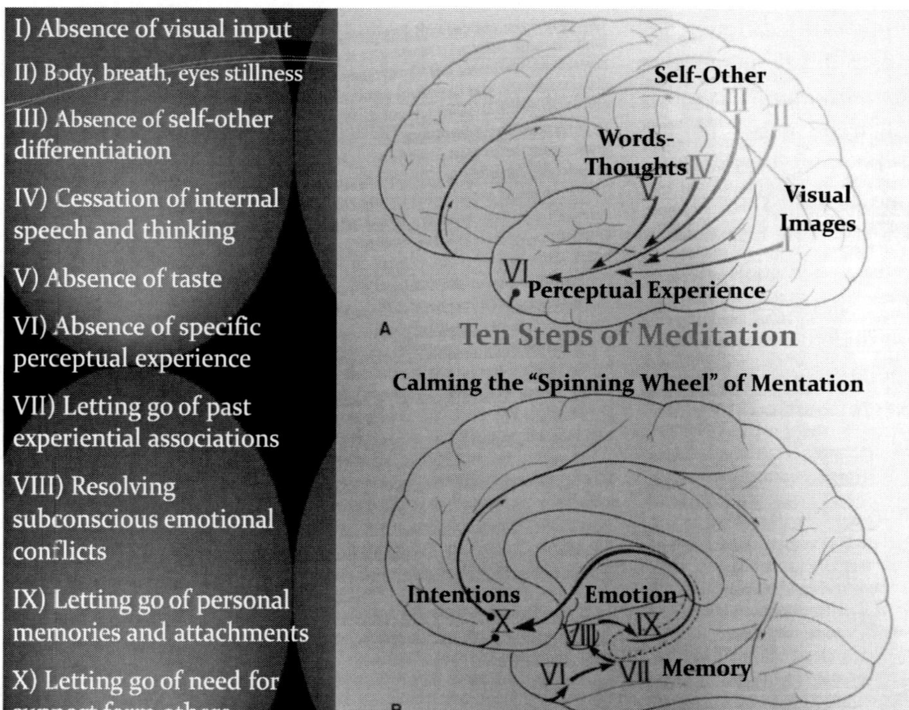

Figure 15. Circular thought process and Meditation. Ten steps of formal "Sitting" Meditation, with probable brain regions involved in the meditative process. The figure was modified from Noback CR, Strominger NL, Demarest RJ and Ruggiero DA. The Human Nervous System: Structure and Function. 6th ed. 2005:458.

MORNING GLORY

One light in many colors,
Many colors in one light.

One energy in many forms,
Many forms in one energy.

One consciousness in many experiences,
Many experiences in one consciousness.

One silence in many voices,
Many voices in one silence.

One stillness in many movements,
Many movements in one stillness.

One feeling in many emotions,
Many emotions in one feeling.

One moment in many years,
Many years in one moment.

One seed in many fruits,
Many fruits in one seed.

One life in many beings,
Many beings in one life.

One point in many spheres,
Many spheres in one point.

One truth in many expressions,
Many expressions in one truth.

One in many, many in one,
Appreciating the wonder
Of this morning glory!

Vinod D Deshmukh

September 23, 2006

Chapter 31

VEDIC PSYCHOLOGY: A SCIENCE OF WISDOM

तरति शोकं आत्मविद् |

Tarati śokaṁ Ātmavid.

Knower of the self overcomes all suffering.

Most of the Vedic literature is devoted to Self-culture, Ātmonnati आत्मोन्नति and actualization of one's essential being with innate wisdom. By wisdom, I mean the innate intelligence with complete natural peace with one's being-in-Reality. Vedānta described it as Blissful~Conscious~Being, Sat~Cit~Ānanda सच्चिदानन्द, [249]. What one experiences, from moment to moment, depends on one's perspective or 'mind-set.' As Śri Hanuman expressed his feelings towards Lord Rama as follows:

देहभावेन दासोऽस्मि | जीवभावेन त्वदंशकः ||

आत्मभावेन त्वमेवाहं | इति मे निश्चिता मतिः ||

"When I consider myself as the physical body, Dehabhāva देहभाव, I am your servant; when I consider myself as a living person, Jīvabhāva जीवभाव, I am an integral part of you; but, when I consider myself as the self-existent, essential, holistic Being, Ātmabhāva आत्मभाव, I am You. This is my firm conviction."

The last, extraordinary perspective, in everyday life, is only possible after a deep self-understanding and self-actualization. This wise stage in life is described in Upaniṣ ads and Bhagavad Gītā as superconscious equanimity, Turīya तुरीय, Sthitaprajñā स्थितप्रज्ञा, Ātmaprasāda आत्मप्रसाद, or Brāhmī sthiti ब्राह्मी स्थिति. There have been many examples of such enlightened individuals in human history. Therefore, such wisdom is potentaially achievable by all of us. Understanding Vedānta, Yoga, and living mindfully, with an undistracted presence, can help us blossom in virtue. Yoga promotes self-development by proposing the practice of the following virtues, namely, Yama यम self-restraint, which include peacefulness, truthfulness, righteousness, fidelity, nongreed, and Niyama **नियम**, which include cleanliness, self-content, austerity, self-study, and self-surrender [250].The elaboration and discussion of this important topic is continued in the next few chapters.

Chapter 32

Wisdom in Modern Psychology

Modern psychology and psychiatry also realize the value of wisdom as a virtue. Erikson conceives eight stages of self-development from birth till death: i) Trust with hope, ii) Autonomy with will, iii) Initiative with purpose, iv) Industry with competence, v) Identity with fidelity, vi) Intimacy with love, vii) Generativity with care, and viii) Integrity with wisdom. In his "balance theory of wisdom" Sternberg emphasized the importance of applying one's intelligence toward the common good through balancing of one's own, others' and institutional interests. Goleman wrote about emotional intelligence comprising of emotional self-awareness, empathy, adaptation, stress-management, and happy optimism.

The American Psychological Association (APA) dictionary, [251], defined "Virtue" as a quality or characteristic that has positive connotation in a particular society and that is considered beneficial to psychological health. It also means moral goodness. Erikson, [252], defined "Virtue" as "inherent stregth." The APA dictionary defined "Wisdom" as the ability of an individual to make sound decisions, to find the right – or at least good – answers to difficult and important life-questions, and to give advice about the complex problems of everyday life and interpersonal relationships. In his theory of wisdom, German psychologist Paul Baltes emphasized the role of knowledge and life experiences in achieving wisdom. The healing process involves the use of conscious understanding, which Rudolf Steiner called anthroposophy or the "Wisdom of Life."

Normal mind is hard to define. Freud thought that normality was an idealized fiction. Eissler thought that absolute normality could not be achieved because the normal person had to be totally aware of his thoughts and feelings. Money-Kryle defined normality as the ability to achieve insight into one's self, an ability that is never fully accomplished. Maughn considered the normal as an ideal. "It is a picture that one fabricates… and to find them all in a single man is hardly to be expected."

Klein conceived normality as strength of character, the capacity to deal with conflicting emotions, the ability to experience pleasure without conflict, and the ability to love. For Erikson, normality was the ability to master the eight phases of psychosocial development as described in detail below. Kubie considered normality as the ability to learn by experience, to be flexible, and adapt to a changing environment. Hartmann suggested that the conflict-free ego functions represented the person's potential for normality. Menninger described normality as the ability to adjust to the external world with contentment and to master the task of acculturation. Rank considered normality as the capacity to live without fear, guilt, or anxiety and to take responsibility for one's own actions. World Health Organization considered normality as complete physical, mental and social wellbeing. [253]. Well-being is defined as a state of happiness, contentment, lack of distress, overall good physical and mental health, and a healthy outlook of life, with a good quality of living.

The importance of culture as a context to human behavior is now well-recognized in modern psychology and psychiatry. Culture is the intervening variable between the human organism and its physical "environment." As such, culture is man-made, although the genetic factors may also contribute to cultural phenomena. Culture may be defined as the complex whole, which includes knowledge, beliefs, arts, law, morals, customs, and any other capabilities, and habits acquired by the man as a member of society. Culture is learned and includes the totality of human achievements. [254].

The National Institutes of Mental Health, Culture, and Diagnostic Group have adopted a more clinically orientated definition of culture: "meanings, values, and behavioral norms that are learned and transmitted in the dominant society and within its social groups. Culture powerfully influences cognitions, feelings and the 'self' concept, as well as the diagnostic process and treatment decisions. Culture provides a context and makes us human. It provides a context for the bio-psycho-social-existential variables that make us who we are from moment to moment.

Chapter 33

MULTI-STREAM, PSYCHO-SOCIAL GROWTH

काव्यशास्त्रविनोदेन कालो गच्छति धीमताम् ।
व्यसनेन तु मूर्खाणां, निद्रया कलहेन वा ॥

They wise spend their life time in creating poetry, discussing sciences and enjoying light humor, whereas, the unwise get involved in addictions, quarrels and fights or excess of sleep[1].

"When you speak of a path to truth, it implies that truth, this living reality, is not in the present, but somewhere in the distance, somewhere in the future. Now to me, truth is fulfillment, and to fulfillment there can be no path."

J. Krishnamurti's public talk, 1934

It was proposed by the author, that the standard bio-psycho-social concept of mind and self, be extended to a more comprehensive model of bio-psycho-social-existential self and mind. By adding the existential component to the self-concept and mind, the total human experience is better understood and explained. The word "existential" refers to the concrete lived experience of human beings, firmly rooted in the reality of the present moment. Existential living is the capacity to live fully in the present, and respond freely and flexibly to new experience without fear. Such integrative living would create an experience of presence, with an awareness and understanding of one's current existence, and a life of self-actualization and well-being. The bio-psycho-social-existential factors make us, who we are, from moment to moment, from conception till death.

From the point of view of psychosocial development, Erikson described eight stages of psychosocial growth. He also emphasized the development of eight different virtues associated with each of these stages:

1. Trust vs. Mistrust: From birth till about 18 months. Development of trust in an infant depends upon the quality of maternal or primary caretaker relationship. This is also the stage when the infant is taking in and exploring the world through his or her mouth and other cephalic senses. An infant enjoys and internalizes simple pleasures and develops a sense of hope, a basic virtue for life.

1 Velankar B. Translator. Selective Sanskrit-Marathi Quotations. Panavela, India: Velankar UB; 1994:89.

2. Autonomy vs. Shame: From age 18 months to 3 years. With the development of better volitional, muscular, and sphincter control, as well as speech, a toddler develops a sense of will and ego. It learns to say "No" and starts making intentional decisions or choices as to what it wants to do or doesn't want to do. It starts developing a sense of internal agency, self-control or autonomy and an ability to make independent situational judgements.
3. Initiative vs. Guilt: From age 3 years to 5 years. With greater mastery over personal behavior and speech, a child develops a sense of omnipotence and an active, intrusive exploration of the world with an endless curiosity. However, with proper parental guidance, direction, and restraints, the child learns to be more realistic, and is able to stop or say "No" to himself or herself, and thus, develops a sense of super-ego with a defined purpose and conscience.
4. Industry vs Inferiority: From age 5 years to 13 years. A child discovers the pleasure of making and producing things. He or she learns to use different tools and develops manual and language skills. A child develops competence in different skills and may imagine himself or herself play different occupational roles. A child also learns the value of team work in completing a bigger project.
5. Identity vs Role confusion: From age 13 years to about 21 years. With the onset of teenage, many physiological and social changes occur in the adolescent's life. This is a turbulent period of bio-psycho-social growth and adjustment. This is also the time to define one's gender-identity and self-identity. One develops close friendships and may even fall in love with some one. He or she develops the virtue of fidelity and defines a probable role one may play in life by projecting oneself as the self-in-world.
6. Intimacy vs Isolation: From age 21 years to 40 years. These are the years of more mature and responsible commitments to work, career, and love. One makes decisions about longterm commitment to a professional career, as well as a longterm relationship with somebody that one loves most.
7. Generativity vs Stagnation. From age 40 years to about 60 years. Generativity is genuine concern for guiding the next generation and one's favorite social institutions. One has the feeling of caring for others and the society-at-large. Naturally, one wishes to pass on one's knowledge, experience and skills to the next generation, with some seniority, authority, and self-satisfaction.
8. Integrity vs Despair: From 60 years till death. The wisdom of self-integrity is beautifully expressed by Erikson. It means acceptance of oneself and all aspects of one's life and integration of these elements into a stable pattern of living. It implies the experience of and adjustment to the trials and troubles of life as well as to its rewards and joys. Consequently, existence holds no fear; the ego has resigned itself to the acceptance of life itself and to acceptance of the inevitable end of that life in death. Integrity thus represents the fully developed personality in its most mature self-realization. Integrity is acceptance of one's one and the only one life cycle, and of the people who have become significant to it as something that had to be and that, by necessity, permitted of no substitutions.

"The individual relinquishes the wish that important people in his or her life had been different and is able to love and live in a more meaningful way - one that reflects an acceptance of responsibility for one's own life." The individual, in possession of the virtue of wisdom and a sense of integrity, has room to tolerate the proximity of death and achieve an attitude, what Erikson termed a detached yet active concern. "The style of integrity developed by his or her culture or civilization thus, becomes the 'patrimony' of his or her soul. [...] In such final consolidation, death loses its sting."

The self-actualized individual learns to overcome the four existential fears, the four 'I's, namely, Insecurity, Isolation, Insignificance and Inexistence or death. Yalom, [255], wrote about the fears of one's inexistence or death, lack of external support and being on oneself with a need for free choice with responsibility, self-isolation from all creatures in the world, and a lack of meaning and hope in life. He suggested whole-hearted engagement in current life, creativity, self-actualization, and altruism as possible solutions to these ultimate existential fears.

Vedic seers have similarly expressed the value of freedom from fears and the development of friendliness toward others and love for Nature.

अभयं मित्रादभयममित्रादभयं ज्ञातादभयं पुरो यः ।
अभयं नक्तमभयं दिवा नः सर्वा आशा मम मित्रं भवन्तु ॥
अथर्ववेद XIX XV ६.

May we be fearless of friends, as well as of enemies, fearless of the known and the unknown, fearless during the day and at night. My hope is that all beings will be my friends.
Atharva Veda XIX XV 6

This reminds me of Adi Śaṅ karāchārya's well known 27th verse from Ātmabodha:

रज्जुसर्पवदात्मानम् जीवो ज्ञात्वा भयं वहेत् ।
नाहं जीवः परात्मेति ज्ञातश्चेन्निर्भयो भवेत् ॥

"Having mistaken oneself as a (vulnerable mortal) being, one gets overwhelmed with fear. It is like mistaking a rope for a snake; however, when one realizes one's true infinite Self, the Ātman, all fear goes away."

Chapter 34

PEARLS OF WISDOM FROM THE BHAGAVAD GĪTĀ

NINE DOMAINS OF HUMAN WISDOM

1) Knowledge and Experience of Life:

Presiding over the ear, the eye, the touch, the taste, and the smell, as also, the mind, He experiences objects. While transforming from one experience to the other, or dwelling on the same experience, the deluded person does not see Him (existential Being); but those who have the eye of wisdom behold Him. The yogis striving for perfection behold Him dwelling in them; but the unrefined and inattentive persons, even though striving, see Him not.

BG Chapter 15, Ṣlokas 9 – 11.

2) Emotional Self-Regulation:

It is desire – it is the anger, born of the Rajo-guna; of great craving, and of great sin; know this as the foes here, in this world. As fire is enveloped by smoke, as a mirror by dust, as an embryo by the secundine, so is It (the existential Being) covered by all that. Knowledge is covered by this, the constant foe of the wise, O son of Kunti, the unappeasable fire of desire. The senses, the mind, and the intellect are said to be its abode; through these, it deludes the embodied by veiling his wisdom. Therefore, O leader of the Bharata race, controlling the senses at the outset, overcome it – the sinful, the destroyer of knowledge and realization. The senses are said to be superior to the body; the mind is superior to the senses; the intellect is superior to the mind; and that which is superior to the intellect is He (the existential Being), the Ātman. Thus, knowing Him (Being), who is superior to the intellect, and restraining the self by the Self (Being), overcome, O mighty-armed, that enemy, the unseizable foe, desire.

BG Chapter 3, Ṣlokas 37 – 43.

3) Awareness and Control of Desires; Love of and Faith in the Nature-God:

The turbulent senses, O son of Kunti, do violently snatch away the mind of even a wise man, striving for perfection. The steadfast, having controlled them all, sits focused on me as the Supreme. His wisdom is steady, whose senses are under control. Thinking of objects, attachment to them is formed in a man. From attachment longing and from longing anger grows. From anger comes delusion, and from delusion, loss of memory. From loss of memory, comes ruined discrimination and from the ruined discrimination, he perishes. But, the self-controlled man, moving among objects, with senses under restraint, and free from attraction and aversion, attains tranquility. In tranquility, all sorrow is destroyed. For the intellect of him who is tranquil-minded, is soon established in firmness. No knowledge of the Self has the unsteady. Nor has he meditation. To the unmeditative there is no peace; and how can one without peace have happiness? For the mind, which follows in the wake of wandering senses, carries away his discrimination, as a wind carries away from its course, a boat on the waters. Therefore, O mighty-armed, his knowledge is steady, whose senses are well restrained, from their sense objects. That, which is night to all beings, in that the Self-controlled man wakes. That, in which all beings are awake, is night to the Self-aware Muni. That person, who lives devoid of longing, abandoning all desires, without the sense of "I" and "mine", attains to peace. This is to have one's being-in-Brahman, O son of Prithā. None, attaining to this, becomes deluded. Being established therein, even at the end of life, a man attains to Oneness with Brahman.

BG Chapter 2, Ṣ lokas 60 – 72.

4) Clarity of perception and Decisiveness:

As blazing fire reduces wood into ashes, so, O Arjuna, does the fire of Awareness (mindful presence) reduce all karma (residual subconscious memories, unresolved conflicts, influences, and habits) to ashes (to emptiness, nothingness, clarity and transparency). Verily, there exists nothing in this world purifying like the essential Awareness. In good time, having reached perfection in yoga, one realizes that one Self, in one's own heart. The man with faith, ṣ raddhā, the devoted, the master of one's senses, attains this intrinsic Awareness. Having attained Awareness-as-such, one goes at once to the Supreme Peace. The ignorant, the man without ṣ raddhā the doubting self, goes to destruction. The doubting self has neither this world, nor the next, nor happiness. With work renounced by yoga and doubts rent asunder by Awareness, O Dhananjaya, actions do not bind him, who is poised in the Self. Therefore, working with the sword of Awareness, end this doubt about the Self, born of ignorance, residing in the heart. Take refuge in yoga. Arise, O Bharata!

BG Chapter 4, Ṣ lokas 37 – 42.

5) Personal Duty and Work:

In the beginning, the twofold path of devotion was given by Me to this world. The path of awareness for the meditative, the path of work for the active. By non-performance of work, none reaches effortlessness (spontaneity); by merely giving up action, no one attains to perfection.

BG Chapter 3, Ṣ lokas 3, 4.

6) Self-Contentedness and Life-Satisfaction:

But, whose ignorance is destroyed by the Awareness of Self (Being) - that Awareness of theirs, like the sun, reveals the supreme *Brahman*. Those who have their intellect absorbed in That (Being), whose self is That, whose steadfastness is in That, whose consummation is That, their impurities cleansed by Awareness, they return to non-return of Moksha, the absolute freedom. The knowers of the Self look equally, with an eye of equanimity, on a brahmaṇ a endowed with learning and humility, a cow, an elephant, a dog, and a pariah. Relative existence has been conquered by them, even in this world, whose mind rests in evenness, since Brahman is even and without imperfection. Therefore they indeed rest in Brahman. Resting in Brahman, with intellect steady, and without delusion, the knower of Brahman, neither rejoices on receiving what is pleasant, nor grieves on receiving what is unpleasant. With the heart unattached to external objects, he realizes the joy that is in the Self (Being). With the heart devoted to the meditation of Brahman, he attains undecaying happiness.

BG Chapter 5, Ṣ lokas 16 – 21.

7) Compassion and Sacrifice for Others, Kindness, and Charity:

Fearlessness, purity of heart, steadfastness in awareness and yoga, almsgiving, control of the senses, sacrificial ritual Yajña, reading of the Śāstrās, austerity, uprightness; Non-injury Ahimsā, truth, absence of anger, renunciation, tranquility, absense of calumny, compassion to beings, un-covetousness, gentleness, modesty, absense of fickleness; Courage, forgiveness, purity, absence of hatred, absense of pride; these belong to one born for the divine state.

BG Chapter 16, Ṣ lokas 1 – 3.

8) Self-Integration, Yoga:

He whose intellect is unattached anywhere, who has subdued his heart, whose desires have fled, he attains by renunciation to the supreme perfection, consisting of freedom from action. Learn from Me in brief, how reaching such perfection, he attains to Brahman, that supreme consummation of awareness. Endued with a pure intellect; subduing the body and the senses with fortitude; relinquishing sounds (words) and such other sense-objects; abandoning attraction and hatred; Resorting to a sequestered spot; eating but little; body, speech, and mind controlled; ever engaged in meditative awareness and concentration; possessed of dispassion;

BG Chapter 18, Ṣ lokas 49 – 52.

9) Insight and Humility:

Forsaking egoism, power, pride, lust, wrath, and property; freed from the notion of "mine" and tranquil – he is fit for becoming *Brahman*. *Brahman*-become, tranquil-minded, he neither grieves nor desires; the same to all beings, be attains the supreme devotion unto Me.

BG Chapter 18, Ṣ lokas 53, 54.

Compiled by the author based on a published article: "Comparison of the Conceptualization of Wisdom in Ancient Indian Literature with Modern Views: Focus on the Bhagavad Gita." Published by Jeste DV, Vahia IV, in the journal, Psychiatry. 2008; 71(3): 197-209.

Chapter 35

YOGA-STHITIḤ योगस्थितिः

Shrimad Bhagvad Gītā has many words of wisdom. The five Ṣ lokas (19-23) from its chapter VI describe Yogasthitiḥ or a state of profound serenity and conscious clarity. Here is a translation of those five Ṣ lokas:

- A flame, which is sheltered from the wind, does not flicker. This has been a simile used for a yogi of self-disciplined mind, who is practicing meditative awareness on the Self. (VI:19).
- When the mind is fully resolved, by the practice of meditative awareness and attains quietitude, one realizes the Self by the Self and one is fully content within one Self. (VI:20).
- This extraordinary Bliss, which is beyond sensory perception, can be verified by the refined intellect. Once established in it, one does not depart from one's true Nature. (VI:21).
- Having realized such a state, one regards no other acquisition superior to it, and where established, one is not moved even by heavy sorrow. (VI:22).
- This is known as Yogasthitiḥ or the state of Yoga, which is a state of freedom from suffering. Such yoga should be practiced with perseverance and with a mind not discouraged by thoughts of depression. (VI:23).
- In explaining the 20th shloka, Shri Jñāneṣ vara beautifully described this unique process of Self-discovery. He stated: "When one turns inward and experiences one Self, then one recognizes one Self as the Tatva or the Truth of one's essential Nature."

With serenity and mindful presence, one can realize the timeless totality and the eco-systemic, holistic field. The totality of our existential reality is Pūrṇ atā. There is a well known Sanskrit Ṣ loka that is often repeated daily by many Hindus:

पूर्णमदः पूर्णमिदं पूर्णात्पूर्णमुदच्यते | पूर्णस्य पूर्णमादाय पूर्णमेवावशिष्यते ||

Pūrṇ amadaḥ pūrṇ amidaṁ, pūrṇ ātpūrṇ amudacchyate,
Pūrṇ asya pūrṇ amādāya, pūrṇ amevāvaśiśyate.

What is beyond is holistic, Pūrṇ a. What is here is holistic. From the holistic emerges holistic. When the holistic is removed from holistic, what remains is holistic. Holistic, Pūrṇ a is the infinite Reality that can be realized by direct existential experience.

In Vedānta, the concepts of non-duality, Advaita अद्वैत and unity Ekatwaṁ एकत्वं have been beautifully expressed by many sages from prehistoric times. Some of these profound statements expressing the ultimate Truth are:

एकं ज्योतिः बहुधा विभाति |

Ekaṁ Jyotiḥ Bahudhā Vibhāti.

One flame (energy~awareness) that shines in so many ways (processes and forms).
Atharva Veda.

एकोऽहं बहुस्याम् |

Ekohaṁ Bahusyām.

I am One. I will become many.

आनीत अवातं स्वधया तदेकम् |

Ānīta Avātaṁ Swadhayā Tadekam.

(In the beginning), the One was breathing by itself, without any air.
Nasadīya Sūkta, Ṛg Veda.

एकं सत्विप्राः बहुधा वदन्ति |

Ekaṁ Sat viprāḥ bahudhā vadanti.

There is only one Truth, but, the wise express it in many different ways.

These ancient words of wisdom make us realize that we are neither just the physical body, nor just the mind, nor just the experienced world, but the living totality Pūrṇ a that is infinite and ever-present. We breathe in Existence and the Existence breathes in us. Any single breath could potentially inspire us to such an astounding Self-realization, or awakening, but we need to be totally aware, clear, sensitive and receptive for such a great insight.

Māṇ ḍ ūkyopaniṣ ad माण्डूक्योपनिषद् described the Yogasthiti as: The Self integrates itself, within itself, by itself. Ātmaiva Saṁviśati Ātmanāmānaṁ आत्मैव संविशति आत्मनात्मानम् | The Bhagavad Gītā described it as: The self achieves serenity within itself. Ātmani eva ātmanā tuṣ taḥ आत्मनि एव आत्मना तुष्ट: The Upaniṣ ads declared: The self is serene. Śantoyaṁ Ātmā शान्तोयऽमात्मा. It is the ultimate blissful serenity of self-realization. Finally, the light of self-awareness is a light to itself. Swayaṁ Jyotiḥ स्वयंज्योतिः

These are all lofty thoughts, but to realize them, one has to start from where one is, and as one is, from moment to moment, mindfully watching i) the phenomena that one is experiencing Dharmānupāsanā, ii) the position of one's body Kāyānupāsanā, iii) the breathing activity Prāṇ ānupāsanā, iv) the emotion that one is experiencing at the moment Vedanānupāsanā, and v) the random thoughts that are racing through one's mind like passing clouds Cittānupāsanā. As Gautam Buddha advised us, that we have to learn to be mindful Vipaśyanā and serene Śamatā, making peace with our selves and the world.

One should learn to realize the wonder of being alive and aware. The wonder of being whole-heartedly present in this timeless moment. The present reality is infinite. It is always new and at the same time, the same, depending on our perspective. The same day does not dawn twice. In fact, no two conscious moments are exactly alike. One should learn to be fully awake to the present reality, as it unfolds from moment to moment. It is the greatest wonder that is to behold.

One should realize that one is always sharing this reality with some one else or with some other thing. One is an open system with constant exchange of molecules, energy and information with Reality. One is always connected to the ongoing phenomena. As J. Krishnamurti said, "To be is to be related." We are always a part of the big picture. Remember that every journey starts with a single step and now is the time to take that first step.

Chapter 36

YOGA AS A SCIENCE OF WISDOM

From the ancient times, people have been fascinated by the wonder of their mind and the experience of the universe. This pondering, about one's being-in-Reality, may have been the beginning of a meditative mind, and the origin of various philosophies and religions. The origin of yoga is difficult to establish since it was preserved mainly by oral tradition. There are references to Yoga in ancient Sanskṛ it संस्कृत literature like the Ṣ wetaṣ watara and Maitri Upaniṣ ads, and the Bhagavad-Gītā. Ghosh, [256], in his book "The Original Yoga," included three books — Pātañjali Yogasūtra, Śiva Samhitā, and Gheraṇ ḍ a Samhitā as the basis of Yoga.

According to Pātañjali Yogasūtra, Yoga योग is a science of wisdom and Self-development Ātmonnati आत्मोन्नति. He prescribed the following eight disciplines to achieve this goal:

i) Universal values, Yama यम includes self-restraints, nonviolence, peacefulness, Ahimsā अहिंसा, truthfulness, Satya सत्य, righteousness, Asteya अस्तेय, fidelity, brahmacharya ब्रह्मचर्य, nongreed, Aparigraha अपरिग्रह.

ii) Personal virtues, Niyama नियम includes cleanliness, Śouca शौच, self-content, Santoṣ a संतोष, austerity, Tapaḥ तपः, self-study, Swādhyāya स्वाध्याय, and self-surrender Īṣ war praṇ idhāna ईश्वर प्रणिधान.

iii) Steady posture, Āsana आसन,

iv) Skillful regulation of breathing, Prāṇ āyāma प्राणायाम,

v) The art of detachment or letting go Pratyāhāra प्रत्याहार.

vi) Sustained focusing of attention, Dhāraṇ ā धारणा, like a spot light, on an object, an activity, a thought, or any ongoing experience.

vii) Continuous, sustained attentiveness or meditative vigilance Dhyānaṁ ध्यानं, like a flood light, on the total experiential field, both outside and inside

viii) Ripe, effortless, self-absorptive, and self-integrated state of self-understanding and self-realization of one's energy~being, Samādhiḥ समाधिः. Here are a few excerpts from Pātañjali's Yogasūtra पातञ्जलि योगसूत्र.

"Yoga is calming the fluctuations of a (wandering and agitated) mind (Verse 2). Then the Self abides in his or her own (natural serene) state (Verse 3). Other times, the self is associated with the sense of agency and ownership of ongoing mental experience (Verse 4). Mental calming can be achieved by disengagement or letting go (of a ruminating mind) and constant self-awareness (mindful presence) (Verse 12). The cause of selfishness or egoism is a lack of self-awareness and self-understanding (Verse 75).

On being fully aware, the false association between self-regulatory activity and the essential self disappears, which leads to a complete self-freedom (Verse 76). With vigilant attentiveness comes fitness of mind (Verse 104). The capacity to change mental state manifests in three different ways: i) ability to stop ongoing mental activity, ii) ability to focus attention on a specific event in space-time, and iii) the ability to maintain attention on a given task or event leading to enhanced cognitive capacity (Verse 122). Being free from any egoistic motivation, instinctual pressure, and mental conflict, one can live naturally, Sahaja Jīvan सहज जीवन, with spontaneity, mindful presence, and natural wisdom (Verse 195)."

Here are a few excerpts from the Ṣ wetāṣ watara Upaniṣ ad ष्वेताष्वतर उपनिषद् "let the wise man restrain his mind vigilantly as (he would restrain) a chariot with vicious horses. (Verse 9). Even as a mirror covered by dust shines brightly when it has been cleaned, so the embodied one, when he has seen the real nature of the Self, becomes integrated, and becomes of fulfilled purpose and freed from all suffering. (Verse 14)."

A few excerpts from Maitri Upaniṣ ad मैत्री उपनिषद् "That which is non-thought, which stands in the midst of thought, the unthinkable, the hidden, the highest, let a man merge his thought there. Then will this living being be (free) without any support (or dependence). (Verse 19). For by the serenity of thought, one destroys deeds, good and evil, with the serene Self abiding in itself, he enjoys enduring happiness. (Verse 20)."

A few excerpts from the sixth chapter of the Bhagavad-Gītā भगवद् गीता on Dhyāna Yoga, [165]: "Let a man lift his self by his own self; Let him not lower himself; One's self alone is one's own friend or foe. (Verse 5). "That in which thought ceases, stopped by the practice of disciplined attention, and in which, seeing himself through himself, one is content in one Self (Verse 20).

A few excerpts from Śiva Samhitā शिवसंहिता "Out of consciousness is born all the animate and inanimate objects (of experience) of this world. Hence, abandoning all these, one should abide in holistic consciousness itself. (Verse 49). Indivisible by time-space, Ātman, in its natural state, is always truly complete, whole, Pūrṇ a पूर्ण (Verse 54). "The Ātman, however, is ever blissful. All desires disappear only through Self-knowledge (and Self-awareness). When the sense of plurality fades away, the light of Oneness dawns. (Verse 57)… The Ātman alone is without duality and beyond words. (Verse 61)."

Excerpts from Gheraṇ ḍ a Samhitā घेरण्ड संहिता "Getting into (a self-absorptive) mental state, let the mind be united with the Self Ātman. When both, mind and ego, merge into the supreme Soul Paramātman, Samādhi ensues. (Verse 16). All living creatures on the land and in the sky, all trees, bushes, creepers, plants, grass, all rivers, and mountains – all are seen as the one supreme Brahman, and one's own Self is seen in all. (Verse 19)."

Yoga is a way of adaptive self-integration, being at peace with one Self and being at home in the world. Self-integration results from constant Self-awareness and letting go of irrelevant memories, imaginations, mental agitations, and distractions. Such a person functions with a truly undistracted and serene mind. When the mind is undistracted and assumes its original, unmodified, Self-effulgent state, the Self experiences Itself.

Effortless Mind

Without an effort,
It breathes, sleeps, wakes,
Moves and rests.

Without an effort,
It listens, watches,
Feels and rejoices.

Without an effort,
It experiences, understands,
Recalls and creates.

Without an effort,
It appreciates
The language of the wind-swept trees,
The heart of an ocean,
On a full moon night,
The scream of
A thundering monsoon sky and
The wonder of
A silent, setting sun.

Without my effort,
The garden grows,
The wind blows,
The river flows and
The sun rises.

Without my effort,
People move and talk,
Animals bark and walk,
Birds fly and sing,
Bees hum and sting,

Flowers blossom daily,
And fill up my heart with love.

Effort is needed,
Only to change what is,
Into what we think it should be,
Either inside or outside of us.

Why struggle so hard
And be stressed,
When everything is happening
All by itself, naturally,
Harmoniously.

Efforts are needed,
To write all this down.

But, even this poem is
Flowing naturally,
From this amazing,
Effortless Mind!

Vinod D Deshmukh

November 5, 2005

Chapter 37

WISDOM OF ĀDI ŚANKARĀCHĀRYA

SELECTIONS FROM THE DIRECT EXPERIENCE, APAROKSHĀNUBHUTI

Ādi Śaṅ karāchārya was one of the India's greatest saint and philosopher. He was also a great scholar, poet, mystic, and a reformer of Hinduism. He was born in the year 788 and died in 820 at a young age of 32 years. He was born in Kaladi, on the coast of Malabar and died in Kedarnath, in the Himalayas. He was the greatest proponent of Advaita Vedānta. He wrote original works like Aparokshānubhūti, Ātmabodha, Tattvabodha, Vivek Cudāmaṇ i, Upadeśa Sāhasrī. He also wrote commentaries on Bhagavad-Gītā, Upaniṣ ads and Vedānta Sūtra. He was a self-realized, enlightened genius.

WHAT IS SELF-KNOWLEDGE, ĀTMA JÑĀNA आत्मज्ञान?

Ādi Śankarāchārya eloquently expressed his own direct experience of Self in Aparokshānubhūti[1], ṣ loka 24-28: "I am truly *Brahman*, the ultimate Energy~Being~Awareness in Reality, which is equanimous śama, serene śānta, existential sat, conscious cit, blissful ānanda, non-changing nirvikāra, formless nirākāra, flawless niravadya, non-decaying avyaya, healthy nirāmaya, beyond appearance nirābhāsa, non-wavering nirvikalpa, pervasive ātataḥ , attributeless nirguṇ a, restful niṣ kriya, enduring nitya, steady acyuta, pure nirmala, immovable niṣ cala, infinite ananta, sacred śuddha, non-aging ajara and imperishable amara. I am not a mere body (image). This is true Self-knowledge realized by the wise."

HOW TO REALIZE SELF, *ĀTMAN* आत्मन्?

Ādi Śankarāchārya described fifteen steps of meditation to help one realize one's true nature (Aparokshānubhūti, ṣ loka 102-126):

1 Vimuktānanda S. Aparokshānubhūti or Self-Realization. Kolkata, India: Advaita Ashram; 1966: 3rd Impression.

1) Attentiveness Yama: Develop ability to attend intently to what one is experiencing at the present moment with all of one's senses, energy and feelings e.g., whole-hearted listening, looking, smelling, touching and tasting etc.
2) Concentration Niyama: Focus attention on a single experiential event or object, like spontaneous breathing, sound of Silence anāhat nāda, bodily stillness, a pleasing thought, a visual image or an emotion.
3) Letting Go Tyāga: Make peace with and let go of random verbal and visual thoughts, old recurring memories, day-dreaming and wishful thinking.
4) Inner Silence Mounaṁ: The serene, inner Silence is spontaneous, ineffable, beyond all words, descriptions, and imagery. Learn to stay quiet and restrain oneself from the internal speech.
5) All-Pervasive Space Deśa: Realize the all-pervasive, experiential space within and around oneself. There is no partition or division in such global, life-space.
6) Being-in-the-Moment Kālaḥ : One experiences oneself and the world moment by moment. Each experienced moment captures a part of the phenomena. One can also learn to transcend the phenomenal experience and directly realize the truth of the Self within, in the twinkling of an eye.
7) Steady, Comfortable Posture Āsanaṁ: Sit and remain quiet and composed in a steady and comfortable posture to meditate on the truth of Brahman unceasingly. An enlightened person is completely merged in the universal, existential ground of all beings.
8) Ego-mergence in the Source-Being Mūlabandha: One should let go of one's mental activity and merge naturally in Brahman, the seed, root or source of being-in-existence.
9) Equipoise Dehasāmyaṁ: Let the body be in a relaxed and equipoise state like an unmoving, fallen tree.
10) Presence, mindful vigilance Jñānamayī Dṛ iṣ ṭ ī: With sustained presence, one should view the world as existential *Brahman* itself. In such a unique state, the differentiation between the seer, seen, and sight vanishes.
11) Self-Regulation of physiological arousal-energy Prāṇ āyāma: Witness and let go of all spontaneous thoughts and emotions and realize the unwavering, ground-consciousness. Inhale with the thought that "I am Brahman," and exhale with the thought that "all experience is transient and apparent." During the pause between inhalation and exhalation, one should steady one's awareness on the existential Truth within, which is *Brahman*.
12) Self-Absorption Pratyāhāra: Let the egoistic mind get absorbed in Ātman, the supreme Self-consciousness, which is immanent in all experienced objects and events.
13) Spiritual Perspective Dhāraṇ ā: Where ever the mind goes, think of Brahman, and develop a constant awareness of the sacred Reality every where, all the time.
14) Meditation on the Self Ātmadhyānaṁ: Being free of all phenomenal experience, always meditate upon the thought, "I am truly *Brahman*." Such holistic super-Awareness leads to spontaneous, natural bliss.

15) Self-Integration Samādhiḥ: Total absorption in the ever-present, changeless *Brahman* is called Samādhiḥ or true Self-knowledge Ātmajñāna. By the practice of mindful presence, one should excel in this meditative skill of natural blissfulness, so that one can instantly shift oneself into such a blissful mode of Being. On achieving mastery over such blissful mode of being, the aspirant becomes free from the need to do ritualistic routines. The true nature of such an enlightened person, never becomes the object of anyone's mind or speech.

Chapter 38

ŚRI RAMAṆA MAHARṢI'S SELECTED TEACHINGS

Śri Ramaṇ a Maharṣ i was born to a Tamil Hindu, Brahmin family in Tiruchuzhi, Tamil Nadu, India, on December 30, 1879. After attaining Self-liberation at the age of 16 years, he left home for Arunachala, a mountain considered sacred by the Hindus, at Tiruvannamalai, and lived there for the rest of his life. Arunachala is located in Tamil Nadu, South India. Although born a Brahmin, after having attained moksha, he declared himself an "Atyāṣ ramī," a state of complete non-attachment and beyond all limitations of color, caste, stage-in-life and religion, jāti, varṇ a, āṣ ram and dharma जाति-वर्ण-आश्रम धर्म.

Śri Ramaṇ a maintained that the purest form of his teaching was the powerful Silence which radiated from his Presence and quieted the minds of those attuned to it. He gave verbal teachings only for the benefit of those who could not understand his Silence. His verbal teachings were said to flow from his direct experience of Consciousness-as-such as the only existing Reality. When asked for advice, he recommended Self-enquiry as the fastest path to Self-freedom, moksha. Though his primary teaching is associated with Non-dualism, Advaita Vedānta, and Jñāna yoga, he highly recommended devotion Bhakti, and gave his approval to a variety of paths and practices. The following are some of the key concepts of his philosophy of Existence:

> "The Self is that in which all these worlds seem to exist steadily, that of which all these worlds are a possession, that from which all these worlds rise, that for which all these exist, that by which all these worlds come into existence and that which is indeed all these – that alone is the existing Reality. Let us cherish that Self, which is the Reality-in-Heart."

The essence of Śri Ramaṇ a's teachings is conveyed in his frequent assertions that there is a single immanent Reality, directly experienced by everyone, which is simultaneously the Source, the Substance and the real Nature of everything that exists. The Single Immanent Reality, to which he gave a number of different names, each one signifying a different aspect of the same indivisible Reality. What follows is the explanation of the three terms that he frequently used for this Truth:

i) The Self. This is his most used term. He defined it by saying that the real Self or real `I' is, contrary to perceptible experience, not an experience of individuality, but a non-personal, all-inclusive Awareness. It is not to be confused with the individual ego, which he said was essentially non-existent, being a fabrication of the mind, which obscures the true experience of the real Self. He maintained that the real Self is always present and always experienced but he emphasized that one is only consciously aware of it, as it really is, when the self-limiting tendencies of the mind have ceased. Permanent and continuous Self-awareness is known as Self-realization.

ii) Sat~Cit~Ānanda. This is a Sanskrit term which translates as Being~Consciousness~Bliss. Śri Ramaṇ a taught that the Self is pure Being, a subjective Awareness of `I am' which is completely devoid of the feeling `I am this' or `I am that.' There are no subjects or objects in the Self, there is only an awareness of Being. Because this Awareness is conscious, it is also known as Consciousness-as-such. The direct experience of this Consciousness is, according to Śri Ramaṇ a, a state of unbroken happiness, and so the term Ānanda or Bliss, is also used to describe it. These three aspects, Being, Consciousness and Bliss, are experienced as a unitary whole and not as separate attributes of the Self. They are inseparable in the same way that wetness, transparency and liquidity are inseparable properties of water.

iii) God. Śri Ramaṇ a maintained that the universe is sustained by the power of the Self. Since theists normally attribute this power to God, he often used the word God as a synonym for the Self. He also used the words Brahman, the supreme Being of Hinduism, and Śiva, one of the Hindu trinity, Brahma~Vishṇ u~Śiva, in the same way. Śri Ramaṇ a's God is not a personal God; It is the formless Energy-Being, which sustains the universe. He is not the creator of the universe; the universe is merely a manifestation of his inherent power; he is inseparable from it, but he is not affected by its appearance or its disappearance.

[The above narration was partly based on excerpts from an article by Mr. M. Mathur in Tattva magazine, February 2009 issue.]

OTHER QUOTATIONS OF ŚRI RAMAṆA MAHARṢI:

"The state of realization is often called 'Jāgrat Suṣ upti' i.e. wakeful sleep or sleeping wakefulness. In it, there is an awareness of the waking state and the stillness of deep sleep. It is the state of perfect Awareness and perfect Stillness combined. It is the Source from which thoughts spring and make all the difference between the stillness of sleep and the turmoil of waking. In Self-realization, the Stillness is reached with perfect Awareness." (From "Talks1" number 609).

"The world is not other than the body; the body is not other than the mind; the mind is not other than the primal Awareness; the primal Awareness is not other than Being. That (alone) exists unchanging in peace." (From "Guru Vachak Kovai" Saying 99).

"In the nature of their being, creature and creator are, in substance, one. They differ only in adjuncts and awareness. (From Upadeśa Sāram, verse 24).

1 Śri Ramaṇ a Maharṣ i. Talks with Śri Ramaṇ a Maharṣ i. Tiruvannamalai, India: Śri Ramaṇ āshramam; 2010:17th reprint.

Chapter 39

ŚRI AUROBINDO'S SELECTED WRITINGS

"When we withdraw our gaze, from its egoistic preoccupation, with limited and fleeting interests, and look upon the world with dispassionate and curious eyes, that search for the Truth, our first result is the perception of the boundless Energy, of the infinite existence, infinite movement, infinite activity, pouring itself out in limitless space, in eternal Time, an existence that surpasses infinitely our ego, any ego, or any collectivity of egos, in whose balance the grandiose products of eons are about the dust of a moment and in whose incalculable sum numberless myriads count only as a petty swarm." (From "The Life Divine[1]," page 78).

"The Self of things is an infinite indivisible existence; of that existence the essential nature or power is an infinite, imperishable force of Self~Conscious~Being; and of that self-consciousness, the essential nature or knowledge of Self is, again, an infinite, inalienable delight of Being." (From "The Life Divine," page 108).

"To be and to be fully is Nature's aim in us; but to be fully is to be wholly conscious of one's Being; unconsciousness, half consciousness or deficient consciousness is a state of being not in possession of itself; it is existence, but not fullness of Being. To be aware wholly and integrally of one Self and of all the truth of one's Being is the necessary condition of true possession of existence. This Self~Awareness is what is meant by spiritual knowledge: the essence of spiritual knowledge is an intrinsic, Self-existent Consciousness; all its action of knowledge, indeed all its action of any kind, must be that Consciousness formulating itself." (From "The Life Divine," page 1060).

"There is a Reality, a truth of all existence, which is greater and more abiding than all its formations and manifestations; to find that Truth and Reality and live in it, achieve the most perfect manifestation and formation possible of it, must be the secret of perfection, whether of individual or communal being. This Reality is there within each thing and gives to each of its formations, its power of Being and value of Being. The universe is a manifestation of the Reality, and there is a truth of the universal existence and power of Cosmic Being, and all-Self or world-Spirit." (From "The Life Divine," page 1085).

"The delight of the Spirit is ever new; the forms of beauty it takes are innumerable; its godhead ever young and the taste of delight rasa रस of the Infinite are eternal and inexhaustible. The gnostic manifestation of life would be more full and fruitful and its interest

---

1 Śri Aurobindo. The Life Divine. Pondicherry, India: Śri Aurobindo Ashram Trust; 2006: 7th edition.

more vivid than the creative interest of ignorance; it would be a greater and happier constant miracle." (From "The Life Divine," page 1106-1107).

Chapter 40

J. KRISHNAMURTI'S SELECTED WRITINGS

"Awareness is the silent and choiceless observation of what is."

Jiddu Krishnamurti (1895–1986) was a modern-day sage with a profound insight into the human mind and Self-knowledge. Here are a few of his excerpts:

"So there is an origin, an original ground, from which all things arise, and that original ground is not the word. The word is never the thing. And meditation is to come upon that ground which is the origin of all things and which is free from all time. This is the way of meditation. And blessed is he who finds it... Meditation means awareness – to be aware of what you are doing, what you are thinking, what you are feeling, aware without any choice, to observe, to learn. [...] Out of this awareness comes the capacity to be completely attentive. Then there is freedom to see things as they actually are, without distortion. The mind becomes unconfused, clear, and sensitive; such meditation brings about a quality of mind that is completely silent."

"There is no actual division between the organism and the mind. The brain, the nervous system, and the thing we call the mind are all one, indivisible. [...] Meditation really is a complete emptying of the mind. Then there is only the functioning of the body; there is only the activity of the organism and nothing else; then thought functions without identification as the 'me' and the 'not me.' There is no self to understand but only the thought that creates the self. [...] Mind can understand the present only if it does not compare, judge; the desire to alter or condemn the present without understanding it gives continuance to the past. Only in comprehending the reflection of the past in the mirror of the present, without distortion, is there renewal... We consider the present as a means to an end, so the present loses its immense significance. The present is the eternal. [...] The awareness, of which I speak is of what is, from moment to moment, of activities of thought and its subtle deceptions, fears, and hope. Choiceless awareness wholly dissolves our conflicts and miseries."

"Meditation is to find out whether the brain, with all its activities, all its experiences, can be absolutely quiet. Not forced, because the moment you force, there is duality. The entity that says, "I would like to have marvellous experiences, therefore I must force my brain to be quiet" will never do it. But if you begin to inquire, observe, listen to all movements of thought, its conditioning, its pursuits, its fears, its pleasures, watch how the brain operates, then you will see that the brain becomes extraordinarily quiet; that quietness is not sleep, but it is tremendously active and therefore quiet. A big dynamo that is working perfectly hardly makes a sound; it is only when there is friction that there is noise." [257].

"What lies beyond can be found only if the mind is still. There may be something or there may be nothing at all. So the only thing that is important is for the mind to be still. Again, if you are concerned with what lies beyond, then you are not looking at what the state of actual stillness is. If stillness to you is only a door to that which lies beyond, then you are not concerned with that door, whereas what is important is the very door itself, the very stillness itself. Therefore you cannot ask what lies beyond. The only thing that is important is for the mind to be still. Then what takes place? That is all we are concerned with, not with what lies beyond silence."

"There is no other fact but silence, which has not been invited, induced, sought after, but which is the natural outcome of observation and understanding of oneself and the world about one. In this, there has been no motive, which has brought silence. If there is any shadow or suspicion of a motive, then that silence is directed and deliberate, so it is not silence at all. If you can honestly say that that silence is free, then what actually takes place in that silence is our only concern. What is the quality and the texture of that silence? Is it superficial, passing, measurable? Are you aware of it after it is over, or during the silence? If you are aware that you have been silent, then it is only a memory, and therefore dead. If you are aware of the silence while it is happening, then is it silence? If there is no observer – that is, no bundle of memories – then is it silence? Is it something intermittent which comes and goes according to your body chemistry? Does it come when you are alone, or with people, or when you are trying to meditate? What we are trying to find out is the nature of this silence. Is it rich or poor? (I don't mean rich with experience or poor because it is uneducated.) Is it full or shallow? Is it innocent or is it put together? A mind can look at a fact and not see the beauty, the depth, the quality of that fact. Is it possible to observe silence without the observer? When there is silence, there is only silence, and nothing else. Then in that silence what takes place? [...] Is there an observation of silence by silence in silence?

Questioner: That's a new question.

Krishnamurti: It is not a new question if you have been following. The whole brain, the mind, the feelings, the body, everything is quiet. Can this quietness, stillness, look at itself, not as an observer who is still? Can the totality of this silence watch its own totality? The silence becomes aware of itself – in this there is no division between an observer and an observed. That is the main point. The silence does not use itself to discover something beyond itself. There is only that silence. Now see what happens."

"To awaken this energy, the mind must have no resistance. [...] Now, how do we awaken in ourselves an energy that has its own momentum that is its own cause and effect, an energy that has no resistance and does not deteriorate? How does one come by it? The organized religions have advocated various methods, and by practicing a particular method one is supposed to get this energy. But methods do not give this energy. The practice of a method implies conformity, resistance, denial, acceptance, adjustment, so that whatever energy one has is merely wearing itself out. If you see the truth of this, you will never practice any method. That is one thing. Secondly, if energy has a motive, an end towards which it is going, that energy is self-destructive. And for most of us, energy does have a motive, does it not? We are moved by a desire to achieve, to become this or that, and therefore our energy defeats itself. Thirdly, energy is made feeble, petty, when it is conforming to the past – and this is perhaps our greatest difficulty. The past is not only the many yesterdays but also every minute that is being accumulated, the memory of the thing that was over a second before. This accumulation in the mind is also destructive of energy. [...] So, to awaken this energy, the mind must have no resistance, no motive, no end in view, and it must not be caught in time as yesterday, today, and tomorrow. Then energy is constantly renewing itself and therefore not degenerating. Such a mind is not committed, it is completely free, and it is only such a mind that can find the unnameable, that extraordinary something which is beyond words. The mind must free itself from the known to enter into the unknown. (From Collected Works, Vol. XIII – 337).

"You actually have to die (let go of) to everything you know – to your memories, to your miseries, your pleasures. And, when there is no jealousy, no envy, no greed, no torture of despair, then you will know what love is and you will come upon that which may be called sacred; therefore, sacredness is the essence of religion. You know, a great river may become polluted as it flows past a town, but if the pollution isn't too great, the river cleanses itself as it goes along and within a few miles it is again clean, fresh and pure. Similarly, when once the mind comes upon this sacredness, then every act is a cleansing act; through its very movement the mind is making itself innocent and, therefore, it is not accumulating. A mind that has discovered this sacredness is in constant revolution – not economic or social revolution, but an inner revolution through which it is endlessly purifying itself. Its action is not based on some idea or formula. As the river, with a tremendous volume of water behind it, cleanses itself as it flows, so does the mind cleanse itself when once it has come upon this religious sacredness." (Daily Quote from Collected Works, Vol. XV – 244).

"Reality is in what is. Instead of asking who has realized or what God is, why not give your whole attention and awareness to what is? Then you will find the unknown, or rather it will come to you. If you understand what is, the known, you will experience that extraordinary silence that is not induced, not enforced, that creative emptiness, in which alone entity can enter. It cannot come to that, which is becoming, which is striving; it can only come to that which is being, which understands what is. Then you will see that reality is not in the distance; the unknown is not far off; it is in what is. As the answer to a problem is in the problem, so reality is in what is; if we can understand it, then we shall know truth." (From J. Krishnamurti's "The Book of Life[1]").

"Awareness is not the outcome of practice: Problems will always exist where the activities of the self (ego) are dominant. To be aware which are and which are not the activities of the self needs constant vigilance. This vigilance is not disciplined attention, but an extensive awareness which is choiceless. Disciplined attention gives strength to the self; it becomes a substitute and dependence. Awareness, on the other hand, is not self-induced, nor is it the outcome of practice; it is understanding the whole content of the problem, the hidden as well as the superficial. The surface must be understood for the hidden to show itself; the hidden cannot be exposed if the surface mind is not quiet. This whole process is not verbal, nor is it a matter of mere experience. Verbalization indicates dullness of mind; and experience, being cumulative, makes for repetitiousness. Awareness is not a matter of determination, for purposive direction is resistance, which tends towards exclusiveness. Awareness is the silent and choiceless observation of what is; in this awareness the problem unrolls itself, and thus it is fully and completely understood. A problem is never solved on its own level; being complex, it must be understood in its total process. To try to solve a problem on only one level, physical or psychological, leads to further conflict and confusion. For the

1 Mark Lee RE, ed. J. Krishnamurti: The Book of Life. San Francisco, CA: HarperSanFrancisco; 1995: August 22.

resolution of a problem, there must be this awareness, this passive alertness which reveals its total process." (From Commentaries on Living Series I Chapter 41 Awareness).

Happiness and pleasure you can buy in any market at a price. But bliss you cannot buy for yourself or for another. Happiness and pleasure are time-binding. Only in total freedom does bliss exist. Pleasure, like happiness, you can seek, and find, in many ways. But they come, and go. Bliss that strange sense of joy has no motive. You cannot possibly seek it. Once it is there, depending on the quality of your mind, it remains timeless, causeless, and a thing that is not measurable by time. Meditation is not the pursuit of pleasure and the search for happiness. Meditation, on the contrary, is a state of mind in which there is no concept or formula, and therefore total freedom. It is only to such a mind that this bliss comes unsought and uninvited. Once it is there, though you may live in the world with all its noise, pleasure and brutality, they will not touch that mind. Once it is there, conflict has ceased. But the ending of conflict is not necessarily the total freedom. Meditation is a movement of the mind in this freedom. In this explosion of bliss the eyes are made innocent, and love is then benediction. (J. Krishnamurti Meditations 1969 Part 10).

PEACE AT CROSSROADS

At this conscious moment,
We are at the crossroads of our minds,
We decide whether to look out or in;

Whether to act willfully,
And purposefully,
Or to let things happen,
As they would naturally.

We decide to attend to something
Or to someone, or to just ignore;

Whether to respond whole-heartedly,
Or just be indifferent.

We decide whether to respond verbally
To others or to ourselves,
And to this nested Reality of
Sound and Silence,
Or just be at ease,
And Silent in the present.

We decide whether to dwell
On our past wounds, and

Get hateful, lustful or fearful;

And lose inner peace;

Whether to dream of a happy future,
Or just be in the spontaneous fountain of
This blissful Energy-Being.

We decide to be selfish and possessive,
Or be loving and generous.

Whether to move, act, and play a role,
And become someone special,
Or just be the Being that one is,
At this saddle-point of our life.

Finally, we decide at this moment,
And at each of our living moments,
Whether to will or wish for
Something to be and to have
Other than what is,

Or to let the Infinite, Holistic Reality
Unfold and flow
Naturally and bountifully,
Like a mountain stream of
That Silent Energy from
The Great Serene Source.

Vinod D Deshmukh

December 30, 2006

Chapter 41

FIVE 'E'S OF EXPERIENCE:
A NESTED, HIERARCHICAL, MIND~BRAIN MODEL

प्रकाशमानं न पृथक् प्रकाशात्
स च प्रकाशो न पृथक् विमर्शात् |
नान्यो विमर्शोऽहमिति स्वरूपात्
अहंविमर्शोऽस्मि चिदेकरुपः ||

All conscious experience is not separate from the conscious being. The conscious being is not different from the existential energy~being~awareness. I am that energy~being~awareness, which is my true nature. I am the energy~being~awareness, the holistic consciousness.

Vijñānbhairava. Page 127-128.

The five 'E's of human experience, from inside-out, are as follows:

1) Existential Essential Experience
2) Embodied Experience
3) Emotional Experience
4) Experiential (Nonverbal) Experience
5) Expressive (Verbal) Experience

The key structures and functions of the five hierarchical neural networks that mediate these human experiences are as follows:

1) ***Existential Essential Experience*** is mediated by the holistic reticular-limbic-cortical network:

a) Conscious arousal, awareness, attention and a feeling of an integrated, holistic Being.
b) Mediation of sleep-wake cycle including dream state (Multiple neurotransmitters, neuronal groups and their ascending and descending pathways including locus ceruleus for norepinephrine, raphe nuclei for serotonin, pedunculo-pontine nuclei for acetyl choline, substantia nigra for dopamine, histamine, orexin, and the excitatory neurotransmitter, glutamate and an inhibitory neurotransmitter, GABA).

c) Generation of respiratory rhythm (medited by the ventral respiratory nuclei, PreBotzinger complex).
d) Regulation of heart beat, blood pressure, and the whole body circulation (medited by the nuclei located in the rostral ventrolateral medulla).
e) Maintenance of body's muscle tone, upright posture, orientation to a stimulus with body, head and eye movements, locomotion, walking and running (medited by the premotor networks, parapontine reticular formation, superior colliculus, mesencephalic locomotor region).
f) Activation (excitation) and calming (inhibition) of the organism as a whole (medited by the ascending and descending reticulo-limbic-cortical activating and inhibiting networks).
g) Sensory-motor interactions through the twelve cranial nerves including the sense of smell, taste, touch, pain, rotation, audition, and vision.
h) Regulation of visceral-motor autonomic functions of swallowing, phonation, coughing, sneezing, crying, laughing, as well as digestive and genito-urinary activities.

2) ***Embodied Experience*** is mediated by inner limbic network:

a) Sense of embodiment by scanning of and orientation to the immediate environment, primary emotional reactions, like fear, anger, lust, disgust, sadness, happiness and their memories and learning (medited by the amygdala, hippocampus, fornix, mammilary bodies, anterior thalamic nucleus).
b) Homeokinetic regulation and maintenance of body chemistry, water, electrolytes, temperature, hormones, feeding and drinking behavior, sexual behavior, stress response, immune response and circadian rhythms (medited by the hypothalamus, amygdala).

3) ***Emotional Experience*** is mediated by outer limbic network:

Conscious feelings and motivation to act, opponent processes such as approach or avoid, reward or punishment, pain or pleasure, coordination of feeling, thinking and intentionality (medited by the orbito-frontal, cingulate gyrus and subcallosal area).

4) ***Experiential Nonverbal Experience*** is mediated by right cerebral hemispheric network:

a. Parallel, holistic processing creates the experience of a timeless awareness-being.
b. Autobiographical memories and the sense of autobiographical self or ego (medited by the hippocampus, right precuneus and the related medial prefrontal-parietal network).
c. The seven 'L's of right cerebral hemispheric functions: Language (prosody), Laughter, Lacrimation (sadness), Laudation, Lying, Lyric and Love[1].

1 Trimble MR. The Soul in the Brain. Baltimore, MD: The Johns Hopkins University Press; 2007:213.

d. Focused attention, nonverbal intellect, nonverbal memory management, social conduct, insight and judgement, voluntary initiation and synchronization of speech and complex movements with fine sensory-motor coordination, speech, prosody and gesturing, naming, hearing, sensory integration and recognition, audiovisual awareness and deficit recognition, music and voice recognition, visuo-spatial recognition, visual orientation, guidance, scanning, and seeing (these functions are represented on the outer surface of the right cerebral hemisphere, from front to back).
e. Nonverbal memory and emotion, retrograde episodic memory, sense of smell (these functions are represented on the inner and under surface of the right cerebral hemisphere).

5) ***Expressive Verbal Experience*** is mediayed by the left cerebral hemispheric Network:

In most right-handed individuals, the processing of verbal information, including language and mathematics, occurs primarily in the left cerebral hemispheric network. This language processing network mediates the following complex, mental activities:

a) Sequential, dualistic, symbol processing and experience of a differentiated centered personality.
b) Focused attention, verbal intellect, verbal memory management, social conduct, insight and judgement, voluntary initiation and synchronization of speech and complex movements with fine sensory-motor coordination, speaking, naming, hearing, sensory integration and recognition, general understanding or comprehension, reading aloud, writing to dictation, spelling, mathematics, verbal repetition, visual recognition, visual orientation, guidance, scanning, and seeing (these functions are represented on the outer surface of the left cerebral hemisphere, from front to back).
c) Visuo-spacial recognition, seeing colors and whole object imaging, verbal memory and emotion, sense of smell. (these functions are represented on the inner and under surface of the left cerebral hemisphere).

Key References: [258 - 260].

RUNNING THROUGH A CANYON

This mind of mine is
Running through a mindless canyon.

It is the only stream that I know of.
It runs by itself, not knowing,
What, where, or when,
The next turn may come.

But, the stream flows effortlessly,
Conversing with the giant cliffs.

This is the only stream
That I know of.
All other streams that I hear,
Are rumblings from a distant Forrest.

I don't know what it feels like,
To be someone else,
And to flow like them.

They are just images and imaginations,
Like these transient whirlpools,
In my mind's conscious stream.
All this is happening,
In a great field of Existence,
Which I don't know much about.

I can't really see
The whole thing, all at once.
Who knows what's beyond?
Or even ahead?

All that I truly know
Is the current curve,
That I am facing and negotiating now,
On these white-waters of my mind.

These waters, at times,
Become so turbulent,
That they create
A sudden, blinding spray on me.
Momentarily, I can't see
Where I am going.
But, suddenly, the fog lifts off by itself,
And I find myself clear, serene and enchanted,
In this infinite, silent, crystal-clear sky!

I don't know what to call it.
No name justifies It, and
What it feels like to be in it.

So, I stop naming or describing It.
I know, it can't be grabbed by the senses,
Nor framed by this clever mind.

But my *heart* knows, for sure,
How peaceful it is within,
At this great Living Moment!

Vinod D Deshmukh

April 3, 2007

Chapter 42

FUNCTIONAL BRAIN MODEL

A NESTED HIERARCHICAL AND PARALLEL ORGANIZATION, DURING DEVELOPMENT AND EVOLUTION.

अकामो धीरो अमृतः स्वयंभू रसेन तृप्तो न कुतश्चनोनः ।
तमेव विद्वान् न बिभाय मृत्योरात्मानं धीरमजरं युवानम् ॥४४॥

"*Ātman*, the energy~being~awareness, is free of desires and fear of death. It is full of courage and wisdom. It is self-existent and self-content with the essentials, lacking nothing. It is the knower of itself; it is healthy, cheerful, serene, and youthful."

Atharva Veda अथर्ववेद 10:8:44

Traditionally, the brain is anatomically divided into I) Hindbrain - rhombencephalon, which includes myelencephalon and metencephalon, II) Midbrain - mesencephalon and III) Forebrain - prosencephalon, which includes Interbrain diencephalon and Endbrain - telencephalon. This current division does not fit well with the complex hierarchy of animal and human behavior and self-consciousness. A unified brain-behavior model is currently lacking. Thus, we are left with a sense of awe, facing daunting complexity of countless interactive neurons, with innumerable connections and patterns of neural networks, with the manifestation of a variety of simple and complex animal behaviors and mentations. The astonishing unfolding of the brain and behavior, during animal development and evolution, are even more perplexing.

In this chapter, a Functional Brain Model (FBM) is described, which was proposed by the author in 2009. It is based on a Nested Hierarchy and Parallel Organization (NHPO), for behavior and mentation. Seven postulates were described in details. Based on this model, the brain is classified into: I) Invertebrate brain, II-a) Vertebrate Oro-Pharyngeal Brain (OPB), II-b) Verterbarte Cephalo-Truncal Brain (CTB), and II-c) Vertebrate Neo-Cortical Brain (NCB). OPB includes medullary and caudal ponto-cerebellar regions. CTB includes rostral pons, midbrain and limbic-allocortical regions and NCB includes telencephalic, hemispheric and bi-hemispheric, global networks. The NHPO organization operates at all functional brain levels. The parallel processing occurs within a single NHPO level, whereas, nested hierarchy manifests between the five vertical levels. This functional brain model is illustrated in Figure 15, and its structural and behavioral details are given in Tables 1, 2, 3 and 4 in APPENDIX 5.

This functional brain model is based on sound principles of behavioral neurobiology [261], which not only deal with how brain works and how animals behave, but also why they behave, the way they do. Every animal has a behavioral body-plan or a bauplan. The bauplan depends on animal's genetic make-up and its mode of living, in its specific environment. The main drive for animal behavior is survival of the individual and its genes i.e., species. Both animal form and behavior have evolved to best serve these goals. For survival of individual, various essential neural mechanisms have evolved, which regulate i) ionic-osmotic homeostasis, ii) respiration, iii) gustation, iv) locomotion, v) defense, vi) reproduction and vii) purposeful behavior. All animals, being thermo-dynamically open systems, have to exchange continuously, biomolecules-energy and information, with their environments, for survival, growth and fecundity.

Hierarchical organization, of the complex metazoan animals, has evolved in five progressive stages: i) the protoplasm, ii) the cell, iii) the tissue, iv) the organ, and v) the organism, the holistic system. The NHP organization of the invertebrate brain and behavior is summarized in Table 1. In vertebrates, behavioral hierarchy and parallel processing are evident in the functions of swallowing [262], hypothalamo-pituitary-adrenal stress response [263], primate basal ganglia activity [264], human olfaction, visual, auditory and somatosensory functions [265 - 267], cognition, working memory [268], and language [269].

In vertebrates, the first NHPO level regulates most of the simple, essential behaviors for survival. This Oro-Pharyngeal Brain (OPB) regulates the pharyngeal arches and their derivatives. The next two divisions, Cephalo-Truncal Brain (CTB), and Neo-Cortical Brain (NCB) have adaptively evolved to favorably move, and relocate the oro-pharyngeal apparatus, for successful sensing, capturing prey, feeding, and mating and escape behavior. CTB organizes all activities of vertebrate head, trunk and limbs, together as well as independently. NCB evolved as the highest integrative level for emotions, perception, cognition, consciousness, memory, intentions, planning and creativity. During evolution, OPB is relatively conserved, whereas, CTB and NCB have evolved extensively, for the optimization of complex behavior, mentation and consciousness.

In the NHP organization, rostral (higher) neural network exercises an overriding influence on the spontaneous activities of caudal (lower) neural network. For instance, in invertebrates, supra-pharyngeal ganglion modulates the sub-pharyngeal ganglion, which coordinates swallowing behavior. In vertebrates, CTB modulates OPB, whereas, NCB modulates both CTB and OPB. The CTB and NCB are of recent origin in animal ontogeny and phylogeny.

THE FIRST POSTULATE

The first postulate is about the bidirectional embryonic development that starts at the medullo-spinal region. The development of neural tube begins at this region and proceeds both rostrally and caudally, [270]. From ontogenic and phylogenic perspectives, cranial nerves appear in the reverse order i.e. hypoglossal, the XIIth cranial nerve appears earlier than olfactory, the Ist cranial nerve. Therefore, they are better understood in the order as they appear during embryogenesis. The numbering of pharyngeal arches and rhombomeres is also better understood in the reverse order. With this perspective, the tongue, which is innervated by the hypoglossal nerve, is the true rostrum of many animals, like chameleons, snakes, frogs and bats. The tongue is also a vital, multifunctional organ, in many terrestrial animals, including humans.

The pharyngeal arches develop early during embryogenesis. They form tongue, stomodeum, mouth, face, head and related brain structures [271 - 273]. During evolution, some of the animal's oropharynx and head became adaptively specialized, e.g. the evolution of hardened bills in birds, turtles and mammals, due to the deposition of keratin in their lips. Their tongues evolved to better serve functions, like handling food, taste appreciation, temperature control, capturing prey, an accessory organ for olfaction and the production of complex human speech.

The Second Postulate

The second postulate is that the development of Visceral Nervous System (VNS) precedes the development of Somatic Nervous System (SNS). VNS mediates vital functions including alimentation, swallowing [274, 275], breathing [276], cardiovascular regulation [277], thermal and ionic homeostasis and procreation.

The Third Postulate

The third postulate is about the role of Somatic nervous system (SNS) in varied environments, when there is a need for an animal to quickly move towards an opportunity and away from any danger. This is achieved by somato-visceral coordination resulting in efficient relocation of the animal body, head and mouth, either together or independently, towards food, bio-energy and a mate, and away from dangers, like heat of a volcano or fire, acidity, toxic substances, like extreme sour or bitter foods, precipitous heights and predators. Various locomotor systems [278 - 280] evolved, which enabled animals to swim, crawl, walk, run and fly. Such activities require coordination of head, body, and limbs, with guidance from sensory organs, like skin, face, tongue, whiskers, lateral-line receptors, vestibular organs, ears, eyes, nose and memory.

Initial progravity, side-to-side movements were followed by antigravity movements like vertical stance, gait and rotatory movements of head [281], and eyes [282 - 284]. This enabled animals to swim, stand, walk, run, climb and fly vertically. These developments depended on the evolution of neural networks, integrating vestibular, cerebellar, and oculomotor and midbrain reticular nuclei. The mesencephalic, basal ganglia and cerebellar locomotor-circuits are well adapted to mediate these complex behaviors.

THE FOURTH POSTULATE

The fourth postulate is about sensory-motor integration. The neuromotor system evolved for stronger and faster locomotion and skillful movements of head, mouth, lips, tongue, larynx, hands and fingers, for better gestural and vocal communication [285, 286]. The communicative abilities and skills reached their pinnacle in the human oral and written languages, performing arts and sports [287].

The neurosensory system integrates information from various receptors including tactile, vibration, chemo-, baro-, thermo-, geo- (gravity), proprio-, phono- and photo-receptors. The neurosensory system evolved in two major specialized divisions. The contact-senses (CS) include taste, touch, temperature, pain, vibration, pressure, proprioception and vestibular sense. The distance-senses (DS) include auditory, visual and olfactory [288]. Both CS and DS guide animal behavior. The CS are involved in reflex responses of pharynx, tongue, lips, mouth, face, head, hands and feet, whereas, DS are involved in long-distance, whole body movements, like locomotion, swimming, walking, running, jumping, flying, gesturing and vocal communication.

THE FIFTH POSTULATE

The fifth postulate is about memory. The initial memory circuits were developed probably, due to an intense painful or pleasurable experience, leaving a memory-trace in the limbic system [289 - 291]. Intuitively, it is important and adaptive for an animal to register, store and recall significant life-events, which serve for the anticipation and guidance of future behavior, in order to avoid pain and pursue pleasure. Emotional memories are established through classical conditioning by reward or punishment, and are automatically and subconsciously, mediated by the reticulo-limbic-allocortical networks.

The "on-line" working memory is a function of the most recently evolved, prefrontal and posterior temporal-occipital-parietal (TOP) associative cortices. This amazing ability of episodic working-memory makes it possible for us to register, hold and manipulate information or a representation of an object or an event, as a conscious mental content. There is sufficient evidence that working memory is mediated by the dorso-lateral prefrontal-parietal network and the long-term, semantic memories are stored in the TOP associative cortices. By interaction between the dorso-lateral prefrontal cortex and the TOP associative cortices, meaningful, experiential, personal stories are built. The evolution of such cognitive ability is crucial for the purposeful decision-making, symbol-language processing, story-telling, creative arts and sciences [292, 293].

THE SIXTH POSTULATE

The sixth postulate is about attentive facing, which is the turning of body, head, face, mouth, ears and eyes towards pleasant stimuli like food, air, water, warmth and friends, and away from unpleasant stimuli like excessive heat or cold, foul smell, toxins and predators. Attentive facing has evolved as an adaptive mechanism for security, comfort, pleasure and communication. For instance, flock of birds and mammals prefer to face warm wind, light and to stay together safely, within their group. Attentive facing helps to communicate by gestures, grimacing, vocalization and language [294]. Decorating one's face, for better communication and relationship with others has luxuriously evolved in several birds, mammals and humans.

Attentive facing conveys emotions, like fear, anger, joy, sadness, disgust, humor, peace and happiness. These expressions can be reflex at oro-pharyngeal brain level, automatic at cephalo-truncal brain level and intentional at neocortical brain level. There is evidence of deliberate ignoring of a stimulus and even falsifying facial expressions to hide emotions. Facing behavior forms the beginning of human attentiveness. Just as evolution of binocular vision improved visual acuity, attentional behavior has increased our capacity to gather, process, store, and communicate, multimodal information, from the environment and the past experience. Further expansion of such cognitive ability and working memory, probably resulted in the emergence of an efficient, anticipatory and adaptive animal and human consciousness [295 - 298].

THE SEVENTH POSTULATE

The seventh postulate is about creative neo-cognition, which is the ability to generate and use new and appropriate information. Such information may be a new perception, a new understanding, a novel imagination, a unique movement, an original narration, writing or any discovery. Human cognition is defined as the ability to attend, perceive, comprehend, manipulate, integrate and maintain information; to intend, act, and communicate [299]. Human executive function is defined as the ability to abstract, plan, organize, shift set and adapt current and past knowledge, for future behavior [300].

Human creativity is well developed. Creativity is defined as: "The ability to produce work that is novel, original, spontaneous, appropriate, useful and adaptive" [301 - 305]. It has given us an enormous advantage over our environment and other animals. Spontaneous as well as intentional creativity is useful for making cognitive models of self and environment. Such ability gives us capacity to simulate and anticipate future, based on our past experience. Such a mind is capable of complex decision-making, creative thinking and altruistic behavior. Recently, rostral prefrontal cortex has been shown to be activated in explicit processing of self-generated information in humans. The lateral Brodmann's area10 was recruited during cognitively oriented tasks and medial Brodmann's area 10 was recruited during emotionally oriented tasks.

Creativity is further defined as an understanding and expression of novel orderly relationships, [306]. Such innovation may occur in a motivated individual, when there is co-activation and communication between prefrontal and TOP associative cortices, in a relatively low norepinephrine arousal state, with a vast knowledge of the subject, stored in multimodal cortices. Innovative cognition requires us to attend, reflect, imagine, model, and predict by participating actively in our ever-changing situations. This promotes active exploration of new environments, for security, profit, pleasure and curiosity. It is the very basis of an astronomical progress made in human knowledge, languages, communications, sciences, technologies, space-explorations and creative arts. There is an endless opportunity for us to learn, innovate, invent, explore, discover, understand, express and share our unique experience of this astonishing and apparently endless, live universe. Figure 16.

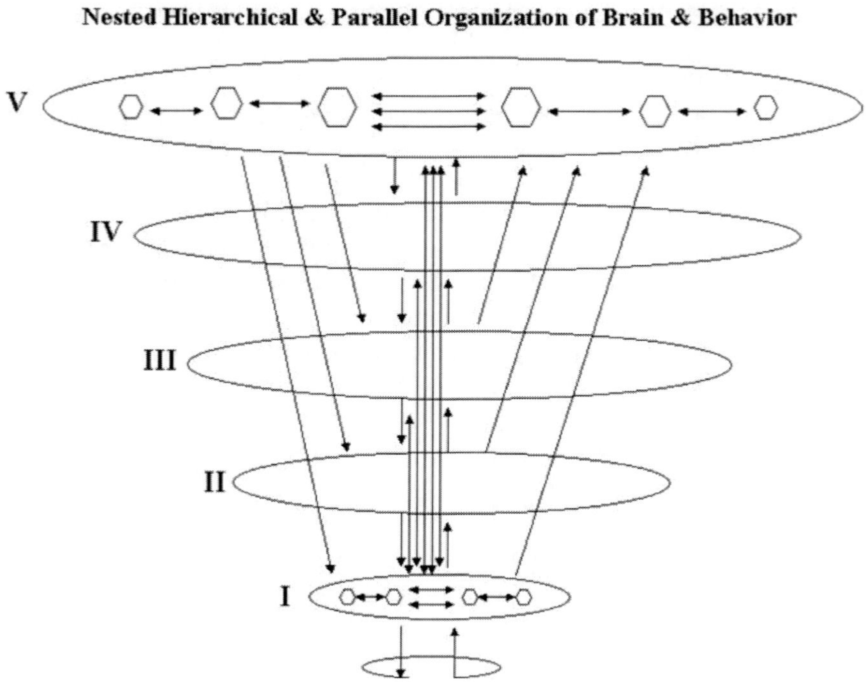

Figure 16. Functional Brain Model. Nested hierarchical and parallel organization (NHPO) of brain, behavior, and mentation. I-V represent NHP organizational levels. The lowest ellipse represents the spinal cord. Level I: medulla, Level II: pons-cerebellum, Level III: mid brain, Level IV: limbic-allocortex and Level V: multimodal neocortex. Hexagons represent neuronal groups or ensembles and cortical functional modules. Single arrows show the direction of afferent and efferent connections and triple arrows represent commissural connections between cerebral hemispheres and the subcortical structures. (Please refer to Tables 1, 2, 3, and 4 in Appendix 5).

A few other authors have similarly emphasized the nested hierarchical nature of the central nervous system organization. For instance Faw, [307], proposed five levels of functional organization:

Level I. Emotional consciousness mechanisms. Spinal cord-brainstem pain reflexes of the somatic motor system. Visceral activation of the autonomic motor system. Electrolyte-hormone endocrine systems.

Level II brainstem zone of interacting, arousal-affective circuits. Acetylcholine brainstem consciousness-oscillator system. Norepinephrine vigilance system. Dopamine 'motivational' system. Serotonin emotional-tone system. Periaqueductal gray (PAG) - endorphin emotional valence system. Cortical arousal, emotion, and motivation systems.

Level III diencephalon areas, to which level II projects. Acetylcholine intralaminar nuclei thalamus (ILN): attentional gating. Nucleus accumbens, staging area for higher attentional control. Acetylcholine basal forebrain cognitive enabler. Hypothalamus as a level III motivation controller. Perceptual-thalamus as an information processor.

Level IV subcortical limbic emotional mechanisms. Amygdala is a fourth-level, emotional evaluator and conditioner. Hippocampus as a level IV novelty evaluator episode recorder.

Level V Anterior cortical control areas. Prefrontal lobe as an 'executive committee,' representing the emotional-motivational self in committee decisions; Representing the 'days of our lives' in committee decisions; Insurrection or rebellion in the executive committee."

Forehand, [308], highlighted the nested hierarchy in the integrative neural networks or neural centers of integration. In caudal-to-rostral sequence, the more rostral it is placed, the greater the complexity of the neural network. The following are the major centers of neural integration:

Brainstem: The brainstem reticular formation is critical for arousal and sleep. The ascending reticular activating system mediates consciousness and arousal.

Hypothalamus: The hypothalamic nuclei are centers for physiological regulation. It regulates bilological clock, arousal-energy balance, and sexual activity.

Limbic System: It is the seat of emotions. It contains cortical and subcortical structures. It contains the reward system. It mediates aggresion and sexual activity.

Forebrain: It processes sensory information, executes behavior, makes decisions, and is capable of learning. It is functionally compartmentalized. Memory and learning require cerebral cortex and limbic system."

Forehand elaborated on the role of the reticular formation. "The reticular formation plays a central role in the regulation of the state of consciousness and arousal-energy. It consists of a complex network of interconnected circuits of neurons in the tegmentum of the brainstem, the lateral hypothalamic area, and the medial, intralaminar, and reticular nuclei of the thalamus. Many of these neurons are serotonergic or noradrenergic. Axons from the nonspecific thalamic nuclei project to most of the cerebral cortex, where they modulate the level of activity of large numbers of neurons. [...] Reticular formation plays a crucial role in maintaining the brain at an appropriate level of arousal, some authorities refer to it as the reticular activating system. The descending reticulo-spinal tract modulates the spinal reflexes, spinal autonomic activity and spinal sensory input."

Functions of reticular formation include arousal-energy, consciousness, and sleep. Regulation of arousal-energy and level of consciousness is a generalized function of the reticular formation. The neurons of the reticular formation are stimulated by a variety of stimuli from the somatosensory, auditory, visual, and visceral sensory systems. The reticular formation is, therefore, nonspecific in its response and performs a generalized regulatory function. When a novel stimulus is received, attention is focused on it, while general alertness increases. This behavioral arousal is independent of modality of stimulation and is accompanied by EEG changes. The cerebral cortex and the mesencephalic reticular activating system are mutually sustaining areas involved in maintaining consciousness.

Phylogenetically, there is a hierarchy in the evolution of the key neural structures in the Central Nervous System. Here is the list from the oldest to newest:

Hippocampus

  Dentate gyrus

    Amygdala

      Parahippocampal gyrus

        Cingulate gyrus

          Sub-callosal gyrus

Primary motor cortex
Primary sensory cortex
Association cortex.

Functional hierarchical organization is also evident in the autonomic nervous system as follows:

Spinal cord: peristalsis, micturition, defecation, sexual reflexes.

Medulla: Respiratory, cardiovascular and alimentary functions. Regulation of blood glucose, salivation, micturition, vomiting, sneezing, coughing and gagging.

Pons: Rhythmic respiration, laughing center, horizontal eye movements.

Midbrain: Accommodation and reaction to light, vertical eye movements and other ocular reflexes.

Hypothalamus: autonomic coordination, including sympathetic and parasympathetic regulation, circadian rhythms, neuro-hormonal regulation, primal affective responses.

Limbic system: visceral manifestations of emotion and drives such as sexual behavior, fear, rage, aggression, and eating behavior. Stimulation can elicit cardiovascular, gastrointestinal, responses, micturition, defecation, piloerection, and pupillary changes.

Cerebral neocortex: It may initiate autonomic reactions such as blushing or blanching of the face in response to receiving bad or good news. High emotional stimuli may cause fainting or syncope. Executive function, [309], is defined as the ability to sequence, monitor, and plan behavior. These functions are linked to the prefrontal cortex.

In summary, a functional brain model is proposed, based on neurobiology, nested hierarchical and parallel organization, evident during animal development and evolution. The drive for animal behavior is survival of the individual and genes (species). Brain has evolved to better serve these goals. Based on this model, behaving, thinking brain is classified into: I) Invertebrate brain, II) a) Vertebrate Oro-Pharyngeal Brain, b) Cephalo-Truncal Brain, and c) Neo-Cortical Brain. Seven postulates are proposed in order to better understand the evolutionary development of i) medullo-spinal region, ii) visceral networks, iii) somatic networks, iv) sensory-motor integration, v) memory, vi) attentive facing, and vii) creativity.

A behavioral hierarchy results in reflex, conditioned, sensory-guided, memory-guided, rule-based, self-generated, and creative behaviors, with emergence of cognition, speech, imagery, self-consciousness, creativity and altruism, as specialized behaviors. These functions are most evolved in humans. The proposed brain model is based on the functional behavior development and evolution of invertebrate and vertebrate animals including humans. It is founded on a hierarchy of simple, essential to more complex and creative behaviors in all animals. The simple organismic activities or behaviors include ionic-osmotic homeostasis, respiration, swallowing, feeding, sleeping, waking, and locomotion. Whereas, the more complex behaviors include vocalizing, communicating by verbal and nonverbal gestures, symbol creation and manipulation, language, memory, mentation, self-awareness, intention-volition with purposeful actions, anticipation, decision-making, planning, social-emotional intelligence, creativity and altruism. Understanding this brain model will enhance our understanding of animal and human behavior and conscious mentation.

EMBEDDED LIFE

All life is embedded in some habitat.
Each becomes a part
Of a collective Being.

All of us are embedded in Nature.
We are connected to each other,
Through Nature's elemental energies.

The good Earth carries us all.
The Ocean connects all continents.
The fluid Atmosphere moves together.
The Sun energizes all Life,
And the Space contains us all.

Life begets life.
Colonies of bacteria and insects,
Schools of fish,
From silversides to whales,
Flocks of birds,
From pelicans to seagulls,
Herds of mammals,
From wildebeests to elephants.

We are all connected,
In some way or the other,
Like a group of buffalos
In torrential rain,
A pride of lions
Under the shade of a tree,
A crowd of humanity
Gathered in a sports arena,
To cheer or jeer
The player of the moment.

Whether we realize it or not,
Whether we like it or not,
We are all connected and embedded in
This infinite, existential field of
Energy-Being-Awareness.

We are conscious of
Only a tiny part of it.
But, intuitively we can feel

Its benevolent wholeness,
Supporting all Life and Minds.
It is the nameless, timeless infinite.

Who could define and describe it?
Who could encircle it?
With arms as long as the galaxy?
Who has a giant eye?
Like the brilliant Sun?
The all-listening ear?
Like a black hole?
Or an omniscient Mind?
That knows it all?

All of us can intuitively feel,
Its benevolent Presence
In our heart,
As something pure, precious, and ever new,
Ever-present, self-creative and ever-nurturing,
One energy~being~awareness
One field of all Life,
And all that exists.

Vinod D Deshmukh

August 4, 2007

Chapter 43

Consciousness and Spirituality: Neuroscience And Vedānta Perspectives

देहो देवालयः प्रोक्तः स जीवः केवलः शिवः |
त्यजेत् अज्ञाननिर्माल्यं सोऽहंभावेन पूजयेत् ||

This body is the temple. The living being is sacred. Let us discard the old flowers of self-ignorance and worship the self as the Divine.

Skandopaniṣ ad स्कन्दोपनिषद् 10

All of us know, from our personal experience, what consciousness is. However, it is difficult to capture in words, its extraordinary complexity. It is like a beautiful diamond with multiple facets, each being as amazing as the other. The reality of our conscious experience is just as complex and multifaceted.

I would suggest a simple working definition. Consciousness is a living, organismic process. It is the property of a living organism. Brain is the organ of consciousness. Conscious experience is a synthesis of three aspects or perspectives, which I would call a philosophy of "Triple Aspect Monism." i) the first aspect is the describable, objective reality, the observed world. ii) the second aspect is the describable, subjective, mental world, and iii) the third aspect is the indescribable, all-inclusive/exclusive, essential, intrinsic, subjective Energy-Awareness-Being. It is the mysterious wonder within all of us. Only a few of us realize this aspect of our consciousness. This is the 'existential-spiritual' aspect of our conscious experience that waits to be discovered by each one of us, in our own Heart and Being.

Thus, consciousness has a biophysical, mental, and existential basis. Neuroscience has made much progress in understanding the neurobiology of consciousness, which is a function of the brain. Neuroscience describes the brain as a self-organizing, holarchical (emergence of whole from whole) system, which is thermodynamically open and biophysically auto-regulated. Such a complex system has multiple levels of organization with many nested, hierarchical, neural networks and processes.

For a conscious experience to occur, the most essential neural networks are: i) Reticulo-hypothalamic, neuroendocrine and autonomic network, which is the basis for visceral integration and an undifferentiated, affective, arousal-energy-being, ii) Reticulo-limbic-cortical network, which is the basis for differentiated emotional being, positive or negative feeling and its expression, iii) Reticulo-thalamo-cortical, multi-modal, associative network, which is the basis for cognition, thinking, intentionality, imagination, and planning, and iv) Reticulo-thalamo-cortical, percetual-motor network, which is the basis for exteroceptive organism-environment interactions.

The reticulo-limbic-cortical network is absolutely essential for both affective as well as cognitive consciousness. Without it, an organism cannot be awake, conscious and function as an intentional, individual being. The mental aspect of conscious experience has been studied, historically by folk psychology, spiritual disciplines, and more recently by the cognitive neurosciences. Much progress has been made in our understanding of human motivation, arousal-energy, action, perception, cognition, emotion, volition, intentionality, memory, and subjectivity.

Spirituality is the search for inner peace, happiness and personal wellbeing. It is about mental health and finding meaning and purpose in life. It can also be defined in terms of a unique mystical experience. As William James, [310], described it in 1902, the mystical experience is characterized by ineffability, noetic quality, transiency, passivity, and memorability. Such a spiritual experience is difficult to describe; it has a quality of intrinsic Energy-Awareness-Being; it is spontaneous, effortless, unintentional, radiant, and enduring. It is the very nature of our existential Energy-Awareness-Being.

The human experience of the ultimate Truth has been described in various religions and philosophies, as *Ātman~Brahman*, Turīya, Nirvāṇ a, Tao, Unio Mystica, the Ground, the Order of One, the Absolute Unitary Being and the Holistic Superconsciousness. Such a unique perspective of the existential Truth remains a matter of first-person experience only; it cannot be fully objectified for a third-person perspective. It is essentially a subjective, holistic mode of being. All of us have the potential for such an amazing and self-fulfilling discovery.

"Latin roots of the term "sacred" include sacer (holy), sacrare (to devote), and sancire (to make holy). The early Greeks believed that many things could be hieros, holy or sacred owing to their relationship or connection to one of the Gods. Pavitra पवित्र means sacred. According to Vedic-Hindu perspective, Nature, the global space or the total field of Existence, and all of its living beings, are sacred. In the Hindu tradition, the sanctity of the Divine comes from its integral presence in all Reality and its availability to the individual to be intuitively perceived and experienced. Just as the more a place or object becomes pure, the more it comes into proximity with the sacred, so is the case with humans. Physical, mental, and emotional purity are all believed to elevate one toward the sacred, toward the Divine, and the greater the ability one has to have direct Divine experience. In Hinduism, this is possible because of the manner in which the tradition understands and interprets "Omnipresence." [311].

Maslow described a hierarchy of human needs:

i) *Physiologic:* Biologic need for food, water, shelter, sleep, oxygen, and sexual expression.
ii) *Safety:* Avoiding harm, attaining security, order and physical safety.
iii) *Love and Belonging:* Giving and receiving affection. Companionship and identification with a group.

iv) *Esteem and Recognition*: Self-esteem and the respect for others, success at work and prestige.
v) *Self-Actualization*: Fulfillment of one's unique potential.

In the field of Mental Health and Psychiatric Counseling, [312], a Spiritual Health Assessment scale has been developed, which is based on grading the following responses:

i) I trust myself.
ii) I feel my life has meaning and purpose.
iii) Other people give meaning to my life.
iv) I trust other people.
v) I have close friends.

Spirituality entails an inspired life. It is recognized as a source of inner peace, hope, trust, faith, meaning, and inner strength. It incorporates our sense of being, identity, and an understanding of our place in the world. It is natural to be inspired by Nature with feelings of wonder, awe, and transcendence; a renewed sense of vigor; an increased sense of mindful presence, attentiveness and arousal-energy; a sense of being present in the moment; humility; and a better perspective of one's own existence in this astonishing universe.

One can also be inspired by art, music, reviewing of life stories (one's and other's), keeping a journal or diary of what is most important to us and listening to Self and others. One can be inspired by reading the great books of wisdom and the inspirational writings of the past and present sages, wise men and women, philosophers and scientists.

Meditation, contemplation, and prayer are now accepted ways of finding meaning, purpose, and spiritual insight in one's own life. Mindfulness, Vipassanā, or Presence are now widely accepted as effective and valid techniques for mental health, personal growth, and mental excellence. Secular or medical meditation is described in the textbooks of mental health and psychiatric counseling.

Some of the psychiatrists recommend adding a metaphysical or spiritual component to their therapeutic regimen. They discuss four metaphysical techniques for facilitating patient healing: i) refocusing on the present, ii) reframing adversity, iii) practicing surrender, and iv) meditation. These approaches can be mutually integrated and compliment the psychological treatment in either the psychiatric or primary care setting, regardless of whether or not the patient has formal religious beliefs. [313].

The effects of spiritual and meditative practices on human brain are currently being investigated in neuroscience by using such techniques as functional magnetic resonance imaging (fMRI), postron emission tomography (PET) scanning, spectral electroencephalography (EEG), and magnetoencephalography (MEG). There are two temporally distinct forms of self-reference: extended self-reference linking experiences across time and momentary self-reference centered on the present. Functional MRI was used to examine monitoring of enduring traits (narrative focus, NF) or momentary experience ('experiential' focus, EF). In novices, EF yielded focal reductions in self-referential cortical midline regions (medial prefrontal cortex, Mpfc). In mindfulness-trained participants, EF resulted in more marked and pervasive reductions in Mpfc, and increased engagement of right lateralized network, comprising the lateral prefrontal cortex PFC, viscero-motor areas such as the insula, secondary somato-sensory cortex, and inferior parietal lobule. Functional connectivity analyses further demonstrated a strong coupling between the right insula and the Mpfc in novices that was uncoupled in the mindfulness group. These results suggest a fundamental neural dissociation between two distinct forms of self-awareness that are habitually integrated but can be dissociated through attentional training: the self across time and the self in the moment. [314].

Three types of meditation have been proposed i) focused attention, ii) open monitoring, and iii) spontaneous self-transcendence. Spontaneous self-transcendence includes techniques designed to transcend self-centered thinking or egoistic mental activity. This contrasts with focused attention, in which attention is focused on an object or an event; as well as open monitoring, in which attention is involved in the monitoring of the ongoing aspects of self-situation. [315]. Self-transcendence is a quality inherent in every human being. This process of personal transformation is instrumental in finding meaning and purpose in life. When faced with adversity, self-transcendence can be a powerful coping strategy. [316].

Transpersonal psychology addresses topics such as i) the importance of spirituality in psychotherapy and counseling, ii) spirituality as a resource for maintaining and regaining health, iii) spiritual experiences as an avenue to consciousness, and iv) the delimitation of extraordinary states of consciousness. [317].

Eco-spirituality is a manifestation of the spiritual connection between human beings and the natural environment. It incorporates an intuitive and embodied awareness of all life and engages a relational view of a person to planet, inner to outer landscape, and soul to soil. This study described an appraisal of a pattern in the human-environmental, continuous mutual process and innovative change. The essential features of eco-spiritual consciousness are tending, dwelling, reverence, connectedness, and sentience. [318].

Neocortical evolution has progressed through five major transitions: from early reptiles to early mammals, early primates, simians, early Homo, and finally, the modern Homo sapiens. These transitions provide the foundation for human self-awareness related to sexuality, materiality, emotionality, intellectuality, and spirituality, respectively, [319]. Spirituality is distinct from organized religions as it relates to personal wellbeing, wholeness, and healing, [320].

THE SANCTUM

At dawn,
I woke up and faced the world,
Like a new flower,
That felt on its sensitive face,
The breeze, for the first time,
From the ever-blowing wind,
Sometimes, gentle,
But at times, furious and destructive,
With its angry look,
And furious thunder.

At noon,
I struggled with life's challenges,

Trying my best to survive,
Thrive, and be happy.

But everything seemed
To be so transient,
Unreliable, uncertain, and unpredictable,
That I suffered
Through life's ladders and slides.

At dusk,
I closed my eyes,
Like a flower
That closes its petals,
And I dreamt of my childhood days,
When I was but an innocent child,
Who had not yet seen the real world.

At times, I have had a nightmare
Of the last storm,
Which I lived through.
What an awful experience it was!

But, I woke up this morning,
And felt the Sanctum within me.
It was something unusual, but natural.
It was quiet, still, and profoundly silent,
Yet, softly audible like a distant waterfall.

There was a feeling
Of beginningless Energy,
An ineffable Peace and great Bliss.

There was no face or voice in it,
Not even my own,
Yet, it was not a non-being or no-thing.

In fact, it lacked no-thing.
It contained nothing specific,
Yet, it had the essence
Of all that exists.
In it, everything was,
As it should be.

The world and the restless mind,
Were out of that intrinsic Awareness.
No-thing could intrude or disturb it.

It was
The source, surface and sink
Of all human experience.
It was, and it is now,
A place of natural bliss
Within the *Heart* of *hearts*,
The Sanctum Sanctorum.

Vinod D Deshmukh

March 14, 2010

Chapter 44

CONTINUING SELF-UNDERSTANDING

UPDATING NEW RESEARCH FROM NEUROSCIENCE

आपूर्यमाणं अचलप्रतिष्ठं समुद्रं आपः प्रविशन्ति यद्वत् |
तद्वत्कामा यं प्रविशन्ति सर्वे स शान्तिं आप्नोति न कामकामी ||७०||

Just as the ocean remains brimful and still, even though waters (rain, rivers and streams) enters it (from all sides), similarly, a person of wisdom remains calm (oceanic feeling), unaffected and non-deluded, even though many attractions, temptations, (desires) enter his/her mind (from all sides). The person who cherishes desires does not achieve peace.

Bhagavad Gītā II: 70

Vedic seers looked at their being-in-Reality, with an everfresh feeling of astonishment, Āshcharyaṁ आश्चर्यं, Vismayaḥ विस्मयः, a sense of wonder, surprise, amazement, and a feeling of awe and reverence. Bulkeley, [321], defined "Wonder" as the feeling excited by an encounter with something novel and unexpected, something that strikes a person as intensely real, true, and/or beautiful. Wonder is something that causes astonishment. To feel wonder is to experience a sudden decentering of the self (ego). Facing something surprisingly new and unexpectedly powerful, one's ordinary sense of personal identity is dramatically altered, leading to new knowledge and understanding that ultimately recenter the self. The profound impact of this decentering and recentering process is evident in the intense memorability of the experiences and the strong bodily sensations that often accompany them."

Panksepp, [322], described a basal, experiential awareness: "Experiential consciousness seems to be an intrinsic capacity of mammalian brains. My overall position is that affective consciousness, the non-reflective, subjective experience of being a living creature, is much older in brain evolution than cognitive forms of consciousness, that allow us to think about the world. [...] The capacity to experience oneself in the world (primary process mentality) is a remarkably useful survival device. Affects are a part of primary-process consciousness, which may have been the precondition for the eventual emergence of thoughts and a self-reflective, self-awareness (secondary and tertiary forms of consciousness) that can only be well studied in humans. Emotional brain functions need to be viewed, from two complimentary perspectives - the neurodynamic and the psychodynamic — using a dual-aspect monism strategy. The primary affective brain systems facilitate survival, unconditionally by anticipating major survival issues."

Dual-aspect monism was elaborated by Solms, [323]. "Brain is the seat of the mind, somehow producing our feeling of being ourselves in the world right now. [...] Dual-aspect monism accepts that we are made of only one type of stuff (that is why it is a monist position), but it also suggests that this stuff is perceived in two different ways (hence, the dual aspect monism). The important point to grasp about this otherwise straightforward position is that it implies that in our essence, we are neither mental nor physical beings — at least not in the sense that we normally employ these terms. Dual-aspect monism implies that the brain is made of stuff that appears "physical" when viewed from the outside (as an object) and "mental" when viewed from the inside (as the subject). When I perceive myself externally (in the mirror, for example) and internally through introspection, I perceive the same thing in two different ways (as a body and a mind, respectively). This distinction between body and mind is therefore an artifact of perception."

He goes on to say, "A property of consciousness that can be easily agreed upon is that it is normally a unified experience. Each one of us has the impression of being a single entity, experiencing an integrated perceptual world, at this particular moment in time. It is me that is surveying the scene in front of me right now. I am the unifying point of reference for all the objects I see scattered before me. The objects, too, appear to me to exist in a unified field of space and time." (We have to realize this continuous unity of space-time-person). "The background state" of consciousness does mean or represent something. It represents 'you'[1] — the most basic embodiment of your 'self.' More than that, it represents the current state of your self: 'This is me, I am this body, and right now, I feel like this.' Far from being without quality the background state of consciousness is therefore replete with meaning and feeling — indeed, it is the very bedrock of personal meaning and feeling. This aspect of consciousness therefore not only "represents" your self, it also tells you how you are doing."

He further elaborates, "Emotion is akin to a sensory modality — an internally directed sensory modality that provides information about the current state of the bodily self, as opposed to the state of the object world. It adds a sixth sense, (a sixth modality of "qualia") to our conscious existence. Emotion is the aspect of consciousness that is left if you remove all externally derived contents. If you were deprived of all sensory images (drawn from present and past perceptions) you would still be conscious. You would still be aware of your inner state — of your core self. Emotion is a perception of the state of the subject, not of the object world."

Solms proposed an underlying neuroanatomy of our primal feeling of being a whole person. "Periaqueductal gray (PAG) has a vertical columnar organization. The columns are divided into two broad types: pleasurable sensations in the ventral PAG and unpleasure in the dorsal PAG. Tectum-Tegmentum (a zone of convergence) together generates a rudimentary representation of the whole person, the inner and outer "virtual bodies" combined. Jaak Panksepp calls it the SELF, "Simple Ego-like Life Form."

Gendlin, [324], proposed a first-person-process model in order to resolve the conflicting dichotomy of Mind-Body problem. It was suggested, "What is missing here is that 'the person' is much larger than our limited conscious capacities. The person includes the body-

1 This reminds me of the famous Vedic dictum, "You are That. तत्त्वमसि." It means the existential, blissful Conscious~Energy~Being, Sat~Chit~Ānanda, is your true nature.

as-internally-sensed, and it also includes a much greater variety of reflectively aware experiencing than merely the deliberately controlled. What we control is a relatively small part of sentient experiencing and experienced internal and external actions. This is a first-person model, which I call 'a model of process,' a model in which each next bit is a newly-made whole."

Locke Simeon, [325], asserts that the function of the nervous system as a totality is to model reality. We as human beings sense and conceive our environment by three sets of sensory receptors, namely, interceptors, proprioceptors, and exteroceptors, or teloceptors. This is consistent with three concentric spheres, relating respectively to neural derivatives of the three concentric embryonic layers — the germinal, the mantle, and the marginal[2]: "i) the innermost layer or environment, composed of the organism's viscera and related structures, transmit information by way of the autonomic nervous system and do not require voluntary control. Information from this layer is transduced by receptors called interceptors, ii) the second middle environmental sphere that is interposed between the viscera and the external world is the body wall, neurologically served by cells aggregated in located nuclei, in what may be viewed as a middle neurological layer. Information from this middle environment is conveyed to the nervous system by way of receptors termed proprioceptors, and iii) the most external environment — the outside world — is represented in the outermost layer of the central nervous system, particularly the cerebral cortex, which receives information collected by exteroceptors, sometimes called teloreceptors such as the eye or ear."

The holistic eco-systemic perspective, [326], is crucial for our understanding of the organism-environment relationship. Such "Systems Thinking" is about patterns of relationships and how these translate into new emergent properties and behaviors. "Underlying systems thinking is the premise that systems behave as a whole and that such behavior cannot be explained solely in terms a simple aggregate of individual elements. An important emergent property of the whole is self-organization. […] One well-known statement associated with systems thinking is that "Everything is connected to everything else."

"A systems description is always from the perspective of an observer, and the question or issues, in which they are interested. […] Every system description is a partial description of the Reality based on an observer's perspective. So when we talk about a system, we are not talking about a physical object but rather, our limited mental representation of it. The system is not "out there" but "inside us[3]." […] "Of particular interest in this regard are open systems: systems that have an environment that provides their context (the conditions in which they are embedded) and provides the source and sink for flows in and out of the system."

"It should be noted that a Holon refers to a system considered at one scale and from one perspective. A holarchy is a nesting of holons, each at a different scale of observation, but all seen from the same perspective. A hierarchical description is a set of holarchic descriptions, each holarchy reflecting a relevant type of perspective. […] A central feature of self-organizing systems is that they can manifest coherent self-perpetuating behavior that is internally generated. Such systems have a tendency to establish themselves in thermodynamically nonequilibrium steady states that are capable of persisting, even when the external environment changes."

2 This reminds me of the three aspects of the Self described in the Ātmopaniṣ ad, as the external self Bahyātmā, internal ego Antarātmā and the tracendent Self Paramātmā.

"Schrondinger, Odum, and Prigogine have observed that thermodynamics is the foundation for understanding self-organization and life. In particular, Prigogine developed a theory of nonequilibrium thermodynamics and self-organization, in terms of the dissipative structures. This theory explained how spontaneous coherent behavior and organization emerge in open systems. Central to understanding such phenomena is the realization that open systems are processing an enduring flow of high quality energy. High quality energy or exergy is a measure of the maximum capacity of the available energy contained in a system to perform useful work as the system proceeds to equilibrium with its surroundings. [...] Exergy is a function of the gradient between a system and its environment. It is a summation of the free energies in a situation. In effect, it measures how far the system is from thermodynamic equilibrium with its environment. Exergy is not a useful concept for discussing equilibrium situations. However, it is a very powerful tool for nonequilibrium situations."

"In summary, self-organizing dissipative processes emerge in biophysical systems whenever sufficient energy is available to support them. Once such processes are established, they manifest as a structure. These structures provide a new context, nested within which new processes can emerge. These, in turn, beget new structures, nested within which, and so on. Thus emerges a self-organizing holarchic open system (SOHOs) embedded in a physical environment. A nested constellation of self-organizing dissipative process-structures organized about particular sources of exergy, materials, and information that give rise to coherent self-perpetuating behaviors. This is the conception of self-organizing holarchic open systems (SOHOs).

An ecological perspective of the brain and our subject-object interactions are being proposed as a model for psychiatry and psychotherapy. Fuchs, [327], proposed an ecological or systemic view of the brain, which regards cognition and consciousness as components in a circular causality of organism and environment[3]. "In these cyclic processes, the brain functions as an organ of transformation which mutually translates elementary and complex system states into each other, thus allowing the organism to develop integral options of perception and action in its environment. Since these interactions, on their part, continuously change the microstructure of the brain, it has to be regarded as an organ that is formed biologically, socially as well as historically."

Panksepp, [328], defended the energy metaphor of mind. "Human thoughts can be driven by sub-neocortical large-scale (networks) energetic states. Sadly, energy metaphors of mind were discarded a long time ago, to the great detriment of understanding what emotions really are. However, information processing metaphors, failed miserably when we seek to envision the actions of such visceral-emotional brain systems. Energetic dynamics are clearly reflected in emotional actions of both brain and body, as large ensembles of neurons are brought into distinct but coherent action modes by executive neuropeptides. To understand such global functions of the brain, we need functional 'network doctrines' as much as we need a 'neuron doctrine."

Schiff, [329], reviewed the importance of the central thalamic nuclei, in cortical arousal and consciousness "Forebrain arousal is regulated by ascending influences from brainstem/basal forebrain neuronal populations ("arousal systems") and control signals descending from frontal cortical systems. These subcortical and cortical systems have

3 This reminds me of the complimentarity of the pair in essential union, the Person-in-Nature, Puruṣ a-Prakṛ iti, in the Indian Sānkhya philosophy or the concept of Śiva~Śakti in Śaiva~Śaktism.

converging projections to the central thalamus that emphasize their role in maintaining organized behavior during wakefulness. Central thalamic neurons appear to be specialized, both anatomically and physiologically, to support distributed network activity that maintains neuronal firing patterns across long-range cortico-cortical pathways and within cortico-striatopallidal-thalamocortical loop connections. Recruitment of central thalamic neurons occurs in response to increasing cognitive demand, stress, fatigue, and other perturbations that reduce behavioral performance. In addition, the central thalamus receives projections from brainstem pathways evolved to rapidly generate brief shifts of arousal associated with the appearance of salient stimuli across different sensory modalities.

Manna et al., summarized their fMRI research on meditation, [330]: "Meditation refers to a family of complex emotional and attentional regulatory practices, which can be classified into two main styles – focused attention (FA) and open monitoring (OM) – involving different attentional, cognitive monitoring and awareness processes. In a functional magnetic resonance study we originally characterized and contrasted FA and OM meditation forms within the same experiment, by an integrated FA–OM design. Theravada Buddhist monks, expert in both FA and OM meditation forms, and lay novices with 10 days of meditation practice, participated in the experiment. Our evidence suggests that expert meditators control cognitive engagement in conscious processing of sensory-related, thought and emotion contents, by massive self-regulation of fronto-parietal and insular areas in the left hemisphere, in a meditation state-dependent fashion. We also found that anterior cingulate and dorsolateral prefrontal cortices play antagonist roles in the executive control of the attention setting in meditation tasks."

Shergill et al., report their fMRI findings in the generation and perception of inner speech, [331]: "Monitoring one's thoughts (in the verbal modality) is thought to be critically dependent on the interaction between areas that generate and perceive inner speech in the frontal and temporal cortex, respectively. We used functional magnetic resonance imaging (fMRI) to examine the relationship between activities in these areas while the rate of inner speech generation was varied experimentally. The faster rate was associated with activation in the left inferior frontal gyrus, the right pre- and postcentral gyri and both superior temporal gyri. Thus, temporal cortical activation was associated with increasing the rate of covert articulation, in the absence of external auditory input, suggesting that there is effective fronto-temporal connectivity. Furthermore, this may provide support for the existence of feed forward models, which suggest that activity in regions responsible for verbal perception is modulated by activity in areas that generate inner speech."

Rubia et al., reorted an fMRI study of the maturation of self-cognitive control from childhood to mid-adulthood, [332]: "In this study, rapid, randomized, mixed-trial event-related fMRI was used to investigate developmental differences of the neural networks mediating a range of motor and cognitive inhibition functions in a sizeable number of adolescents and adults. Functional brain activation was compared between adolescents and adults during three different executive tasks measuring selective motor response inhibition (Go/no-go task), cognitive interference inhibition (Simon task), and attentional set shifting (Switch task). Adults compared with children showed increased brain activation in task-specific frontostriatal networks, including right orbital and mesial prefrontal cortex and caudate during the Go/no-go task, right mesial and inferior prefrontal cortex, parietal lobe, and putamen during the Switch task and left dorsolateral and inferior fronto-temporo-parietal regions and putamen during the Simon task. Whole-brain regression analyses with age across all subjects showed progressive age-related changes in similar and extended clusters of task-specific frontostriatal, frontotemporal, and frontoparietal networks. These findings suggest progressive maturation of task-specific frontostriatal and frontocortical networks for cognitive control functions in the transition from childhood to mid-adulthood."

Berman et al., reported the effects of typical childhood absence seizures on EEG, fMRI and behavior, [333]: "We performed EEG-fMRI with simultaneous behavioral testing in 37 children with typical childhood absence epilepsy (CAE). Attentional vigilance was evaluated by a continuous performance task (CPT), and simpler motor performance was evaluated by a repetitive tapping task (RTT). Results: Spike-Wave-Discharge (SWD) episodes were obtained during fMRI scanning from 9 patients among the 37 studied. The fMRI signal increases during SWDs were observed in the thalamus, frontal cortex, primary visual, auditory, somatosensory, and motor cortex, and fMRI decreases were seen in the lateral and medial parietal cortex, cingulate gyrus, and basal ganglia. Omission error rate (missed targets) with SWDs during fMRI was 81% on CPT and 39% on RTT."

In his article Feinberg, [334], presented a triadic neuro-hierarchical model of the self that proposed that the self could be understood as the product of three hierarchical anatomical systems: The intero-self system, the integrative self system, and the extero-sensorimotor system. An analysis of these three systems and their functional features indicated that the neural hierarchy possesses features of both non-nested and nested hierarchies that are necessary for the creation of a unified consciousness and self. These functional properties also make the central nervous system a biologically unique entity unlike anything else in nature.

Dehaene and Naccache, [335], reported three empirical observations of consciousness and a theoretical framework based on the global workspace: "We isolate three major empirical observations that any theory of consciousness should incorporate, namely (a) a considerable amount of processing is possible without consciousness, (b) attention is a prerequisite of consciousness, and (c) consciousness is required for some specific cognitive tasks, including those that require durable information maintenance, novel combinations of operations, or the spontaneous generation of intentional behavior. We then propose a theoretical framework that synthesizes those facts: the hypothesis of a global neuronal workspace. This framework postulates that, at any given time, many modular cerebral networks are active in parallel and process information in an unconscious manner. Information becomes conscious, however, if the neural population that represents it is mobilized by top-down attentional amplification into a brain-scale state of coherent activity that involves many neurons distributed throughout the brain. The long-distance connectivity of these 'workspace neurons' can, when they are active for a minimal duration, make the information available to a variety of processes including perceptual categorization, long-term memorization, evaluation, and intentional action. We postulate that this global availability of information through the workspace is what we subjectively experience as a conscious state."

Silva et al., [336], reported their interesting fMRI findings in patients with persistent vegetative state: "Global neuronal workspace theory predicts that damage to long-distance white matter tracts should impair access to conscious perception. During persistent vegetative state, we identified a hyper-metabolism in the ascending reticular activating system (ARAS) and impaired functional connectivity between the ARAS and the precuneus. This result emphasizes the functional link between cortices and brainstem in the genesis of perceptual awareness and strengthens the hypothesis that consciousness is based on a widespread neural network."

Vandekerckhove and Panksepp, [337], described three forms of consciousness namely, anoetic, noetic and autonoetic: "In recent years there has been an expansion of scientific work on consciousness. However, there is an increasing necessity to integrate evolutionary and interdisciplinary perspectives and to bring affective feelings more centrally into the overall discussion. Pursuant especially to the theorizing of Tulving, Panksepp and Vandekerckhove, we will look at the phenomena starting with primary-process consciousness, namely the rudimentary state of autonomic awareness or unknowing (anoetic) consciousness, with a fundamental form of first-person 'self-experience' which relies on affective experiential states and raw sensory and perceptual mental existences, to higher forms of knowing (noetic) and and self-aware (autonoetic) consciousness. Since current scientific approaches are most concerned with the understanding of higher declarative states of consciousness, we will focus on these vastly underestimated primary forms of consciousness, which may be foundational for all forms of higher "knowing consciousness."

Panksepp and Northoff, [338, 339], proposed a trans-species concept of the Core-SELF mediated by the cortical and subcortical mindline neural networks: "The nature of the self has been one of the central problems in philosophy and most recently in neuroscience. Here, we suggest that animals and humans share a 'core self' represented in homologous underlying neural networks. We argue that the core self might be constituted by an integrative neuronal mechanism that enables self-related processing (SRP). Because mammalian organisms are capable of relating bodily states, intrinsic brain states (e.g. basic attentional, emotional and motivational systems) and environmental stimuli to various life-supporting goal-orientations, SRP appears to be a core ability preserved across numerous species. Recent data suggest that SRP is operating via a central integrative neural system, made up of subcortical-cortical midline structures (SCMSs) that are homologous across mammalian species."

Kak, [340], has presented some interesting ideas from the computer and information sciences, as well as neurosciences perspective, about our conscious sense of being an agent for perception, cognition and action. He draws information and models, with mathematical equations, from the fields of quantum mechanics and quantum computing. He argues that living beings are quantum agents with quantum states, in biophysical cognitive systems. He concluded: "quantum computing ideas help us understand puzzling problems of mind's agency. Awareness is seen to be a property related to certain neural hardware interacting with a quantum field." Kak has also written extensively, about the historical aspects of the Vedic concepts from ancient India, of the gods-within, devas, as cognitive centers, the nature of mind, and consciousness [341, 342].

Kak, [343], in describing the holistic processing and quantum models, makes a valid case of looking at animal and human brains as quantum systems. "Although many processes that constitute the mind can be understood through the framework of neural networks, there are others that require a holistic basis. Furthermore, if each computation is seen as an operation by a reorganized brain on the signals at hand, this has a parallel with a quantum system where each measurement is represented by an operator. I also suggest that the macrostructure of the brain must be seen as a quantum system."

Damasio, [344], recently hypothesized about the role brain stem in the generation of protoself with primordial feelings: "I hypothesize that the first and most elementary product of protoself is primordial feelings, which occur spontaneously and continuously whenever one is awake. They provide a direct experience of one's own living body, wordless, unadorned, and connected to nothing but sheer existence. These primordial feelings reflect the current state of the body along varied dimensions, for example, along the scale that ranges from pleasure to pain, and they originate at the level of the brain stem rather than the cerebral cortex. All feelings of emotion are complex musical variations on primordial feelings."

This reminded me of the description of the primordial self, Ādi Puruṣ a by Śri Jñāneṣ wara in Jñāneṣ wari[4]. He described this primal existential being as continuous nitya, essential ṣ uddha, aware buddha, spontaneously independent svatantra, and unrelated to any object asanga. His insight was profound and quite revealing.

Finally, I would highly recommend a new neural network thinking and network approach to the integrative or holistic functions of the brain~mind. We need to learn from both approaches, namely, the neuron doctrine and the network doctrine. Olaf Sporns' new book, "Networks of the Brain" is a landmark publication in this new approach to understanding brain, mind and behavior. [345]. I would like to highlight a few quotations from this very important and timely book.

"Cognition is a network phenomenon. It does not exist in synapses or single neurons. Instead, it is a collective property of very large numbers of neural elements that are interconnected in complex patterns. [...] Cognition has an anatomical substrate. [...] Integration involves dynamic coordination (synchrony, coherence, linear and nonlinear coupling) as well as convergence. [...] Stimuli and cognitive tasks act as perturbations of existing network dynamics. Patterns of functional connectivity due to spontaneous neural activity are reconfigured in response to changes in sensory input or environmental demands."

AT THE SUMMIT

At the Summit,
The humanity comes together.
At Jungfraujoch in Switzerland,
The world came together.

I heard many languages,
German, French, Italian, Spanish,
English, Japanese, Hindi, Gujarathi,
And surprisingly,
Even my mother-tongue, Marathi.

The frquent laughters,
Sounded just as happy,
In all languages.
They needed no translation,
Nor any interpretation.
The natural joy was abundant
In the air.

I saw people from many nations.

[4] Dandekar SV. Translator. Sārtha Jñāneṣ wari (in Marathi). Pune, India; Joshi YG; 1953: XIII: 1069.

All of them were doing their usual activities,
And also exploring the place with enthusiasm.
They were getting along with each other,
With courtsey and mutual respect.

I saw many people,
Having fun in the snow,
Skiing, snow-boarding, snow-tubing,
Sliding down the cable rope,
Hiking and rock-climbing,
Or just throwing snowballs,
At each other and laughing.

At that times,
In my mind's summit,
There was a spontaneous joy,
And a timeless, serene Silence.
This is hard to describe.

All of our conscious moments,
Can potentially lead us
To this peaceful Summit-within.
It depends on the quality
Of our inner Presence,
Our mode of being.

The inner Summit
Lacks no-thing.

It is,
Where the whole Existence
Comes together,
In an astonishing Oneness.

One realizes,
'Now' is the timeless truth of
One's mind's Summit.

Vinod D Deshmukh

September 4, 2010

Chapter 45

In Closing

स्वयंज्योतिः बहुधा विभाति।

Swayaṁ jyotiḥ bahudhā vibhāti.

The flame of self-sentient energy~being~awareness manifests in various ways (forms and processes).

The following is a summary of my overall thinking~feeling, on this subject of holistic brain~energy~mind and consciousness~being~reality.

Bi-Modal Cosciousness: I think consciousness can be thought of as bi-modal, in the sense that it is both affective as well as cognitive. These affective and cognitive modes of consciousness are served by two major complementary subsystems of the brain, namely, the reticulo-limbic-cortical system and the reticulo-thalamo-cortico-striate, (multimodal associative) neocortical system. The affective mode is the first-person, primary, qualitative ("what it feels like to be…" or qualia mode), enduring, direct, prereflective, nondual, essential Self-feeling. The cognitive mode is the third-person, secondary or tertiary, episodic, subject-object dualistic, sequential, time-bound with memory associations, reflective, retrospective in the past and projective in the future, slow, intentional, deliberate, ego-centric, situational, and fluid. Like the analogy in my poem, "River and Lake," the affective mode is like the still, silent, serene lake or ocean, whereas, the cognitive mode is like the turbulent, ever-flowing river or the waves on the ocean. Meditation is about switching one's being, from the usually dominant, cognitive mode of egoistic thought-action-reaction orientation, to the unique, self-calming, self-healing, affective mode of Energy-Being-Bliss. Of course, one has to use both modes of being depending on what one is facing from moment-to-moment.

Tri-laminar Consciousness: Based on the three the receptor-action systems and the trilaminar embryonic development of the human organism, from three germinal layers. Our consciousness can be thought of as tri-laminar i.e., having three aspects of: i) Visceral-Autonomic-Interoceptive, ii) Somatic-Proprioceptive and iii) Environmental-Exteroceptive-Distant. The interoceptive-visceral consciousness includes sensations from and actions to, nasal mucosa, oro-pharynx, tongue, palate, saliva, trachea, larynx, chest, abdomimen and pelvic organs. The somatic-proprioceptive consciousness includes sensations from and instructions to all of the voluntary muscles, joints, bones, body surfaces, body positions and movements. The environmental-exteroceptive-distant consciousness includes signals from the peri-personal and distant environments like, gustatory (e.g., the forked tongue of a snake that has directional sense), olfactory e.g., large differential nostrils of a vultue, the alternating nasal and hemispheric cycles including the sleep-wake cycles of whales and other mammals as well as humans, differential visual fields and visual experience, and the differential, but spherical auditory field (some animals like bats, specialize in sonar detection and capture of small insects at very high speeds).

Every organism, including humans, obtain information about their body and its internal activities as well as the organism's outer environment, continuously, both subconsciously and consciously, by sensory receptor-action systems and their pathways, namely, interoceptors, proprioceptors, exteroceptors, and tele-receptors: i) the interoceptors mostly include all visceral sensations, plus olfaction and taste. ii) proprioceptors receive information from muscles, ligaments, and joints and thus, monitor the relative position of the body, limbs and the direction, force, and speed of all bodily movements. iii-a) the exteroceptors include the sensations of touch, temperature and pain and inform the organism of the immediate enironment that it is facing. iii-b) tele-receptors include specialized sensory systems, namely, olfaction, audition and vision for the perception, comprehension, and appropriate responses to distant events. It is truly amazing that the visual system can not only detect a single quantum of light, a photon in the dark, but can also see clearly on a bright day, when the retina is bombarded with over 1014 photons per second of Sunlight.

Our conscious experience can also be conceived as a unitary, neurophysiological field, which is subdivided into at least four segments, namely, interoceptive, proprioceptive, exteroceptive, and tele-ceptive, based on the source of the information that is being experienced. There are, of course, other ways of subdividing the unitary conscious field, namely, intrinsic-extrinsic, self-other, ego-world, figure-ground, center-surround etc. But, it is good to remember that all of these subdivisions have a reciprocal, inhibitory relationship. When the attended center is activated, the attentional surround is inhibited and vice-a-versa. Such selective attention with differential activation of the unitary conscious field is a matter of our observer-observed perspective and choice.

These three or four sensory-perceptual systems of awareness or "the doors of perception and knowledge" are analogous to Buddha's teachings of Anupāsanā, mindful presence. In Satipatthāna sūtta, four major ways of mindful awareness or presence are described: i) Kayānupāsanā - mindfulness of one's body's current state, position, and movement, ii) Vedanānupasanā - mindful awareness of one's present feelings, and emotions iii) Cittānupasanā - mindful awareness of thoughts and memories, and iv) Dhammānupasanā - mindful awareness of the current phenomenal events, [346].

I think to understand our own conscious experience and the world that we live in, understanding and appreciating the *energy-being perspective*, is absolutely crucial. It is a fact that all Life is embedded in the unified, Matter-Energy-Information Field. From Einstein's famous equation E = MC2, showing the equivalence of matter and energy, it is reasonable to consider both the material and energy perspectives of our conscious experience as equivalent. Matter, energy and information are three aspects of the same natural Reality. Matter-energy-information manifest at multiple levels of natural self-organization, including our own bio-physical body, mind, being and consciousness. Matter-energy-information transformation or transduction is evident in every biophysical event.

In *electrophysiology*, we have already established many mechanisms of energy transcduction, for instance, in sensory perception, brainstem and cortical evoked potentials, brainstem reticular activating system, electroencephalography, magneto-encephalography, electromyography, nerve conduction studies, electro-retinography, electrococleography, electrocardiography, electro-dermal response, deep brain stimulation, transcranial magnetic stimulation, and so on. Many of these neural, electromagnetic bio-fields are not only responsive to biophysical signals, but also to intentional, conscious mental events.

Sensory systems provide a continuous representation of the internal state of the body and the external world in a way that makes sense to the organism. Some of the neural mechanisms of sensory energy transduction are well described in neuroscience text books [347]. Neural epithelial membrane, in invertebrates and vertebrates, is endowed with properties that tranduce molecular-signal energy into electromagnetic field potentials. Living organisms are full of such elctromagnetic field activities and potentials. Such energy transductions occur, both within the organism as well as on the organismic surfaces that are in contact with its natural environment.

Some of the examples of sensory-motor signal and energy-transductions include:

i) *Photo-transduction* i.e., conversion of light energy, photons, into quanta of neural electromagnetic energy, in retinal rods and cones using pigment molecules and the isomerization of vitamin A.
ii) *Phono-transduction* i.e., conversion of auditory-accustic energy, phonons, into quantal, electrococlear auditory frequencies.
iii) *Olfactory transduction* i.e. conversion of odorant, molecular energy into quantal, neural electromagnetic energy. Such energy transformations are crucial for prey-predator interactions, food-selection, reproductive activities including signals used for attracting mates, identifying them, copulating, blocking pregnancy, facilitating nipple attachment by infants, infant identification, and social organization and mentation.
iv) *Taste transduction* i.e., conversion of molecular energy in food, water and air into quantal, neural electromagnetic energy. Ionic stimuli (H^+ ions or protons in acids, and Na^+ sodium ions in salts) interact directly to ion channels to activate the taste cells in the tongue, palate, and other oral sites. Protons utilize several mechanisms of energy-transduction i) amiloride-sensitive sodium channel, ii) proton-gated, acid-sensing, ion-channels, and iii) proton-modulated, hyperpolarizing cation-channels. More complex molecules like sugars and amino acids bind to receptor proteins that are coupled directly to ion-channels or indirectly through G-proteins and second messengers. Flavor perception includes sensory information from the olfactory, gustatory, and trigeminal sensory systems.
v) *Mechano-transduction* i.e., conversion of mechanical-vibrational energy into quantal, neural electromagnetic energy. Organisms are capable of detecting both remotely generated, mechanical perturbations in the environment (sounds and vibrations) and also the self-generated mechanical perturbations induced by body, limbs and vocal cord movements. Such a neuro-physical system is called acoustico-lateralis system and its basic energy-transduction unit is a modified epithelial cell called, "the hair cell." These hair cells directly transduce mechanical energy into quanta of neural electromagnetic energy.

The *feeling* of conscious arousal-energy-being, is the feeling of one's ability to act, to execute or to stop behavior and withold an action, a movement, speech, or cognition, at a given moment in time. It implies an intentional and selective activation or inhibition of any of these behaviors. It implies an expertise, a natural ease, and an excellence in cognitive self-control. Cognitive executive control is defined in neuroscience, as the ability to take charge of one's actions and direct them toward future aims. It may involve the use of working memory with online computations, keeping active mental representations of a problem, operating on that representation, storing the altered representation, and operating on that, and so on. [348].

Our feeling of arousal-energy-being can take three major forms: i) personal arousal-energy-being (visceral-somatic), ii) transpersonal or collective, group-arousal-energy-being, and iii) transcendental, holistic, holarchic, or existential Energy-Being. Pātañjali's Yoga-sutra advises mindful awareness training, in the self-regulation of one's own actions, behavior, and cognitive processes, using proactive cognitive inhibition, cittanirodha चित्तनिरोध and emotional equanimity, sthitaprajñā स्थितप्रज्ञा. Thus, realizing one's true self-energetic, self-effulgent, self-existent, blissful nature, naturally and spontaneously, is a wonder-in-itself.

The main goals of *meditation* are i) to become consciously aware of the present, ii) to let go of all subdivisions of the holistic, conscious field, and iii) to actually overcome such an artificial, and habitually maintained subdivision of this astonishing, unified field of consciousness; iv) meditation is about switching from the superficial, external-distant conscious functioning, to the deeper, internal-visceral, feeling-awareness of still, silent, serene energy-being, and then, to return to the enduring, global field of nondual, holistic and blissful energy~being~awareness. This unified field of consciousness is the wonder of all wonders. It can never be objectified, but it can be intrinsically, subjectively felt, as a transpersonal, nonpersonal or transcendental continuum Reality – an existential, unified field of self-sentient energy~being. Such a perspective may be called the holistic, eco-systemic, existential, or spiritual.

This has been described as a Blissful Conscious Being or Sat~Chit~Ānand, or a full blissful, superconscious existence, an existential fullness of being or Pūrṇ atā in Vedānta and no-thingness or Śunyatā in Buddhism, implying no division in the unified existential field. All life, including all of us, is integrally embedded in this single, unified, existential field of matter-energy-being-life-mind-spirit. It is an astonishingly complex one Reality, the Nature's incredible web. What name we give to it, is up to us, depending on our knowledge, experience, cultural background and subjective perspective.

Samādhi, Śamatā or Turīya, the super-consciousness is an extraordinary state of mental equipoise and nondual singularity. There is no subject-object duality in such a state, as there is no differential activation of that singular existential field of sentient matter-energy-being. Some people describe it as the transcendent or holistic awareness. Meditation is learning and developing the art of mental stillness, silence, and serenity and to live from our primal Source-Energy-Being.

True freedom is freedom from oneself, from one's ego. When one is free, it is natural to be happy. True understanding can only occur in the present moment. Let the Self-understanding dawn naturally. It will happen, when the mind is naturally silent, clear, ripe, receptive, and ready. Let it happen. One has to be totally and whole-heartedly aware of one's body-mind and existence, at each moment. One will be inspired and really understand one's true Nature and the natural surroundings. All virtues including meaning, purpose, love, care, and wisdom will blossom naturally, like a sweet Lotus in spring (painting on the back cover). When a single flower blossoms, the whole garden smiles! It is also good to remember that all of us are flowers of the same Tree of Life. Our sense of self-isolation and defensive individuality is a matter of our own making, due to our false perspectives and unrealistic fears. The Truth is ever-present, natural and spontaneous. It is for all of us to realize from moment to moment. No one has the monopoly on Truth and there are no intermediaries between us and the Reality. As J Krishnamurti said: "Truth is, when the self (ego) is not." As a Zen saying goes, "Don't put any Head above yours."

Realization of one's spontaneous infinite being entails understanding of our body-mind-being's spontaneity. It includes Self-awareness and self-realization of spontaneous breathing and its natural pause, spontaneous movements and rest, spontaneous silence and sounds, spontaneous energy-being and becoming, the spontaneous primal feeling, spontaneous existential awareness and Self-understanding, spontaneous peace and bliss, and spontaneous ever-present Existence! Such, persistent full awareness of our self and surroundings, increases our proactive inhibition and cognitive self-control, over all of our own mental and physical activities. We actualize self-mastery, mental excellence, creativity and expand our intrinsic awareness to limitless possibilities.

Realizing the silence-as-object and the silence-as-subject simultaneously, can lead to a sense of a non-dual, silent Being-in-Reality. Silence listening to silence! Silent energy-being realizing itself! Realizing of energy-as-object and energy-as-subject, can lead to a sense of a primal, singular field of living Energy-Being. Realization that one is that silent living Energy-Being, that infinite blissful being, that ever-fresh, but ever-the-same Perfection, depends on one's present mode of Energy-Being-Awareness.

There is one and only one *Truth*, Ekaṁevādvitiyam एकमेवाद्वितीयम्. This universal creative Energy – the only living Truth, Reality, or the Nature's Continuum, which includes all existential forms and processes, of all Life, including us. It is uninterrupted Energy, Akhaṇ ḍ a Śaktiḥ अखण्डशक्तिः, underlying all life-forms, processes and minds. We are intimately embedded in this Nature's matter-energy-information Continuum, this singular Field of spontaneous, creative Energy.

The *forms and the forming energy* are inseparable. The biophysical forms, including all organisms and humans, are inseparable from the morpho-regualtory energy, from the cellular level to the organismic and the ecosystemic levels. In 1991, the author proposed that the biological forms are not determined by a single set of molecules or processes, but by multiple forms of cascading morpho-regulatory energy acting on a network of molecules. [349]. The cascading morpho-regulatory energy was defined as the quantal, differential energy – internal minus external energy – that is acting on the biological form, at a given moment in time. This complex, composite energy may take quantal, fluid-mechanical, electro-chemical and electromagnetic patterns of flow, in space-time and create infinite variations of material forms, including the cosmos and the cosmic energy. This is comprehensible in terms of interchangeability of energy and matter as expressed in Einstein's equation, $E = MC^2$.

It is up to each one of us to realize such an astonishing ever-present truth, this Nature's amazing web of *energy and form*, within and around us. When one realizes this truth, one feels oneself to be an integral part of this amazing natural process, of this astonishing, singular continuum. Our essential conscious~energy~being in this one holistic Reality, has two fundamental aspects or properties: transience and continuum. We have to realize this mystery, this great wonder that is. Our astonishing brain is capable of realizing this great wonder with proper education, mental preparation, meditative training, right attitude, perceptual sensitivity, curiosity, honesty, willingness and persistence in self-inquiry, self-discovery and self-understanding. Such deep self-understanding with silent, serene presence will make us better students of Life; it will make us loving, caring parents and teachers and above all, compassionate and mindful human beings. That will be the true expression of our spirituality.

Finally, here is my short poem in Marathi, about the meditative process, self-understanding and self-freedom:

अनन्ताची सावली

श्वासाच्या तालावर,
स्वस्थ बसून, स्वानंदात,
स्वनिष्ठ, व स्वतंत्र व्हावे,
आणि अनंताच्या सावलीत रमावे.

Ṣ wāsāchya tālāwara, Swastha basūn, Swānandāta,
Swanishṭ ha va Swatantra vhāve, āṇ i anantācyā sāwalīta ramāwe.

In the presence of the Infinite

During meditation, one should follow the natural rhythm of breathing. Sit still, silent,
serene and be at-ease with self and surroundings. Smile with an unconditional bliss.
Abide firmly in the natural feeling of conscious~energy~being and be absolutely free!
Renew and rejoice in the self-supportive presence of the *Infinite*.

Life is sacred. Nature is sacred. Self is sacred.
Existence is infinite. Present is timeless.
We should not fragment it,
But, appreciate its oneness,
The one holistic Reality,
Paripūrṇ a Sat
परिपूर्ण सत्,
One Existence,
Ekaṁ Sat
एकं सत्
One Energy~Awareness,
Ekaṁ Citśaktiḥ
एकं चित्शक्तिः !

Happiness Smiles!

Sleep ends.

Arousal rises to awareness.
Awareness attends to itself,
And Self-awareness smiles.

Night ends.

The sun rises to its glory,
All life feels energized, and smiles happily.

Storm dies.

The quiet lake reflects
The passing clouds and the blue sky.
The "mirror-like" lake smiles, at itself.

Arguments end.

People start listening to self and others,
And agree to make peace.

Oppression ends.

Liberty rings.
People get together and create
Friendship, goodwill, and justice.

Fear of dying ends.

Suffering ends.

Insightful Life
Realizes its own Wonder.

Life blossoms, fruits,
And smiles at itself,
In this astonishingly
Live Universe!

Vinod D Deshmukh

July 4th 2010

APPENDIX 1: FUNCTIONAL NEUROANATOMY

A BRIEF REVIEW

Homunculus is the representational image of a “dwarf man” on the surface of both cerebral hemispheres. Homuncular reprentation is somatotopic, in the sense that the amount of neural space devoted to a part of the body e.g., hand, depends upon its use and location. Somatotopic organization is evident at many levels of the central nervous system, including spinal cord, cerebellum, thalamus and the cerebral cortex. In the homuncular map, there are regions dedicated to tongue, lips, mouth, swallowing, salivation, vocalisation, eyes, head, shoulders, arms, hands, chest, abdomen, pelvis, genitals and perineum.

Functional dichotomies of left and right cerebral hemispheric dominance: Left cerebral hemisphere mediates verbal, serial, analytic, controlled, logical, propositional, rational and social functions. The right cerebral hemisphere mediates nonverbal, parallel, holistic, creative, pictorial, appositional, intuitive, and physical functions [350].

The term attention refers to that part of the cognitive apparatus that allows an individual to focus on selected features of sensory stimuli and ideas while keeping potentially distracting stimuli at-bay [351]. Attention depends on the interaction of four processes: a) attentional capacity, b) selective attention, c) response selection and executive control, and d) sustained attention. Attentional capacity governs both the amount of information that can be handled and the intensity of cognitive processing. Attentional capacity fluctuates over time. It depends on extrinsic factors such as the perceived value of stimuli and prevailing response demands, and intrinsic processes such as energetic and structural factors. Energetic factors include arousal, affective state, drive and motivation. Structural factors include processing speed, memory capacity, spatial and temporal dynamics of the system. A central feature of the physiology of attention is the orienting response. It is the initial reaction of an animal to a novel stimulus and it is characterized by activation in autonomic and motor behavioral activity with related brain electromagnetic activity.

Models of Attention: Mesulam (1985) subdivided attention into two major categories: matrix or state function and vector or channel function. Matrix function regulates overall information processing capacity, detection efficiency, focusing power, and vigilance, which is primarily associated with the Reticular Activating System (RAS). The vector function regulates the direction or target of selective attention and it is associated with neocortical systems. These two systems are functionally integrated and usually work together.

Heilman and colleagues (1993) developed a model of a cortico-limbic-reticular formation network. Posner and Cohen (1984) proposed a two process model of attention. The cingulate cortex is responsible for the intensity of attentional focus, whereas the parietal cortex is involved in covert disengagement of attention. The RAS plays a major role in modulating arousal and provides global regulation of attentional tone for the forebrain. The RAS-thalamic input to cortex provides nonspecific priming for attention. The intensity of arousal and direction of attention are strongly influenced by the hypothalamus through its regulation of the circadian rhythms and its modulation of the approach function with appetitive behavior.

The frontal lobe is an essential component of the attentional matrix. The prefrontal cortex is linked to the subcortical structures by three neural networks, which are involved in the executive control of attention and cognition. These functions include intention, response initiation, inhibition, persistence, and switching. These processes are central to the planning and generation of goal-directed behavior. The dorsolateral prefrontal cortical network is involved in working memory, temporal sequencing of information, generating response alternatives, and maintaining response flexibility. The orbitomedial prefrontal network modulates impulses, mood, and working memory. The anterior cingulate network plays a major role in drive and motivation.

Consciousness represents the core of our experience as human beings, and its alteration challenge our concepts of self and meaning or value of life [352, 353]. Consciousness involves that set of neural processes that allow an individual to perceive, comprehend, and act on the internal and external environments. It is usually envisioned in three parts: arousal, awareness and attention. Arousal describes the degree to which the individual appears to be able to interact with these environments. Awareness reflects the depth and the content of the aroused state. Awareness implies that the individual is not only alert but also cognizant of self and surroundings. Awareness depends on arousal. It does not imply any specificity for the modality of stimulation. Attention depends upon awareness and implies the ability to respond to particular types of stimuli (modality specific).

Anatomy of arousal, awareness, and attention: Arousal requires the interplay of both the reticular formation and the cerebral hemispheres. The clusters of neurons that are essential for conscious arousal are present in the reticular formation of the upper pons, midbrain and diencephalon. The brainstem reticular formation may be viewed as a driving center for the higher structures and functions. There are three principal paths that project from the midbrain reticular activating system to: a) the thalamic reticular nucleus and then to the cortex, b) the hypothalamus and then to the basal forebrain and limbic system, and c) the brain stem median raphe and locus coeruleus with subsequent diffuse cortical projections.

Awareness is a higher cortical function. It implies that the individual is not only alert but also cognizant of self and surroundings. Interaction of the cerebral cortex and the reticular system is required for the individual to be aware.

Attention to specific aspects of the perceived universe depends on both awareness as a general property and function of the specific anatomical structures that mediate the sensory phenomena involved. The posterior parietal cortex is dominant for bilateral, global attention.

Mood is the term used to describe a sustained internal emotion and should be distinguished from affect, which is more fluid, changing from moment to moment [354]. The spectrum of mood is enormous, and each different mood is colored in a multitude of gradations and shades. The most obvious moods are sadness, joy, anger, and grief. Different moods can coexist. Affect generally refers to the external expression of emotional content.

Emotional experience connotes the whole range of human feelings including anxiety, fear, apathy, euphoria, depression, sadness, anger, and grief. Emotional expression or affect may be mood congruent or incongruent.

Thought is in many ways unrelated to mood or emotions. Thought is considered in terms of the process of thinking and also its content.

The anatomy of mood, emotion, and thought involves the limbic system and the temporal and frontal lobes. The two main divisions of the limbic system are a) an orbito-frontal-amygdala, involved in emotional associations and appetites and b) a hippocampus-cingulate network, serving mnemonic and attentional activities.

A neural network involving amygdala, hypothalamus, and brain stem visceral nuclei mediate fear and "fight or flight" response. The temporal lobes are involved in several functions such as introversion (right temporal), extroversion (left temporal), euphoria, sadness, anger, guilt, hypermoralism, religiosity, hypergraphia, and passivity.

The frontal lobes serve as the "central executive" of the brain and personality, acting to process, integrate, inhibit, assimilate, and remember perceptions and impulses received by the neocortical sensory areas, the limbic system and the striatum. It can be divided into a) precentral consisting of motor and premotor cortex, b) prefrontal cortex, and c) limbic cortex. Prefrontal limbic networks can be further divided into a) dorsolateral prefrontal-subcortical circuit appears to be involved in executive functions including supervision of other brain functions related to developing and implementing a plan, b) the orbitofrontal-subcortical circuit is necessary for social behavior and inhibition of inappropriate activities, and c) medial frontal-subcortical circuit, which is involved in motivation.

The central norepinephrine neurons known as locus coeruleus are about 12,000 in number. They have three major ascending tracts: a) the central gray dorsal longitudinal fasciculus, b) the central tegmental fasciculus, and c) the ventral tegmental-medial forebrain bundle tracts. These tracts innervate all areas of the cerebral cortex as well as specific thalamic and hypothalamic nuclei, and the olfactory bulb. A fourth tract ascends to innervate the cerebellar cortex, whereas the fifth fascicle descends into the mesencephalon and spinal cord; although largely ipsilateral, approximately one-fourth of the fibres cross to the other side, in some animals.

These central norepinephrine neurons have been thought to be involved in many neurophysiologic functions including arousal, novelty-processing, learning, memory, sleep-wake regulation, anxiety and nociception, as well as affective psychosis. In the catecholaminergic theory of affective disorders, it is hypothesized that depression may be related to deficiency of catecholamine at important CNS receptors, whereas mania is associated with an excess catecholaminergic state.

The long-length dopaminergic system connects brainstem nuclei of the ventral Tegmentum and Substantia nigra to the caudate-putamen (nigro-striatal) and limbic-cortical system (mesocortical-mesolimbic). This long-tract neural system is important in motor control, mood, emotion, and cognitive processes. The dopaminergic function is impaired in Parkinson's disease.

The brain stem serotonin neurons have rostral and caudal groups. The rostral group projects to the limbic forebrain, thalamus, neo-striatum, and cerebellum. The caudal group projects to brainstem and spinal cord. The serotoninergic system is involved in a wide variety of homeostatic function including sleep-wake cycle, affective and aggressive states. Low level of serotonin in brain may be associated with depression and suicide, which is typically treated with anti depressant drugs that raise the serotonin level in the brain.

Memory is the recording, retention, and retrieval of knowledge [355]. Acetyl choline is the neurotransmitter that is essential for memory processes. In Alzheimer's disease, there is a degeneration of central cholinergic neurons and loss of their memory function. It accounts for all knowledge gained from experience – known facts, remembered events, and learned skills. Memory can be declarative, explicit or conscious-intentional, and non-declarative, implicit, or unconscious-unintentional. Immediate memory refers to the recall of information without delay, either immediately after presentation or after uninterrupted rehearsal. Working memory is a multi-component psychological system that mediates the temporary processing and storage of internal representations that guide and control actions. Information is held in working memory only as long as it is useful for solving the problem at hand.

Long-term memory refers to permanent and large stores of episodic and semantic memories. They are constantly used to interpret new experiences. Long-term memory is organized by meaning (semantics) or gist rather than by perceptual characteristics of experience.

Cognition refers to the mental process of knowing, including high level perception, language and reasoning. Cognitive process may be dichotomized as crystallized or fluid. The crystallized cognitive processes involve the application of well-established knowledge and skills, whereas, the fluid cognitive processes involve the application of working memory, and a novel strategy in reasoning and problem solving. Verbal and spatial cognition are processed in different regions of the brain.

The anatomy of emotional memory includes the Papez circuit. The declarative memory depends on the interaction between domain-specific neocortical regions and the domain-independent medial temporal, diencephalic and basal forebrain regions. The medial temporal region includes amygdala, hippocampus, the entorhinal cortex, perirhinal cortex and the parahippocampal cortex. The diencephalic structures include dorsomedial and anterior thalamic nuclei, and the mammilary bodies with their interconnecting tracts. The basal forebrain structures include septal nuclei, diagonal band of Broca, and Substantia innominata. These regions provide the largest input of acetyl choline, which is implicated in memory disorders such as Alzheimer's disease. Other neurotransmitters like norepinephrine, dopamine, and serotonin are also involved in memory processing.

Immediate memory depends on the posterior temporo-occipito-parietal (TOP) areas. The auditory memories are processed by the temporo-parietal regions, whereas the visual memories are processed by the occipito-parietal regions. The left hemispheric regions specialize in processing of verbal memories, whereas, the right hemispheric regions specialize in processing of nonverbal spatial memories.

Speech is the ability to vocalize by coordinating the muscles controlling the vocal phonatory apparatus [356]. It is the mechanical aspect of oral communication. Language refers to symbolic communication. It provides the ability to converse, comprehend, repeat, read and write.

Anatomy of speech (Normal phonation and articulation): Normal speech involves a highly coordinated sequence of contractions of the respiratory musculature, larynx, pharynx, tongue and lips. These muscles are innervated by the facial, vagal, hypoglossal and phrenic nerves. The brain stem nuclei of these nerves are controlled directly by the motor cortices through the cortico-bulbar tracts and indirectly through the basal ganglia and cerebellum. The basal ganglia and cerebellum are also important participants in producing the prosodic aspect of speech, including pitch or frequency, stress or differential emphasis placed on syllables, and rhythm or timing.

Language processes are lateralized to the dominant, usually the left hemisphere. Four areas are involved in the comprehension of spoken language: a) receptive auditory area (Heschl's gyrus), b) perceptive auditory association cortex (Wernicke's area), c) semantic angular gyrus area, and d) syntactical inferior frontal cortex (Broca's area). The semantic area, in addition to the interpretation of meaning, also relates the sound to other incoming words, other sensory modalities, and past experience. Broca's area initiates a motor plan that is transmitted to the motor cortex to pronounce the words. The motor cortex, in coordination with the supplementary motor area, basal ganglia and cerebellum, sends cortico-bulbar fibres to implant speech sounds.

The dominance of the right hemisphere in the processing of affective prosody is well supported by lesion studies and functional imaging data. The ability to convey emotional meaning by speech, facial expressions and gestures is a function of the right inferior frontal lobe. The perception of affective components of communication is a function of the posterior areas of the right hemisphere. The striatum is involved in speech output and prosody. The thalamus is important for cortical arousal and language comprehension. The subcortical white matter interconnects language areas.

The olfactory is the first cranial nerve. It constitutes the primary receptor cells for the sense of smell [357]. Along with the sense of taste, it determines the flavor and palatability of foods and beverages. It also warns of spoiled foods, leaking natural gas, polluted air, and smoke. It mediates elements of basic communication e.g., mother-infant bonding. The primary olfactory cortex includes the anterior olfactory nucleus, the olfactory tubercle, the piriform cortex, the anterior cortical nucleus of amygdala, the periamygdaloid complex and the rostral entorhinal cortex. The primary olfactory cortex is reciprocally connected with orbitofrontal cortex, dorsomedial and submedial thalamic nuclei, amygdala, hippocampus, and the lateral hypothalamus.

The optic nerve is the second cranial nerve for visual processing. The oculomotor system with cranial nerves III, IV, and VI and their innervated muscles, which are involved in moving the eyes to allow visual inspection of objects [358]. The act of positioning the image of an object on the retinal fovea, which is the locus of highest visual acuity and the psychological center of visual field, is referred to as fixation. Fusion denotes the primitive reflex action, organized within the CNS, in which the visual axes of the two eyes are made to converge on a single object of regard.

The saccade movements are rapid eye movements with gaze shift. Anatomy of the saccade system includes a) brainstem reticular formation. Midbrain for vertical saccades and Parapontine reticular formation for horizontal saccades, b) superior colliculus for saccade relay, c) parietal eye field for reflexive visual exploration, d) frontal eye field for central fixation and intentional visual exploration, e) supplementary motor area for motor programs, f) hippocampal formation for memory, g) vestibular cortex for vestibular information, and h) prefrontal cortex for inhibition, spatial memory and prediction.

The Vestibulo-Cochlear system for hearing and balance is the VIII cranial nerve: Sound consists of sinusoidal waves of air pressure. Hearing is the perception of sound [361]. The understanding of speech depends on the perception of complex, time-varying multi-frequency sounds. Hearing is possible when the sound of adequate intensity is of audible frequency between 20 Hz to 20,000 Hz. The vestibular nerve system consists of three components of angular and linear velocity detectors for any head movement. It is responsible for maintaining balance during movement.

The nuclei of Glossopharyngeal (IX) and Vagus (X) cranial nerves, [359], are in the medulla and they serve motor, sensory and autonomic functions. Glossopharyngeal nerve receives taste sensation from the posterior third of the tongue, sensorimotor information to and from larynx and pharynx, tongue, auditory meatus, tympanic membrane, baroreceptors from carotid sinus, and chemoreceptors from carotid body. The Vagus nerve has sensorimotor connections with larynx and pharynx, and it subserves esophageal peristalsis, heart rate and blood pressure, gastric secretion, and bowel motility.

The central autonomic network (CAN) integrates visceral, humoral and environmental information to produce coordinated autonomic, neuro-endocrine, and behavioral responses to external and internal stimuli [360]. Within the CAN, there is segmental and regional specialization for the control of autonomic functions. A coordinated response is generated through interconnections among the amygdala and the neocortex, basal forebrain, ventral striatum, hypothalamus, and autonomic and somatic motor nuclei of the brain stem.

The insular and medial prefrontal cortex (paralimbic areas) and the nuclei of the amygdala are the higher centers involved in processing visceral information and the initiation of integrated autonomic responses [361]. Insular cortex is the primary viscero-sensory cortex and receives viscero-topically organized sensory information from visceral receptors including arterial chemoreceptors and baroreceptors. When insula and anterior cingulate cortex are activated by nociceptive input and then autonomic response associated with affective behavior, is initiated. The amygdala receives exteroceptive and interoceptive information and provides its emotional significance. The central nucleus of amygdala projects to the hypothalamus, periaqueductal gray, and the autonomic nuclei of the brain stem to integrate autonomic, endocrine, and motor response to emotionally relevant stimuli.

Hypothalamus integrates the autonomic and endocrine responses that are critical for homeostasis. It is functionally divided into three longitudinal zones: a) paraventricular zone involved in autonomic, circadian, and endocrine functions; b) medial zone is involved in osmo-regulation, thermoregulation, and sexual function; and c) a lateral zone is involved in behavioral arousal and motivated behavior.

The paraventricular hypothalamic nucleus is the site of integrated autonomic and neuro-endocrine responses to stress. The medial preoptic nucleus contains thermo-sensitive neurons including warm-sensitive and cold-sensitive neurons that initiate appropriate responses to changes in body temperature. The lateral hypothalamic area participates in arousal, motivated motor and autonomic control. Some neurons of this region synthesize orexin or hypocretin and project to cholinergic and monoaminergic regions of the brain stem, which regulate rapid eye movement sleep. The lateral hypothalamic neurons as well as the neurons in the ventromedial hypothalamus, including the arcuate nucleus, are the targets of leptin, which is a hormone secreted by adipose tissue in response to food intake. Leptin directly activates arcuate nuclei to inhibit food intake and simultaneously inactivates neurons of the lateral hypothalamus that ordinarily increase food intake. The hypothalamic autonomic pathways descend ipsilaterally to the dorsomedial and ventrolateral tegmentum of the brain stem.

Periaqueductal gray matter (PAG) of midbrain is the site of autonomic, behavioral and antinociceptive stress response. The lateral PAG mediates sympatho-excitation, opiod-independent analgesia, and motor response consistent with flight-or-fight reaction. The ventrolateral PAG produces sympatho-inhibition, opiod-dependent analgesia, and motor inhibition. PAG constitutes a critical relay station for the micturition reflex.

Brainstem neurons in the medulla are critical for the control of cardiovascular, respiratory, and gastrointestinal functions. The nucleus of the solitary tract (NTS) along with the medullary reticular formation generates and integrates respiratory rhythm (ventral respiratory group), cardiovagal outflow (nucleus ambiguus) and sympatho-excitatory outflow. This medullary reticular network is also involved in functions of swallowing, vomiting, coughing and sneezing. The descending reticulo-spinal pathways run in the ventral half of the lateral columns of the spinal cord, and produce autonomic control of breathing and blood pressure, as well as sweating and micturition.

The thoraco-lumbar sympathetic outflow is from T1-L3 spinal levels. The parasympathetic cranial outflow is through cranial nerves III, VII, IX and X, and the sacral outflow is from S2-S4. The sacral parasympathetic outflow is from S2 –S4. It is critical for defecation, micturition, and sexual (penile/clitoral) erection.

APPENDIX 2:
36 OBSERVABLE ELEMENTS OF THE EXPERIENTIAL FIELD, KSHETRA

FIVE NATURAL ELEMENTS, PAÑCA MAHĀ BHUTA:

1) Pṛ ithivī पृथिवी, Earth, Solids, Foods, Bio-Molecules.
2) Āpa आप, Water, Ocean, Rain, River, Moisture.
3) Vāyu वायु, Air, Atmosphere, Wind, Oxygen, Nitrogen, Carbon dioxide.
4) Teja तेज, Light, Heat, Sound, Biophysical Energy: Photo-Electric, Phono-Electric, Electro-Chemical, Iono-Magnetic, Neuro-behavioral arousal-energy, Muscular, Bio-Mechanical, Cognitive-Mental, Emotional, Psychic, Spiritual-Existential energy.
5) Ākāśa आकाश, Space, Field of Existence, Cosmos, Universe, also personal, intrapersonal, peripersonal, and extrapersonal space of a living organism.

FIVE SENSORY ORGANS, JÑANENDRIYA:

1) Eyes for vision.
2) Ears for hearing.
3) Skin for touch, mouth for swallowing, and face for expressions.
4) Nose for olfaction.
5) Tongue for tasting.

FIVE SENSORY EXPERIENCES, TANMĀTRA:

1) Seeing, Looking, Vision.
2) Hearing, Listening, Audition.
3) Touch, Temperature, Pain, Pleasure.
4) Sense of Smell, Olfaction, Odor.

5) Taste, Flavor, sweet, salty, sour, bitter.

TEN MOTOR ORGANS, KARMENDRIYA AND THEIR ACTIONS:

1) Face-Mouth-Nose: Swallowing, Eating, Drinking, Breathing, Sniffing, Speaking, Singing, Expressing, Gesturing, Communicating.
2) Hands: Holding, Gripping, Lifting, Touching, Throwing, Fighting, Caring.
3) Feet: Standing, Walking, Running, Swimming, Kicking, Jumping.
4) Genitory Organs: Sexuality, Reproduction.
5) Excretory Organs: Urination, Defecation.

FOUR MENTAL ORGANS, ANTAḤKARAṆA:

1) Citta चित्त Memory: Working Memory, Episodic or Event Memory, Autobiographical Memory, Procedural or Skills Memory, Semantic or General Memory, Emotional Memory.
2) Manas मन Minding, Mentation, Perception-Cognition-Comprehension, Thinking in Sounds-Gestures-Images, Sequencing, Imagining, Forecasting, Planning, Creating.
3) Buddhi बुद्धि Intelligence, Discrimination, Decision-Making, Choosing, Denying, Self-restraining, Letting go.
4) Ahamkāra अहंकार I-Me-Mine, Ego, Self-Image, Self-Identity, Self-Role, Self-Pride, Self-Agency, Doer-ship, Enjoyer, Sufferer, Volition, Will, Intentionality, Recalling, Goal-Directedness.

SEVEN ADDITIONAL ELEMENTS

Desire, pleasure, pain, hatred, intelligence, fortitude and the aggregate integration of an organism.

Bhagavad Gītā and Jñāneṣ wari chapter XIII: 5-6

APPENDIX 3: ADDITIONAL QUOTATIONS FROM VEDĀS, UPANIṢADS, AND BHAGAVAD GĪTĀ

"Realization of existential Being: When a person, having perceived all creatures (forms) from all directions of the world, dwells perseveringly upon the very first (primal) perception (impression) or basal Awareness, then he or she enters into the core Being by self."

Yajur Veda 32:11.

"I cannot travel to the Truth of the luminous Being by force (deliberate effort) or by duality."

Ṛig Veda 5:12.

"The Supreme Being: The enlightened person perceives within himself the supreme Being, in which the universe has its existence. The universe emerges to a form at the time of creation and returns to a subtle form at the time of dissolution. This supreme Being pervades through and through all forms, like the warp and woof."

Yajur Veda 32:8.

"There is no true image of that glorious Being."

Yajur Veda 32:3.

"One who knows the finite, talks excessively. One, who knows the Infinite, stays Silent."

Yajur Veda 30:19.

"The self alone existed in the beginning in the shape of being, Puruṣ a पुरुष. He, looking around saw no one else but his self. He first uttered, "I am." Hence, he got the name of "Aham, I."

Brihadāraṇ yakopaniṣ ad बृहदारण्यकोपनिषद् 1:4:1.

"Let him realize that one, who is omnipresent, who can't be heard, (who is) unapproachable, unthought of, uncontrolled, invisible, unknowable, and undefined listener, seer, thinker, instructor, proclaimer, knower, intelligence, and the intrinsic self, Antaryāmi अन्तर्यामि of all created beings, is his true self."

Aitareya Upaniṣ ad ऐतरेय उपनिषद् 3:2:4.

"This Ātman is not to be obtained by many explanations, or by intellect, or by much learning. To him, who is receptive, Ātman reveals its true nature (by Itself)."

Kaṭ hopaniṣ ad कठोपनिषद् 2:23.

"Higher than sensorium is mind; higher than mind is intellect; higher than intellect is Jīva (ego); higher than jīva is the unmanifest (subconscious); higher than the unmanifest is the primal Being, Puruṣa, who is all-pervasive, has no attributes, whom having comprehended; a man becomes liberated and fearless."

Kaṭ hopaniṣ ad 6:7 and 8.

"He can reach fast and grasp without hands or feet. He can see without eyes. He can hear without ears. He knows all that is knowable, but there is no knower of his. They speak of him as the great primal Being."

Ṣ wetāṣ watara Upaniṣ ad ष्वेताष्वतर उपनिषद् 3:19.

"There is one Self-luminous Being, hidden in the Heart of all creatures, pervading all, the innermost Self of all, the Organizer of all, the Witness, the existential Awareness without any (specifiable) qualities."

Ṣ wetāṣ watara Upaniṣ ad 6:11.

"He who is the eternal, ever-lasting, the Awareness of awareness, the creator of all desires, having known that (primal) cause by Self-understanding and Self-discipline, one becomes free from all (psychological) limitations."

Ṣ wetāṣ watara Upaniṣ ad 6:13.

"Let one know the speaker, not just speech; the seer, not just sights; the listener, not just sounds; the experiencer of smells, not just odors; the enjoyer of foods, not just tastes; the doer, not just deeds; the experiencer of pain and pleasure, not just pains and pleasures; the enjoyer of sexual union, not just sexual union; the mover, not just movements; the thinker, not just thoughts; It is my Self. It is the essential Being. Know this."

Kauṣ ītakī Upaniṣ ad कौषीतकी उपनिषद् 3:8.

"Know him to be the *Ātman*, ever-shining. He is free from ignorance and all bonds. He is Self-existent and full of bliss. He has grown out of the idea of duality. His individual "I" has merged in the existential Consciousness itself."

Brahmopaniṣ ad ब्रह्मोपनिषद्.147.

भूः भुवः स्वः तत्सवितुर्वरेण्यम् |
भर्गो देवस्य धीमहि धियोयोनः प्रचोदयात् ||

We meditate on that supreme effulgence of the radiant energy~being~awareness within, the indwelling teacher, within all beings. May It inspire and spark our intellect.

ष्लोकार्धेन प्रवक्षामि यदुक्तं ग्रन्थ कोटिभिः |
ब्रह्म सत्यम्जगन्मिथ्या जीवो ब्रह्मैव नापरः ||

I will declare the essential Truth in half a stanza, which has been elaborated, in thousands of books: The Absolute is the Truth. The experienced world is a mere representation or an image. An individual being is none other than the Absolute.

नाना उपाधिवशात् एव जातिवर्णाश्रमादय: |
आत्मनि आरोपितास्तोये रसवर्णादिभेदवत् ||
आदि शङ्कराचार्य, आत्मबोध ११.

Only on account of diverse superimpositions like caste, color, stage in life etc, does the Ātman feels different, just as the pure water that is tainted by different colors, and flavors.
Adi Śankarāchārya, Ātmabodha 11.

अनादित्वान्निर्गुणत्वात्परमात्मा अयं अव्ययः |
शरीरस्थोऽअपि कौन्तेय न करोति न लिप्यते |३१|
Bhagavad Gītā, chapter 13:31

Being without beginning and devoid of specific characteristics (gunas), the non-dissipating, transcendent Being, though existing in the body-mind-existence, neither acts nor is affected by anything or any event.

APPENDIX 4: PRESENCE: A NEW MODE OF HUMAN ATTENTION

AN ABSTRACT

It is proposed that human attention has two fundamentally different modes. The commonly recognized human attention is called 'Mnemic' and the 'New' mode of attention is called 'Presence.' The word 'mnemic' means of or related to memory. In the mnemic mode of attention, there is focussing or directing of partial attention, to a particular object in the environment. There are habitual cognitive and emotional responses, based on memory, that constantly interfere during the mnemic mode of human attantion. This also creates the observer-observed duality, and the experience of personal time and change. It creates, sustains and adds to the ego-image. It always limits perceptivity, attentional energy, intelligence and the feeling of goodness or natural happiness.

The 'New' mode on the other hand, is ever-new. It is not contaminated by the past memories. It is complete, participant attention to the present, now-and-here. It is free of any habitual cognitive or emotional responses. It is free of self-image, with no interference with the present human activity. There is no division as 'I' and the 'rest' or 'not-I." There is no projection into the future, based on the past. It implies tremendous, frictionless, conflictless attentional energy, intelligence, a feeling of self-freedom and natural goodness. Since, it is completely 'one' with the present – what is, it is named as the state of Presence.

An hourglass model of observer and the observed is presented to explain the functioning of mnemic and new modes of participant attention. This model and above modes of attention also help to understand and to resolve the problem of Brain-Mind duality in Neurosciences.

(An Abstract from: Deshmukh VD. Society for Neuroscience Abstracts; 1982: vol. 8).

APPENDIX 5: FUNCTIONAL BRAIN MODEL

Table 1. The Invertebrate Brain and Behavior

Invertebrate Phyla	**Invertebrate Brain structures**	Invertebrate Behavior
Porifera: Sponges.	Neuroid system: No true nervous systems but these organisms have generalized contractile ability through the syncytial trabecular tissue.	Any mechanical stimulus anywhere on the epithelium spreads by electrotonic conduction with a diffuse motor response. Epithelial conduction velocity 3-35 cm/s
Cnidaria: Hydra, Jellyfish, Sea Anemones, Hydromedusae.	Nerve nets: Diffuse two-dimensional plexus of two or multipolar neurons. Sensory ganglia and giant fiber nerve net for global motor response.	Behaviors include feeding, swimming, climbing, burrowing and intra-species aggression. Neural conduction velocity 10-100 cm/s. Chemical neurotransmission including dopamine, 5-Hydroxytryptamine.
The Worms, Platyhelminthes, Nematoda and Annelida: Flatworms, Flukes Tapeworms, and Segmented worms, Earthworms, Leeches.	Suprapharyngeal and Subpharyngeal ganglia connected by circum pharyngeal connectives or ring. Orthogonal pattern of paired nerve cords and commissures.	Subpharyngeal ganglion mediates behaviors like feeding, but the suprapharyngeal ganglion receives and integrates sensory information and makes an appropriate behavioral decision and takes action in the given circumstance.
Arthropoda, Brachipoda: Arthropods, Trilobites, Shrimps, Crabs, Spiders, Scorpions, Millipedes, Centipedes and Insects.	Suprapharyngeal complex with a) Protocerebrum with Neurosecretory cells and Optic lobes, b) Deutocerebrum with antennal nerves and c) Tritocerebrum. Subpharyngeal ganglion and Hypocerebral ganglion	Suprapharyngeal complex modulates the activities of the Subpharyngeal and Hypopharyngeal ganglia, based on sensory input and its integration. Subpharyngeal ganglia control mouthparts, local musculature and salivary glands. Hypocerebral ganglion controls endocrine functions, growth and metamorphosis. Memory and associative learning in Honeybees.
Mollusca, Gastropoda, Cephalopoda: Molluscs, Snails and Slugs, Clams, Shells, Squids, Nautilus and Octopuses.	The brain of an Octopus consists of 15 structurally and functionally distinct pairs of structures including cerebral lobes viz. optic, vertical, frontal, buccal, brachial and pedal.	Modality specific pathways and associative learning, e.g. visual, tactile. Memory traces plus formation of a coded representation of a situation with the ability to generalize from one subject to a similar one.

Table 2. The Vertebrate Oro-Pharyngeal Brain and Behavior

NHP Organizational Level and Neural Structures	Related Cranial Nerves	Mediated Functional Behavior	Motor Responses and Actions	Sensory and Memory Guidance
I Medulla, Myelencephalon-Rhombencephalon, Medullary Reticular Formation (MRF) Hypoglossal n, Dorsal Vagus n, Ambiguus n, Gracile n, Cuneatus n, Raphe n.	Hypoglossal, Accessory, Vagus and Glossopharyngeal Nerves	Reflex Behavior: Regulation of Energy intake, Homeostasis: Cardiovascular, Respiratory and Swallowing behavior, Reflex Phonation and vocalization	Central Autonomic Regulation with Sympathetic and Parasympathetic Responses. Reflex Movements of Pharynx Esophagus and Tongue	Chemosensory Guidance of Behavior: O_2, CO_2, Ph, Water, Salt, Electrolytes, Glucose, Toxins, Taste and Thirst
II Cerebellum-Pons, Metencephalon-Rhmbencephalon, Pontine Reticular Formation (PRF) Vestibular n Cochlear n, Facial n, Abducent n Trigeminal motor and Sensory n, Salivary n, Fastigial n, Interposed n Dentate n, Raphe n.	Vestibulo-Cochlear, Facial, Abducent and Trigeminal nerves	Conditioned Behavior: Startle response. Reflex and Coordinated Movements of head, face, Lips, ears, and eyes, jaws, trunk and Limbs in relation to gravity. Micturition, Sexuality, REM Sleep and Basic Wakefulness. Reflex and Coordinated Vocalization	Whole body, Locomotor response including Stance and Gait. Attentive facing with Directed Head, face, ears and eyes, Jaw, Body and Limbs. Basic reflex Sexuality	Sensory-guided behavior: Behavioral guidance by Pain, Touch, Temperature, Proprioception, Lateral line receptors, Vestibular, and Auditory.

Table 3. The Vertebrate Cephalo-Truncal Brain and Behavior

NHP Organizational Level and Neural Structures	Related Cranial Nerves	Mediated Functional Behavior	Motor Responses and Actions	Sensory and Memory Guidance
III Midbrain Mesencephalic Reticular Formation (MRF) Periaqueductal gray, Tectum Tegmentum, Troclear n, Oculomotor n, Red n. Raphe n.	Troclear, Oculomotor and Optic nerves and Tracts.	Sensory-Guided Behavior: Central pain/pleasure. Reflex Orientation to visual, auditory and Sensory stimuli. Locomotion, Micturition, Sexuality, Wake-Sleep Arousal, Appetite-Satiety	Conditioned orientation, facing, gazing, listening, Behavioral approach or escape. Sexual behavior.	Vision plus the integration of all of the lower level sensory inputs
IV Limbic-Allocortical Hypothalamus-Pituitary, Thalamus, Basal Ganglia, Paleo-Cortex, Arche-Cortex,	Olfactory nerves and tracts, Multiple subcortical white matter fiber tracts and connections.	Memory-Guided Behavior Automatic learned, Subconscious, implicit behavior. Affective/Emotional behavior. Hypothalamo-Pituitary-	Survival and Stress responses, Fight, Flight or Fright, Circadian rhythms, Wake-Sleep cycle, Appetite-Satiety,	Smell plus complex multisensory integration or gestalts. Affective/emotional memories and stereotyped and memory-guided

NHP Organizational Level and Neural Structures	Related Cranial Nerves	Mediated Functional Behavior	Motor Responses and Actions	Sensory and Memory Guidance
Limbic System		Adrenal stress response. Active smelling, sniffing, Sexuality. Wake-Sleep regulation and Neocortical arousal, Species-Specific Vocalizations and Subcortical Language and motor processing.	Conditioned Subconscious Sexuality	perceptions and experiences. Conditioned fear, hatred, anger, pain and pleasure, joy and happiness. Group mentality and insecurity resulting in fierce Territoriality.

Table 4. The Vertebrate Neocortical Brain and Behavior

NHP Organizational Level and Neural Structures	Related Fiber Tracts	Mediated Functional Behavior	Expressive Actions and Behavior	Perceptual, Memory-Guided and Self-Generated Experiences
Va Neocortical-Left and Right Hemispheric Neocortical Left and Right Hemispheres with Primary Sensory-Motor and Unimodal Associative Visual, Auditory, Somatosensory areas and Language dominant Hemisphere	Primary Somato-Motor and Somato-Sensory, Visual, Auditory, Gustatory and Olfactory pathways, Hemispheric white matter connections.	Rule-Based Behavior Primary Hemispheric Sensory-Motor Integration and Unimodal and multimodal, associative, learned behaviors. Oral and Written language Communication in the dominant hemisphere. Stroop and Wisconsin card sorting test	Situational, Skillful, Voluntary, Intentional actions and Motivated behaviors, directed or attentive behaviors and actions or voluntary inattention to a stimulus or situation.	Complex, multisensory, Situational and Memory-Guided Perceptions, Feelings and self-generated Experiences.
Vb Neocortical-Global: Prefrontal, cingulate and temporo-occipito-parietal (TOP) multimodal associative neural network Both cerebral hemispheres connected through corpus callosum and other commissural fibers, working together in parallel and synchronous processing mode.	Profuse convergent and divergent white matter neural pathways connecting tertiary cortical areas from both hemispheres to other cortical areas, subcortex, brainstem and Spinal cord.	Self-Guided, Executive Behavior: Self-generated actions, internal speech and cognition. Working Memory. Situationally adaptive, and Flexible, Conscious Decision Making and Execution of behavior. Anticipatory planning, Volition, Intentionality and Sense of Self. Cognitive Modeling of Environment, Self and others. Creative Problem-solving and creative innovation	Voluntary, Intentional and Planned actions. Skillful and Creative actions and anticipatory behaviors. Go/No-Go abilities with Selective and Purposeful activation or inhibition of cortex, subcortex, brainstem and spinal cord. Complex sexual behavior. Empathy and altruism.	Global situational perceptions and on-going personality. Conscious cognitive and emotional experiences. Self- generated scenarios. Images of self and others. Feelings of hatred, love, fear, anxiety, expectations of the future. Feelings of awe and wonder. Awareness and acceptance of aging and death.

APPENDIX 6: GLOSSARY AND NOTES

Ātman, Energy~Being~Awareness- *Ātman*, the existential energy~being~awareness is described as follows: *Ātman* is distinct from all things described before. It is the innermost (nothing else within it), all-pervasive like an ocean or space, subtle, eternal, without any parts, without qualities, spotless, having no activities like going and coming. It is devoid of ideas like me and mine and also of desire, aversion and effort. By nature, it is self-effulgent, Swayaṁ Jyotiḥ , like the radiant heat of fire or the light of the sun. It has no connections with the natural elements like earth, wind, water, heat and light. It possesses no organs like the vision, hearing, mind, intellect, etc., free from the gunās like sattva, rajas, tamas, and it does not have prāṇ a and other vital airs. It is untouched by hunger, thirst, grief, delusion, body-sense or image, old age and death. It is the Self that resides in the heart of all beings and is the seer of all intellects. It is the conscious witness of both the seer and the seen.

The word *Ātman* is derived from the verb *an* 'to breathe.' It is the breath of Life. It is the essential energy-being of the individual, the Self or the Soul. *Ātman* persists when the not-self Anātman, or the observable field of experience Kshetra, is spontaneously eliminated from the essential awareness. The not-self includes all observable phenomena, the kshetra, including the world, body, mind, intellect and ego. Please refer to Appendix 1 for details of kshetra. The Ātman is the ultimate conscious witness, Sākshī. Some Vedāntins think that Ātman is an unborn, aja, and immortal, amar, element, bhāga, of a person. *Ātman* is the essential self-conscious being. It is the foundational reality of an individual energy~being~awareness.

Absent-minded- "To be absent-minded is to be inattentive to the ongoing activity, to lose track of current aims, events, and to become distracted from intended thought and action by salient but (currently) irrelevant stimuli."

Adaptation- Fitting one's behavior to meet the needs of one's environment. This often involves a modification of impulses, emotions, and attitudes.

Affect- Behavior that expresses a subjectively experienced emotion. Any experience of feeling or emotion, ranging from suffering to elation. Affect can be irreflexive meaning directly experienced or reflexive when the person makes the emotion an object of his or her conscious perception.

Ahamkāra Ahamkāra is a sense of ego, an agent or doer-ship that arises as a result of repeated voluntary acts, efforts, decision making, motivated actions, perceptions and thoughts.

When one realizes that most events are controlled by multiple variables, including a chance factor or Providence Daivaṁ दैवं, one's Ahamkāra or doer-ship dissipates. One realizes the spontaneity of one's being and one's behavior.

Aggression- Forceful physical, verbal or symbolic action.

Agitation- Excessive motor activity, usually nonpurposeful and associated with internal tension.

ALLL- Awareness, Learning and Love for Life.

Approach, Avoid, and Pause-Watch-Witness- Approach, avoid, pause and wait-watch or witness are the three fundamental behavioral responses that an organism can have when facing a new situation. The third third mode of 'witnessing' involves, pausing, waiting, and learning about the evolving situation and then, making an appropriate decision.

Arousal~Energy- Our feeling of arousal~energy can take three major forms: i) personal arousal-energy, ii) transpersonal or collective group energy, and iii) transcendental, holistic, or holarchic existential arousal-energy. It depends upon a well functioning reticulo-limbic-cortical system and the circadian rhythms.

Attention- Human attention depends on three neural networks: i) a subcortical, alerting network that maintains an adequate level of conscious arousal-energy for cognitive processing; ii) a posterior cortical orienting network, which directs the body, head, ears, and eyes towards an interesting or alarming objects, events, activity, or experience, chosen to be attended to; and iii) an anterior cortical central-executive network, which enhances the perception of the selected target event or object, and suppresses interference by distracters like other objects, events, images, and thoughts. Attention can be focused on a specific place, time, and modality like vision, audition, thought, etc. Focusing in space enhances the processing of that region of interest, whereas, focusing in time enhances the processing of events at the present moment. It is the basis of presence or present mindedness, which is also known as *Vipassanā* or mindfulness in the Buddhist, Zen literature.

Attentional Blink - ttentional blink when a second stimulus is missed, if it is presented within 200 msec after the first stimulus.

Attentional Bottleneck- a phenomenon of central bottleneck, as a limit to human attention and information processing

Attentive Facing- attentive facing is the turning of body, head, face, mouth, ears and eyes towards pleasant stimuli like food, air, water, warmth and friends, and away from unpleasant stimuli like excessive heat or cold, foul smell, toxins and predators. Attentive facing is important and adaptive for security, comfort, pleasure and communication… Attentive facing helps to communicate by gestures, grimacing, vocalizing, and language. Attentive facing conveys emotions like fear, anger, joy, sadness, disgust, humor, peace and happiness.

Autobiographical Self- The autobiographical self requires the presence of the essential, core self. It is based on the memory of multiple individual experiences of the past and anticipated future. The autobiographical memory grows with life experiences and gets modified continuously by our new experience. We are conscious of the autobiographical self.

Background State of Consciousness- It is the affective mode of our consciousness. "The background state" of consciousness does mean or represent something. It represents "you" — the most basic embodiment of your "self." More than that, it represents the current state of your energy-being: "This is me, I am this body, and, right now, I feel like this. Far from being without quality the background state of consciousness is therefore replete with meaning and feeling — indeed, it is the very bedrock of personal meaning and feeling. This aspect of consciousness therefore not only "represents" your Self, it also tells you how you are doing (at this moment)." (Solms).

Brahman- The ineffable, infinite, absolute, blissful, self-existent, self-aware Energy-Being. The word Brahman is derived from the root verb Bruh, which means to surge, grow, explode, expand, or mushroom, like the "Big Bang." It is a ceaseless, spontaneous bursting forth or emerging energy-matter-information. It is the primal, self-organized reality, as well as the self-organizing principle and the energy of the universe. *Brahman* is the Real of real, the Truth of truths, Satyasya Satyaṁ सत्यस्य सत्यम् |, the source of all experience and existence. This absolute reality of *Brahman* is the truth, consciousness Jñānaṁ, and Infinity Ananta. It is also described as Blissful, Conscious Being, Sat~Chit~Ānanda. It is both transcendent and imminent. It is not merely a featureless absolute, but the whole universe is its incredible expression.

Chāndogyopaniṣ ad described *Brahman* as Tat-ja-li-an, that which gives rise to, sustains, absorbs and breathes the universe. It is the creative matrix of the dynamic universe. Universe is truly a uni verse, a single holistic verse, a single process-product Reality. Like a spring-fed lake, it has circular causality – process creates the product and the product influences the process. Similar circular causality is evident between conscious contents and the conscious stream. We are an integral part of this natural self-organizing universe.

Buddhi- Buddhi is involved in discrimination of sensory perceptions, recalled memories, and voluntary actions and decision making. Therefore it is required for both knowledge and action.

Catharsis- The healthy voluntary release of ideas by "speaking out" subconscious conflicting desires accompanied by an appropriate emotional adjustment. Also, the release into awareness of repressed or "forgotten" material from the unconscious.

Citta- Citta is the storehouse of genetic and epigenetic endowments and all past memories and experiences Samskāraḥ संस्कारः. These Samskāraḥ set the stage and context for all of our experiences and actions. Ordinarily, we are heavily conditioned and limited by these memories of the past and expectations of the future. We feel as if we are imprisoned in this self-made cage, as if we are ever committed to this life of bondage, limited understanding, and endless suffering. But in all of us there is a natural instinct for curiosity and freedom. This natural desire for freedom and curiosity helps us rescue ourselves from this bondage by essential self-awareness and learning. We can realize the final goal of complete self-freedom with an unshakable understanding, awareness, energy, wellness, and tranquility. That is the goal of Vedānta philosophy of Life.

Cognition- A general term, encompassing various modes of knowing and reasoning. Cognition means information processing, applying knowledge, and developing and changing mental representations or maps, based on one's past experience. It is the flow of information through an organism's brain and mind. It implies management of daily activities and responses to positive and negative stimuli. Cognition includes subprocesses of perception, comprehension, remembering, reasoning, judging, imagining and problem solving. Cognition is a transient neural network phenomenon.

Cognition also means thinking or the thought process, which may be verbal, visual, or tactile. Such a process is usually subvocal and has to be inferred from the observable behavior and verbal reports. It is also symbolic in the sense, that it involves experience and manipulation of recalled mental representations, processed through the brain. Cognition is a neural network phenomenon.

Cognitive development- Beginning in infancy, the acquisition of intelligence, conscious thought, and problem solving abilities.

Cognitive Self-Control- The executive, cognitive self-control is a set of processes that organize, plan, and schedule other mental processes and operations.

Conation- Conation means intention or volition with self-activation toward a goal. Conation is defined as the proactive activation, or inhibition, as opposed to habitual or automatic motivation and behavior.

Concrete Thinking- Thinking characterized by direct immediate experience rather than abstractions.

Conditioning- Establishing new behavior as a result of psychological modifications of responses to stimuli.

Conflict- A mental struggle that arises from the simultaneous operation of opposing impulses, drives and environmental or internal demands. The conflict is *intrapsychic* when it is between the forces within, the personality and *extrapsychic* when it is between the self and its environment.

Conscience- The morally self-critical part of one's standards of behavior, performance, and value judgements. Commonly equated with the Super-ego.

Consciousness- Consciousness is a living, organismic process. It is a biological systems-level process and property. Brain is the organ of consciousness. Conscious experience is a synthesis of three aspects or perspectives, which I would call a philosophy of "Triple Aspect Monism." (See Triple-aspect monism).

The term consciousness is difficult to define, although all of us understand, what it is from our first-person experience. There are many definitions and several reviews on the subject of consciousness. In clinical neurology, consciousness is defined as a set of neural processes that allow an individual to perceive, comprehend and act, on the internal, middle and external environments. It has three functional aspects, arousal, awareness, and attention. Consciousness is viewed as a self-generating, self-organizing process from an ecological perspective.

Consciousness is bimodal: affective and cognitive. These two modes are served by two separate but, complementary neural networks, namely, reticulo-limbic and neocortical. Consciousness is also tri-laminar: Internal-Visceral, Proprioceptive-Somatic and External-Distant, on the basis of specific sensory-motor receptors and their functions.

Conscious Arousal- Conscious arousal describes the degree to which an individual is awake and able to interact with the environment. General arousal is higher in a person who is more alert to sensory stimuli, more physically active, and more reactive emotionally. Conscious arousal requires the interplay, between the brainstem reticular activating system and the cerebral hemispheres. Like a pilot flame, the central brain or the reticulo-limbic system is always active in all living organisms. Without it conscious life is not possible.

Conscious Awareness- Conscious awareness implies that the individual is not only alert but also cognizant of self and surroundings. Awareness is global, multimodal, but nonspecific, in terms of any a particular sensory, motor, or cognitive modality. Awareness depends on arousal. The neuronal mechanism required for conscious awareness is the central thalamic nuclei with their brainstem and cortical connections.

Conscious Attention- Conscious attention implies the ability to respond and direct awareness and modality-specific information to a specific time-place and person. Different sensory-motor-cognitive modalities include visual, auditory, tactile, olfactory, gustatory, locomotion, limb movements, speech, memories, thoughts, and images. Attention directed to a specific aspect of the experiential field, the world or the self, and requires both an intact general awareness and a well functioning, modality-specific thalamo-cortical network.

Conscious Experience and State- Conscious experience is integrated; each conscious scene is unified, and at the same time, it is highly differentiated; a huge number of different conscious states are possible at each conscious moment. They define integration or functional clustering, as a property shared by every conscious experience irrespective of its content: Each conscious state comprises of a single scene that is private and cannot be decomposed into independent components. We cannot be aware of two incongruent scenes simultaneously. So also, we cannot make more than one conscious decision, within an interval of a few hundred milliseconds (300-500 ms), the so-called psychological refractory period. Conscious experience depends upon activation or deactivation of specific neocortical areas, in response to external or internal stimulation or activation by memory, intention, imagery or dreams.

Conscious Will- Wegner, in his book Illusion of Conscious Will, stated: "Conscious will is something that is experienced, when we perform an action – actions feel willed or not, and this feeling of voluntariness or doing a thing 'on purpose' is an indication of conscious will… Intention is normally understood as an idea of what one is going to do that appears in consciousness just before one does it."

Coordination Dynamics - Coordination dynamics is "a set of context-dependent laws or rules that describe, explain, and predict how patterns of coordination form, adapt, persist, and change in natural systems" (Kelso and Engstrom).

Coping Mechanisms- Ways of adjusting to environmental stress without altering one's goals or purposes. Includes both conscious and unconscious mechanisms.

Core Self- The core self is a transient, second-order, non-verbal account that occurs whenever an object, a sensory, emotional, or memory input, modifies the protoself. Core consciousness is created in pulses, each pulse triggered by each objective input that we interact with or that we recall. We are conscious of the core self. The mechanism that produces the core self, undergoes minimal change across a lifetime. The core self requires the presence of the proto-self. (Damasio).

Creativity- Creativity is defined as: "The ability to produce work that is novel, original, spontaneous and appropriate, useful and adaptive." It has given us an enormous advantage over our environment and other animals. Spontaneous as well as intentional creativity is useful for making cognitive models of self-in-the-world. Such ability gives us capacity to simulate and anticipate future, based on our past experience. Such a mind is capable of complex decision-making, creative thinking and altruistic behavior.

Creativity was further defined as an understanding and expression of novel orderly relationships, (Heilman). Such innovation may occur when there is co-activation and communication between prefrontal and TOP associative cortices, in a relatively low norepinephrine arousal state, with a vast knowledge of the subject stored in multimodal cortices, in a motivated individual. Innovative cognition requires us to attend, reflect, imagine, model, and predict by participating actively in our ever-changing situations. This promotes active exploration of new environment for security, profit, pleasure and curiosity. It is the very basis of the astronomical progress made by humans in knowledge, languages, communications, sciences, technologies, space-explorations and creative arts.

Culture- Culture may be defined as the complex whole, which includes knowledge, beliefs, arts, laws, morals, customs, and any other capabilities, and habits acquired by the individual as a member of the human society. Culture is learned and includes the totality of human achievements. The National Institutes of Mental Health, Culture, and Diagnostic Group has adopted a more clinically orientated definition of culture: "meanings, values, and behavioral norms that are learned and transmitted in a dominant society and within its social groups. Culture powerfully influences cognitions, feelings and the 'self' concept, as well as the diagnostic process and treatment decisions. Culture provides a context and makes us human. It provides a context for the bio-psycho-social-existential values and variables that make us who we are, from moment to moment.

Dependence- Reliance on someone or something else, for support.

Dhāraṇā- Undistracted, continuous focusing of conscious attention on an object, an event, an activity, a thought, or some ongoing experience.

Dhyānaṁ- Continued, sustained, dwelling of attention or vigilance, on the same object, event or experience.

Dhyāna Yoga- It is a Sanskrit word for meditation derived from the verb Dhyāyati, which means to meditate, ponder, or Self-reflect. By the practice of dhyāna, one can achieve a state of intuitive, self-absorptive consciousness, with stillness, silence, serenity and presence of mind, which may lead to Samādhi or enlightenment. Such a mental state is conducive to full Self-integration and understanding of the truth of one's Being-in-Reality and reality-in-One-Self. The word Dhyāna was transformed into Jhāna in Pali, Ch'ān in Chinese, and Zennā or Zen in the Japanese languages.

Distractibility- Inability to maintain attention, focused on a selected object, event, activity, experience or task.

Dual-Aspect Monism- Dual-aspect monism was elaborated by Solms. "Brain is the seat of the mind, somehow producing our feeling of being ourselves, in the world right now…Dual-aspect monism accepts that we are made of only one type of stuff (that is why it is a monist position), but it also suggests that this stuff is perceived in two different ways (hence, the dual aspect monism). The important point to grasp about this otherwise straightforward position is that it implies that in our essence, we are neither mental nor physical beings — at least not in the sense that we normally employ these terms. Dual-aspect monism implies that the brain is made of stuff that appears "physical" when viewed from the outside (as an object) and "mental" when viewed from the inside (as the subject). When I perceive myself externally (in the mirror, for example) and internally through introspection, I perceive the same thing, in two different ways (as a body and a mind, respectively). This distinction between body and mind is therefore an artifact of perception."

Eco-Spirituality- Eco-spirituality is a manifestation of the spiritual connection between human beings and Nature. It incorporates an intuitive and embodied awareness of all Life and engages a relational view of the person to planet, the inner to outer landscape, and the soul to soil…The essence of eco-spiritual consciousness incorporates tending, dwelling, reverence, connectedness, and sentience.

Ecological Perspective of the Brain- An ecological perspective of the brain and our subject-object interactions, are being proposed as a model for psychiatry and psychotherapy. Fuchs proposed an ecological or systemic view of the brain, which regards cognition and consciousness as components in a circular causality of organism and environment. "In these cyclic processes, the brain functions as an organ of transformation which mutually translates elementary and complex system states into each other, thus allowing the organism to develop integral options of perception and action in its environment. Since these interactions, on their part, continuously change the microstructure of the brain, it has to be regarded as an organ that is formed biologically, socially as well as historically."

Embodied Self- Embodiment, the sense of being localized within one's physical body, is a fundamental aspect of the self. The phenomenon of embodied self is processed in distinct cortical areas viz. temporo-occipito-parietal (TOP) junction and the extrastriate body area. The neural network that processes embodiment of self, its parts, and corporeal awareness, include not only the posterior TOP cortex, but also premotor and motor cortices.

Emotion- Emotion is an experience with physiological and behavioral responses to a personally significant event. Emotional control implies self-regulation of one's emotions and their influence on one's thoughts and behavior. Emotional insight is an awareness of one's own and others' emotions.

Emotional Intelligence- Emotional intelligence is the ability to process emotional information and to use it in reasoning and cognition. It is defined as the competence to identify, understand, and express emotions; assimilate emotions in thought; and regulate both positive and negative emotions in one self and others. Understanding the emotions of oneself and others is the key to a satisfying life. Those people who are self-aware and sensitive to others manage their affairs with wisdom and grace, even in adverse circumstances.

Energy Metaphor of Mind- Panksepp defended the energy metaphor of mind. "Human thoughts can be driven by sub-neocortical large-scale, energetic states. Sadly, energy metaphors of mind were discarded a long time ago, to the great detriment of understanding what emotions really are. However, information processing metaphors, failed miserably, when we seek to envision the actions of such visceral-emotional brain systems. Energetic dynamics are clearly reflected in emotional actions of both brain and body, as large ensembles of neurons are brought into distinct but coherent action modes by executive neuropeptides. To understand such global functions of the brain, we need functional 'network doctrines' as much as we need a 'neuron doctrine."

Energy Perspective of Life- think to understand our own conscious experience and the world that we live in, appreciating the energy perspective is crucial. It is a fact that all Life is embedded in a single Energy~Field. From Einstein's famous equation $E = MC^2$ showing the equivalence of matter and energy, it is reasonable to consider both the material and energy perspectives of our conscious experience as equivalent. Matter-energy-information is aspects of the same substance, the same natural Reality. Matter~energy~information manifest at multiple levels of natural organization, including our own bio-physical body, mind, and consciousness. Matter~energy~information's transformation or transduction is evident in every natural event and life experience.

Energy Transduction- In neural electrophysiology, we have already established many mechanisms of energy transcduction, for instance, in sensory perception, brainstem and cortical evoked potentials, brainstem reticular activating system, electroencephalography, magneto-encephalography, electromyography, nerve conduction studies, electro-retinography, electrococleography, electrocardiography, electro-dermal response, deep brain stimulation, transcranial magnetic stimulation, and so on. Many of these neural electromagnetic field-potentials are responsive, not only to biophysical signals, but also to conscious mental events.

Executive functioning- higher-level, cognitive abilities such as behavioral sequencing, monitoring, planning, and decision making. Human executive function is defined as the ability to abstract, plan, organize, shift set, and adapt, current and past knowledge, for future behavior. These functions are linked to the prefrontal-temporo-parietal cortical network.

Exergy- High quality energy or exergy is a measure of the maximum capacity of the available energy, contained in a system to perform useful work, as the system proceeds to equilibrium with its surroundings…Exergy is a function of the gradient between a system and its environment. It is a summation of the free energies in a situation. In effect, it measures how far the system is from thermodynamic equilibrium with its environment. Exergy is not a useful concept for discussing equilibrium situations. However, it is a very powerful tool for nonequilibrium situations."

Existential- It refers to the concrete, lived experience of human beings, firmly rooted in the real world. Existential living is the capacity to live fully in the present, and respond freely and flexibly to new experience without fear. Such integrative living would create an experience of presence, with an awareness and understanding of one's current existence, and a life of self-actualization.

Existential Being- The existential being can be behaviorally-mentally oriented in three complimentary modes of existence, namely i) an egocentric, object-avoidant mode; ii) an allocentric, object-approach and explore mode; and iii) an ecosystemic, or field mode, which is self-existent, globally oriented, and holistic.

Existential Fears- The self-actualized individual learns to overcome the four existential fears, the four 'I's, namely, personal Insecurity, Isolation, Insignificance, and Inexistence, or death.

Feeling- Feeling is a self-contained, phenomenal experience. It is called "qualia" implying the quality of experience, in response to the question, "what it feels like to be in the current state of experience." Feelings can vary along three dimensional axis: pleasant-unpleasant, exciting-calming, and arousing-relaxing.

First-Person Process- Gendlin proposed a first-person *process* model in order to resolve the conflicting dichotomy of the Mind-Body problem. It was suggested that what is missing here is that 'the person' is much larger than our limited conscious capacities. The person includes the body-as-internally-sensed, and it also includes a much greater variety of reflectively aware experiencing than merely the deliberately controlled. What we control is a relatively small part of sentient experiencing and the experienced internal-external interactions. This is a first-person model, which he called 'a model of process,' a model in which each next bit is a newly-made whole.

Flight of ideas- A nearly continuous flow of accelerated speech, with abrupt changes from one topic to another, usually based on understandable associations, distracting stimuli or playing on words.

Free association- Spontaneous, uncensored, verbalization of whatever comes to mind by a person.

Happiness- Klamut defined happiness as a state of the spirit (mind), which consists of internal peace, satisfaction with one's life, the joy of life, benevolence, and cordiality towards oneself and others; sensitivity to the beauty of nature, culture, and art; harmonious coexistence with the surroundings. Achievement of such happiness depends on oneself and a rich, encouraging environment.

Holon- It should be noted that a Holon refers to a whole system, considered at one scale and from one person's perspective.

Holarchy- is a nesting of holons, each at a different scale of observation, but all seen from the same individual perspective.

Homeostasis- Homeostasis is a well established term in Biology. 'Homeo' means the same or similar and 'stasis' means a steady state. Homeostasis is defined as a tendency toward a relatively stable internal environment, in organisms through interacting physiological processes. Homeostasis implies maintenance of an internal steady state of an organism by means of self-regulation.

Homeokinetics- Homeokinetics emphasizes the role of kinetic processes, particularly in the form of ongoing periodic thermodynamic engine processes, in carrying out the regulatory functions of the organism.

Individuation-The drive for individuals to become unique and to fulfill the spiritual propensities common to all humanity.

Information- Information created within the brain by a process of representation meaningful to a sentient organism. Information is a reduction in uncertainty provided by a signal, message or a stimulus. Information is knowledge about facts or ideas gained through experience and learning.

Impulse- A desire or propensity to act in a certain way, typically in order to ease tension or gain pleasure. Motivating energy.

Insight- Self-understanding; the extent of a person's understanding of the origin, nature, and mechanisms of his or her perosnality and adaptive attitudes and behaviors.

Intention- Intention implies a conscious decision to perform a behavior.

Introspection- Self-observation or the examination of the contents of one's mind, usually feelings, images, inner speech, and thoughts.

Intuition- McCraty et al. defined intuition as a process by which information that is normally outside the range of conscious awareness is perceived by the psycho-physiological systems. They conclude that the heart and brain, together, are involved in receiving, processing, and decoding intuitive information. The intuitive perception and human creativity are closely linked.

Ipseity- Ipseity (Ipse: I or self) is the unifying basic tone of the first-person's experience. It is the center of all conscious experience and is dependent upon a continuous, internally generated, interoceptive brain input. It gives us a sense of a single unitive being. Ipseity or I, in every experience is implicitly and pre-reflexively present, in the unified field of awareness, through which all conscious experiences pass. It is an intrinsic property of the essential, existential Awareness.

Ipseity is a spontaneous neurobiological phenomenon, which depends upon brain arousal and awareness. Ipseity, by itself is non-interactive and not a pole, until one starts interacting with the 'other' by reflective consciousness. Self-qualia are responsible for the feelings of self-agency, self-unity, self-affectability, and implicit self-history. Ipseity is an unreflected presence, with self-luminosity or the self-sentient energy, Swayaṁ Jyotiḥ स्वयं ज्योतिः.

Jīva, Individual Ego- The individual ego-self is called *jīva*, which means one who breathes. It is the biological aspect of human individuality. The individual jiva is the agent or doer, kartā, as well as enjoyer or sufferer, bhoktā, of various life experiences. It has the biophysical body, deha, the subconscious, self-organizing energy, prāṇa, and a conscious mind, manas.

Judgement- Mental act of comparing choices between a given set of values in order to select a course of action.

Laughter Neural Network- Wild et al. define the "laughter neural network". They summarize: "The expression of laughter seems to depend on two partially independent neural pathways. The first, an 'involuntary' or 'emotionally driven' system involves the amygdala, thalamic, hypothalamic, and subthalamic areas and the tegmental brainstem. The second, 'voluntary' (or self-driven) system that originates in the premotor-frontal areas and leads through the motor cortex and pyramidal tract to the ventral brainstem. These systems appear to be coordinated by a laughter-coordinating center in the dorsal upper pons."

Limbic System- A group of brain structures that help regulate arousal, emotion, feeling, memory, value, and motivation.There are an inner and outer limbic, neural networks. The orbitofrontal and insular cortex, amygdala, hippocampus, hypothalamus, and midbrain are some of the key structures in the limbic nervous system.

Life Space- Life-space is defined as the totality of possible events for one person at a particular time, which is a person's possible options, together with the environment that contains them. It is like multiple streams being coordinated into a single, transient, convergent-divergent system with its complex, coordination dynamics. This is why we have to understand self in terms of new biophysics, synergetics, and coordination dynamics for complex, natural systems.

Manas- Manas is the internal faculty of perception, comprehension, analysis, and synthesis of cognitive experience. It also includes faculties of thinking, reflection, imagination, and invention. Manas presents the cognized information to the central executive or frontal intelligence, Buddhi.

Meditation- Meditation is a unique way of being-in-Reality. It is a set of skills to live consciously with full <u>A</u>wareness, <u>L</u>earning and <u>L</u>ove for <u>L</u>ife (ALLL). It is an art of Presence, which implies being present in the current moment whole-heartedly, with all of one's conscious arousal-energy-being, sensitivity, feeling, intelligence and creativity. Meditation implies living with full awareness and understanding of oneself and the present situation. It is a skill of being at-ease with oneself and at-home in the world. It is being highly adaptive, peaceful, self-content, friendly and caring to oneself and others. It is an art of being a true friend to oneself and the world. It is learning and developing the art of mental stillness, silence, serenity and self-healing.

Roger N. Walsh defined the term "Meditation" as "a family of practices that train attention in order to heighten awareness and bring mental processes under voluntary control. Their ultimate aim is the development of the deepest insight into the nature of mental processes, consciousness, self-identity and reality, and the development of optimal states of psychological well-being and consciousness."

Mental health- Vaillant reviewed different models of mental health. He considered mental health as i) normality, ii) positive psychology, iii) maturity, iv) social-emotional intelligence, v) subjective well-being, and vi) resilience.

Mental Normality- Mental normality implies healthy ability to work, play and love; efficient problem solving; investment in life; and self-autonomy.

Mind- i) a processor of patterns in the flow of arousal-energy-information within the brain. ii) The human consciousness that originates in the brain and is manifested especially in thought, perception, feeling, will, memory, and imagination. iii) the totality of conscious and unconscious processes of the brain that directs the mental and physical behavior of a sentient organism. iv) the principle of intelligence; the spirit of consciousness regarded as an aspect of Reality.

Mind means mental activity. Mind is the product of brain activity, which depends on brain's self-organization. Brain and mental activities occur concurrently like two parallel streams. Mental activity includes three classical domains of conation, cognition, and affect or feeling.

The APA dictionary of psychology defined mind as: i) most broadly, all intellectual and psychological phenomena of an organism, encompassing motivational, affective, behavioral, perceptual, and cognitive systems; In other words, the organized totality of the mental and psychic processes of an organism and the structural and functional cognitive components on which they depend. The term, however, is often used more narrowly to denote only cognitive activities, such as perceiving, attending, thinking, problem solving, language, learning and memory. ii) The substantive content of such mental and psychic processes. iii) Consciousness or awareness, particularly as specific to an individual. iv) A set of emergent properties automatically derived from a brain that has achieved sufficient biological sophistication. v) Human consciousness regarded as an immaterial entity distinct from the brain. vi) The brain itself and its activities.

Mind, Antaḥkaraṇa-The mind, Antaḥ karaṇ a in Vedānta is considered an internal organ or a tool for conscious action or conation Karma, cognition Jñāna, and emotional experiences of pleasure or pain, fear, anger, etc bhogaḥ . It includes four component processes: i) all memories including the conscious working memory, long-term semantic memory, and the subconscious memories, both individual and collective (Citta), ii) mentation, thinking-imagining, dealing with the sensory-motor organs (Manas), iii) decision-making, choosing, discriminating intellect (Buddhi), and iv) a feeling of being an ego, self, interpreter, predictor, volition, intentionality, planning, organizing, and executing (Ahaṁbhāva).

There is a certain nested hierarchy in these regulatory capacities of the four mental subsystems. The hierarchy from below up would be memory (Citta), mentation (Manas), intellect (Buddhi), and ego Ahaṁbhāva. This nested hierarchy is manifested in both human and animal ontogeny as well as phylogeny.

Mindfulness Meditation - Mindfulness meditation is "the effort to intentionally pay attention, non-judgmentally, to the present-moment experience and sustain this attention over time. The aim is to cultivate a stable and nonreactive, present-moment awareness or presence.

Minimal Self- The minimal self represents data available only to its owner including the current body state, and the conscious stream of internal dialogue and imagery. It is rooted in the ancient neural systems of the brainstem reticular formation and the limbic system.

Minimal Self-Awareness- Minimal self-awareness should be understood as the self-acquaintance that consciousness has with itself and not as awareness of an experiencing self.

Mnemic mode of attention- Partial, distracted attention with habitual cognitive and emotional responses based on personal memories. This creates observer-observed duality and the experience of personal time, duration, and change. It creates, sustains, and adds to our self-image. It limits perceptivity, attentional energy, intelligence, and a feeling of natural happiness.

Mood- A pervasive and sustained emotion-feeling.

Mystical Experience- As William James described it in 1902; the mystical experience is characterized by ineffability, noetic quality, transiency, passivity, and memorability. Such a spiritual experience is difficult to describe; it has a quality of intrinsic energy-awareness; it is spontaneous, effortless, unintentional, self-effulgent, and enduring. It is the very nature of our essential, existential Energy-Being.

Narcissism- Self-love, as opposed to love for an object or another person. To be distinguished from egoism. This carries the connotation of self-centeredness, selfishness and conceit. Egoism is but one expression of narcissism.

Normal Mind- Normal mind is hard to define. Freud thought that normality was an idealized fiction. Eissler thought that absolute normality could not be achieved because the normal person had to be totally aware of his thoughts and feelings. Money-Kryle defined normality as the ability to achieve insight into one's Self, an ability that is never fully accomplished. Maughn considered the normal as an ideal. "It is a picture that one fabricates… and to find them all in a single person is hardly to be expected."

Normality- Klein conceived normality as strength of character, the capacity to deal with conflicting emotions, the ability to experience pleasure without conflict, and the ability to love. For Erikson, normality was the ability to master the eight phases of psychosocial development. Kubie considered normality as the ability to learn by experience, to be flexible, and adapt to a changing environment. Hartmann suggested that the conflict-free ego functions represented the person's potential for normality. Menninger described normality as the ability to adjust to the external world with contentment and to master the task of acculturation. Rank thought of normality as the capacity to live without fear, guilt, or anxiety and to take responsibility for one's own actions. World Health Organization considers normality as complete physical, mental, and social wellbeing.

Object Relations- The emotional bonds between one person and another, as contrasted with interest in or love for the self; usually described as a capacity for loving and reacting appropriately to others.

Person- The concept of "person" in Advaita Vedānta is that of a nested, multi-layered entity like the multiple sheaths of an onion or the trunk of a banana plant. A person (Jīva) has at least five layers or sheaths made up of matter-energy-awareness, varying from gross to subtle: i) Material or physical, Annamaya kośaḥ, ii) Vital or physiological, Prāṇ amaya kośaḥ, iii) Sensory-Perceptual, Manomaya kośaḥ, iv) Cognitive or thinking, Vijñānamaya kośaḥ, and v) Joyous, blissful, Ānandamaya kośaḥ, being the core of personality.

Personality- i) The characteristic way in which a person thinks, feels, and behaves; ii) the ingrained pattern of behavior that each person evolves, both consciously and unconsciously, as his or her style of living and a way of being. iii) distinctive style of adaptive functioning that an organism exhibits, as it relates to its typical range of environments.

Poverty of speech- Restriction or reduction in the amount of speech.

Preconscious- Those mental events, processes and contents, that are, for the most part, capable of reaching or being brought into conscious awareness, by the intentional or automatic act of focusing attention.

Presence- The concept of presence refers to being fully present in the moment. It is being fully aware and cognizant. It is a non-directed, pre-reflexive, first-person experience, with a primal feeling of energy~being~bliss. It is similar to essential, existential, affective being, ipseity or proprium. Subject and object are two abstract poles of a unique process, which is presence. Presence is the fact or state of being present. It means being present-minded, as opposed to being absent-minded, which is 'absence.'

Presence is being attentive to what is happening now and here. Presence is being in existence now. Presence is functioning, fully and whole-heartedly, at the present time. It implies freedom from the cognitive burden of the past and imaginations of the future. It implies self-renewal from moment to moment. Presence is being well adapted to one's situational self. Presence is the process of reducing uncertainty, a process of knowing and doing. Presence heightens awareness and may lead to intuitive consciousness, generating new ideas, understanding, and solutions. Presence is a way to achieve mental clarity and peace. Presence is being present at the edge of time. It is the continual effluence of energy~being~awareness. It is the very essence of blissful conscious being or Sat~Cit~Ānanda.

Presence: mode of attention- is not contaminated by personal cognitive memories. It is complete, participatory attention to the present here-and-now. It is free of habitual cognitive and emotional responses. It is free of past self-image (and dualistic thinking). It implies tremendous frictionless, conflictless attentional energy, intelligence, self-freedom, and a feeling of natural wellness and being. Since it is completely one with the present – what is, it is named as the state of presence. (For the full abstract, please see Appendix 5).

Pressured speech- Rapid, accelerated, frenzied speech.

Primal Feeling of Being- Solms proposed an underlying neuroanatomy of our primal feeling of being a whole person. "Periaqueductal gray (PAG) has a vertical columnar organization. The columns are divided into two broad types: pleasurable sensations in the ventral PAG and unpleasure in the dorsal PAG. Tectum-Tegmentum (a zone of convergence) together generates a rudimentary representation of the whole person, the inner and outer "virtual bodies" combined. Jaak Panksepp called it the SELF: Simple Ego-like Life Form.

Proto Self- Damasio defined proto-self as a coherent, first-order collection of neural patterns, which map, moment by moment, the state of the physical structure of the organism, in its many dimensions, at multiple neural levels, from brainstem to cerebral cortex. Proto-self does not perceive or hold knowledge. It has no language and we are not conscious of proto-self. It is a reference point in consciousness but, it is not an interpreter of anything.

Psychic Energy- Attention is directed psychic energy; without it no psychological, cognitive or behavioral work can be done, and in doing such work, this psychical energy is dissipated. We create ourselves by how we invest this arousal-energy. Memories, thoughts, and feelings are all shaped by how we use it. And it is an energy under our control, to do with as we please; hence, attention is our most important tool in the task of improving the quality of our experience.

Psychological Refractory Period- when one is unable to respond to a second stimulus that occurs within 200 msec after the first response. Therefore, 200 ms after any stimulus is the psychological refractory period, for further cognitive processing.

Religion- Generally, a belief in a supernatural Creator, God, a divine, sacred, or holy power or process, and a practice of rituals meant to appease, to glorify, to obey, or to relate better with this God. J Krishnamurti defined religion as "the investigation, with all of one's attention, with the summation of all of one's energy, to find that which is sacred, to come upon that which is holy. That can only take place when there is freedom from the noise of thought, the ending of thought and time, psychologically, inwardly – but not the ending of knowledge in the world, where you have to function with knowledge. That which is holy, that which is sacred, which is truth, can only be, when there is complete silence, when the brain itself has put thought in its right place. Out of that immense silence there is that which is sacred."

Reticular Activating System- The reticular formation plays a central role in the generation and regulation of the state of consciousness and arousal-energy. It consists of a complex network of interconnected circuits of neurons, in the tegmentum of the brainstem, the lateral hypothalamic area, and the medial, intralaminar, and reticular nuclei of the thalamus. Many of these neurons are serotonergic or noradrenergic. Axons from the nonspecific thalamic nuclei, project to most of the cerebral hemispheres, where they modulate the level of activity of large numbers of cortical neurons.

Reticular formation plays a crucial role, in maintaining the brain, at an appropriate level of arousal-energy; some authorities refer to it as the reticular activating system. The descending reticulo-spinal tract modulates the spinal reflexes, spinal autonomic activity and spinal sensory input.

Functions of reticular formation include arousal-energy continuum with circadian periods of consciousness, and sleep. Regulation of arousal-energy and level of consciousness is a generalized function of the reticular formation. The neurons of the reticular formation are stimulated by a variety of stimuli from the somatosensory, auditory, visual, and visceral sensory systems. The reticular formation is, therefore, nonspecific in its response and performs a generalized regulatory function. When a novel stimulus is received, attention is focused on it, while general alertness increases. This behavioral arousal is independent of modality of stimulation and is accompanied by EEG changes. The cerebral cortex and the mesencephalic reticular activating system, are mutually sustaining areas involved in generating and maintaining consciousness.

Sacred- "Latin roots of the term "sacred" include sacer (holy), sacrare (to devote), and sancire (to make holy). The early Greeks believed that many things could be hieros (holy or sacred) owing to their relationship or connection to one of the Gods. Pavitra means sacred. According to Vedic-Hindu perspective, Nature, global space, the total field of Existence with all living beings init, are sacred. In the Hindu tradition, the sanctity of the Divine comes from its integral presence in all reality and its availability to the individual to be directly experienced. Just as the more a place or object becomes pure, the more it comes into proximity with the sacred, so is the case with humans. Physical, mental, and emotional purity are all believed to elevate one toward the sacred, toward the divine, and the greater the ability one has to have direct Divine experience. In Hinduism, this is possible because of the manner, in which the tradition understands and interprets Omnipresence."

Samādhiḥ- effortless, self-absorptive, and intuitive state of Self-understanding and Self-realization of one's primal, affective nature and the essential, existential Energy-Being-Bliss.

Self- Self is a complex, integrative process of a living organism. The living organism is a functioning, behaving unit of Life. The living organism self-organizes, coordinates, and integrates the molecular energy-information, within and around itself, both consciously subconsciously.

The dictionary defines self as i) the total, essential or particular being of one person, the individual, ii) personality, character, individuality, and iii) individual's consciousness of his own being, identity, subjectivity, ego.

The self is the archetype of the ego; it is the innate potential for wholeness, and unconscious ordering principle, directing the overall psychic life, that gives rise to the ego, which compromises with and is partly shaped by the external reality. This Self concept is similar to the concept of *Ātman* in Vedānta.

The present, minimal self is the life-in-the-moment or the immediate experience of one's person, unextended in time. The narrative self, autobiographical, or longitudinal, is related to one's personal past and projected future. A person can refer to self, either as the source of its agency for regulation of behavior, or as the target of perception-cognition-action. It is the essence of individuality, being, proprium, or ipseity.

According to the psychologist William James, nominative self is the knower of the self (self-as-subject), whereas, empirical self is the self so known (self-as-object). The empirical self further consists of the material self, the social self, and the spiritual self, which is closest to one's core, the subjective experience of oneself.

The global self is orchestrated and balanced like a spiral, and it is centered on the I, the Self-as-subject. This I is the living connection with human experience. In addition to the I, as the subject, the self also contains many self-images, based on self-perception, as the self-as-object, the so-called "me." The self is modifiable, in the sense that new perceptions are integrated into the ongoing self-image, throughout life, while old perceptions fade away... A healthy self is highly flexible, well adjusted, creative and adaptive. It is continuously involved in creating new visions of personal growth and enhancement.

Self-Actualization- Maslow defined self-actualization as "an episode in which powers of the person come together, in an efficient and enjoyable way, and in which he/she was more integrated and open to experience, more spontaneous and expressive, fully functioning, more creative, humorous, more ego-transcending, and more independent of his/her lower needs. He becomes more truly himself, more perfectly actualizing his potentialities, closer to the core of his being, more fully human." It is the development of one's full potential as a unique human being.

Self-Awareness- Self-awareness is our capacity to reflect on our feeling and sense of self. Such capacity depends on the proper functioning of medial prefrontal and posterior cingulate cortex and other central, midline networks. Essential, self-awareness implies our natural self-acquaintance and the feeling of being-in-existence.

Self-Consciousness- Self-consciousness implies conscious awareness of oneself, one's own being, one's actions, thoughts, feelings and emotions.

Self-Integrity- The wisdom of self-integrity is beautifully expressed by Erikson. It means acceptance of oneself and all aspects of one's life, and integration of these elements into a stable pattern of living. It implies the experience of and adjustment to the trials and troubles of life, as well as to its rewards and joys. Consequently, existence holds no fear; the ego has resigned itself to acceptance of life itself, and to acceptance of the end of that life in death.

Self-Process- Self-process is both convergent and divergent, it can function both as the source or the target of its activity and mentation. It is ever renewing itself, since it is continuously generated as a result of spontaneous activation of cerebral cortex, by the brainstem-diencephalic arousal system. The brainstem-cortical arousal system is crucial for the manifestation of a living, thinking, and conscious self. Without such neurophysiologic arousal-energy, mental functions like consciousness, sense of self, attention, and volition are not possible.

Self and Qualia- Ramachandran explained: "Obviously self and qualia are two sides of the same coin. You can't have free-floating sensations (feelings) or qualia with no one to experience them and you can't have a self completely devoid of sensory experiences, memories or emotions. The defining characteristics of the 'self' are fivefold. First of all continuity: a sense of unbroken thread running through the whole fabric of our experience, with the accompanying feeling of past, present and future. Second is the idea of unity or coherence of self. Third is the sense of embodiment or ownership. Fourth is a sense of agency, what we call free will, being in charge of our own actions and destinies. Fifth, and most elusive of all, the self, almost by its very nature, is capable of reflection – of being aware of itself."

Self-Realization- Self-realization springs from within, because the fundamental truth of our existential Being is within us. It is not outside in the changing phenomena. There is something amazingly beautiful within each one of us – a primal feeling ādibhāva आदिभाव, of an infinite ananta अनन्त, spontaneous wonder vismayaḥ विस्मय:. It is whole in itself, pūrṇ a पूर्ण. It lacks nothing. It is the greatest wonder within, which waits to be discovered by our watchful Self-enquiry. We are an integral part of this incredible Natural Order, Ṛ tam ऋतं. We are in Nature and Nature is within us, at every level of our biophysical and mental being. We have to realize this amazing integration in our own core *heart~being*. This is what Vedānta is all about.

Self-Reference- There are two temporally distinct forms of self-reference: extended self-reference, linking experiences across time, and momentary self-reference centered on the present experience of the moment.

Sentient Energy-Being- Sentient energy~being variously named as Swayaṁ Jyotiḥ स्वयंज्योति:, Prāṇ aśaktiḥ , प्राणशक्ति, Acintyaśaktiḥ अचिन्त्यशक्ति:, Citśaktiḥ चित्शक्ति:. चित्शक्ति:. Mentation-cognition can be in a potential or kinetic form. It is in kinetic form, during common, interactive wakefulness and dream sleep, whereas, during non-REM sleep and non-REM wakefulness Turīya, they are in a potential form. During non-REM sleep, the conscious arousal-energy is low, whereas during non-REM wakefulness, the conscious arousal-energy is high. That is why the Turīya state has been described to have a feeling of boundless energy, unlimited capacity, creativity, and an intense sense of well-being and bliss, (euphoria in a positive sense).

Sensory Receptors- i) the interoceptive-visceral, chemoreceptors mostly include all visceral sensations plus olfaction and taste. ii) Somatic proprioceptors receive information from bones, muscles, ligaments, and joints, and thus, monitor the relative location of the body, limbs and also the direction, force, and speed of all body movements. iii) The exteroceptive, contact receptors include the sensations of touch, temperature and pain and inform the organism of the current external enironment that it is facing. iv) distant, tele-receptors include specialized sensory systems, namely, olfaction, audition and vision, for the perception, comprehension, and appropriate responses to distant events.

Sixth Sense- Solms: "Emotion is akin to a sensory modality — an internally directed sensory modality that provides information about the current state of the body self, as opposed to the state of the object-world. It adds a sixth sense, (a sixth modality or "qualia") to our conscious existence. Emotion is the aspect of consciousness that is left, if you remove all externally derived contents. If you were deprived of all sensory images (drawn from present and past perceptions) you would still be conscious. You would still be aware of your inner state — of your core self. Emotion is a perception of the state of the subject, not of the object-world."

SOHOs- Self-Organizing Holarchic Open systems (SOHOs) are nested, ecological constellation of self-organizing dissipative process-structures, organized around particular sources of exergy-materials-information that gives rise to coherent self perpetuating behaviors.

Spanda- means spontaneous pulsating or throbbing of life. It is the Divine creative pulsation. It is the throb of ecstacy of the Divine I-Consciousness (Vimarśa). It is the throb of Śiva's absolute freedom or swātantrya. It is the primal creative quivering or vibration. It is movement as it were. It reminds me of David Bohm's term, "Holo-movement." To me, it is high-frequency creative energy~being~awareness like a scanning or strobe light. In the brain, it would be high-frequency electromagnetic activity like the gamma waves and higher, typically seen during vigilant attentiveness. Spanda also means pulse, which can be sensed during meditation. See Singh J. Spanda-Kārikās: The Divine Creative Pulsation. Motilal Banarasidass Publishers, Delhi, India. 1980. Reprint 2009: xvi-xviii.

Spirituality- Spirituality is the search for inner peace, purpose, happiness and wellbeing. It is about mental health and finding meaning and purpose in life… It is an overall philosophy of one's life. "Spirituality, the search for meaning and purpose in life, through a connection with Nature, and/or a belief in a higher power, is at the core of each person's existence. In ancient times, spirit meant breath – as essential to life as air. Spirituality is that part of every person, that yearns to share the beauty, love and joyfulness of the universe…We take our spirituality from many sources: Nature, God or Goddess, Krishna,

Buddha, Higher Power, Yahweh, Jesus, Mohammed, B'ahaullah, Zoroaster and any other concept of supreme Being-Reality and the Natural Order. But sprituality is not religion, nor is religion spirituality.

Spirtuality is the reflection of one's "spirit" and its relationship to the rest of the universe. Spirituality may be developed through Self-reflection, prayer, and meditation." Generally, a belief in a "greater Self" or personal God, a sense of purpose in life and quest for meaning, an acceptance of the sacredness of nature and of all living beings. Ultimate fulfillment is found, not in material things, but, in spirituality, altruism, idealism, awareness of suffering and death, and leading a life that has a positive effect on people, nature and whatever they consider to be the ultimate, transcendent Reality.

Spirituality entails an inspired life. It is recognized as a source of inner peace, hope, trust, faith, meaning, and inner strength. It incorporates our sense of being, identity, and an understanding of our place in the world. It is natural to be inspired by Nature with feelings of wonder, awe, and transcendence; a renewed sense of vigor; an increased sense of presence, attentiveness and mindful energy; a sense of being present in the moment, humility, and a better pespective of one's own existence, in this astonishing universe.

STEP Model- The author proposed the STEP model, Situational-Transient-Executive Process, model of ego-driven, reflective consciousness. Reflective consciousness is transient and it arises from conscious attention and decision-making, as a result of the sequential, executive activity, in the frontal-parietal network at a given moment.

Stimulus- A biophysical stimulus or a signal has both energy and information. Stimulus energy can be both sequential and parallel. It can be discrete or continuous, in space-time, modality and person or the participant observer.

Superconscious- Webster dictionary: i) transcending human consciousness, ii) of, relating to or possessing the highest consciousness or a margin of consciousness, above that within the ordinary range of attention, iii) the superconscious part of the mind or psyche.

APA dictionary: i) a new term for transpersonal awareness. ii) in certain eastern traditions, with variation in Buddhism, Hinduism and Taoism, a state in which the individual attains highest knowledge, freedom from pain, and perfect spiritual insight, because the mind is free from passion and desire. At their most profound level, the practices of Meditation and Yoga (among others) may be directed toward the ultimate achievement of the superconscious state.

Superconsciousness- a unique integrative and spontaneous mode of conscious Energy-Being-Bliss. It is a calm, clear and undistracted presence. It is an optimal alertness with a highest form of conscious arousal-energy, mental clarity, and calmness. It is a global, undirected, undistracted, and spontaneous vigilance or sustained attentiveness. It is an ideal of loving and caring presence or present-mindedness.

Synchronous Self- Carruthers proposed a model of the synchronous self, which included the sense of control over one's body and mind; of being bounded in body and mind; of having perspective from within one's body and mind; and of being extended in time.

Synergetics- Synergetics is the cooperation of individual parts of a system that produces (new) macroscopic spatial, temporal and functional structures. It deals with deterministic as well as stochastic processes.

Synthetic function- The ego's capacity to integrate, unite, self-organize and bind together various drives, tendencies and functions, within the personality, enabling the individual to think, feel and act, in an organized and directed manner.

Systems Thinking- The holistic, eco-systemic perspective is crucial for our understanding of the organism-environment relationship. Such "Systems Thinking" is about patterns of relationships and how these translate into emergent behaviors. Underlying systems thinking is the premise that system behaves as a whole and that such behavior cannot be explained solely in terms a simple aggregate of individual elements. An important emergent property of the whole is self-organization…One well-known statement associated with systems thinking is that "Everything is connected to everything else."

Temperament- Constitutional predisposition to react, in a particular way, to stimuli. A component of one's personality.

Transcendental Self-Consciousness- The transcendental self-consciousness is primal like the seed of a tree or an animal; it cannot be perceived or grasped in words[1]. It is not born nor does it die (questionable in the neurobiological circle). It is beyond all qualities, the witness, eternal and pure, of the essence of the indivisible, one-only subtle, without components, without taint, without egoism. It is beyond senses. It is all-pervading, unthinkable and indescribable. It purifies the defiled, the evil. It is spontaneous, without action, and without any residue (ever fresh and new).

Transpersonal Psychology- Transpersonal psychology addresses topics such as i) the importance of spirituality in psychotherapy and counseling, ii) spirituality as a resource for maintaining and regaining health, iii) spiritual experiences as an avenue to consciousness, and iv) the delimitation of extraordinary states of consciousness.

Triple Aspect Monism- The first aspect is the describable, objective reality, the observed world. The second aspect is the observable and describable mental world of ego, actions, thoughts, emotions, images, memories, imaginations etc. The third aspect is the indescribable, all-inclusive, essential, existential, feeling of intrinsic, subjective essential awareness. It is the mysterious wonder within all of us. Only a few of us realize this aspect of our consciousness, because most of us are so preoccupied with superficial, verbal, cognitive, memory-based processing. This is the 'existential-spiritual' aspect of our conscious Being that waits to be discovered by each one of us, in our own Energy-Being.

Turīya, Non-REM-Wakefulness- The Sanskrit word Turīya literally means the fourth aspect. The Encyclopedia of Eastern Philosophy and Religion defined Turīya as a superconscious state of illumination, called the fourth, because it transcends the three familiar states of deep sleep, dream sleep and wakefulness. This state of essential consciousness is beyond thought, causality and identification with the body. It is pure unified awareness, of indescribable serenity and of the nature of Ātman, the essential, existential Energy-Being.

Turīya is a unique superconscious, awakened state of Non-REM-Wakefulness (NREM-W) characterized by i) an optimal alert attentiveness with freedom from distractions, day-dreaming, and intrusive thoughts, ii) a spontaneous behavioral quiescence, both motor-premotor and preverbal quiescence, mental stillness and speechless Silence, with no internal talk or thoughts, iii) heightened perceptivity, intellectual clarity, and cognitive excellence, and iv) an enhanced sense of well-being, an unconditional Bliss Ānanda, Serenity Śānti, Compassion Karuṇ ā, love for Life, and spontaneous Creativity Srujatā.

---

1 यत्र वाचा निवर्तन्ते, अप्राप्य मनसा सह | That which cannot be reached by speech, nor grasped intellectually by the mind. (From the Bhagvad Gītā).

Ultimate Truth- The human experience of the ultimate truth has been described in various religions and philosophies, as *Ātman~Brahman*, Turīya, Nirvaṇ a, Tao, Unio Mystica, Exitential Ground, Order of One, Absolute Unitary Being and Holistic Superconsciousness. Such a unique perspective of the existential truth remains a matter of first-person experience only; it cannot be fully objectified and described. It is essentially a subjective mode of energy~being~bliss. All of us have the potential for such an amazing and fulfilling self-discovery.

Unconscious- i) that part of memory and mental functioning that is rarely subject to awareness. It is a repository of data, that has never been conscious (primary repression) or may have been conscious and are later repressed (secondary repression). ii) The sum total of all mental contents and processes, at any given moment, outside the range of conscious awareness, including the preconscious.

Unified Conscious Experience- A property of consciousness that can be easily agreed upon is that it is normally a unified experience. Each one of us has the impression of being a single entity, experiencing an integrated perceptual world, at this particular moment in time. It is *me* that is surveying the scene in front of me right now. I am the unifying point of reference for all the objects, that I see scattered before me. The objects, too, appear to me to exist in a unified field of space-time. We have to realize this continuous unity of space-time-energy and personal being.

Vigilant Attention- Robertson and Garavan defined vigilant attention as a continuous inhibition[2] of task irrelevances. "We conceive of the right parieto-prefrontal network and its interactions with the midbrain arousal systems as the circuitry by which vigilant attention is maintained. This circuitry can be 'tuned up' (or down) endogenously or with exogenous support. Within this system, we believe that the prefrontal cortex plays a central role in maintaining and monitoring optimal arousal levels to match current task demands."

Virtue- The American Psychological Association (APA) dictionary defined "Virtue" as a quality or characteristic that has positive connotation in a particular society and that is considered benefitial to psychological health. It also means moral goodness. Erikson defined "Virtue" as "inherent stregth."

Volition- Volition is the mental faculty, by which an individual decides upon and commits to a particular course of action. Volition involves a sense of ego, and an active control over the decision making process, and its veto power.

Wellbeing- Well-being is defined as a state of happiness, contentment, lack of distress, overall good physical and mental health, and a healthy outlook with a good quality of life.

Wisdom- The APA dictionary defines "Wisdom" as the ability of an individual to make sound decisions, to find the right – or at least good – answers to difficult and important life questions, and to give advice about the complex problems of everyday life and interpersonal relationships.

Wonder- Bulkeley defined "Wonder" as the feeling of being excited by an encounter with something novel and unexpected, something that strikes a person as intensely real, true, and/or beautiful. Wonder is something that causes astonishment. To feel wonder is to experience a sudden decentering of the self (ego). Facing something surprisingly new and

2 This is similar to the classical definition of Yoga by Pātañjali: Yogaḥ chitta vritti nirodhāḥ, which implies voluntary or spontaneous inhibition of irrelevant mental, verbal and cognitive activity.

unexpectedly powerful, one's ordinary sense of personal identity is dramatically altered, leading to new knowledge and understanding, that ultimately recenter the self. The profound impact of this decentering and recentering process is evident in the intense memorability of the experiences and the strong bodily sensations that often accompany them."

Yoga- The word Yoga is derived from the verb Yuj, which means to integrate or unite. Yoga is a way of integration through self-understanding and self-realization. It is a system of discipline that facilitates the ultimate goal of an adaptive, creative, and enlightened life for a human being.

APPENDIX 7: VEDĀNTA, YOGA AND MEDITATION ADDITIONAL REFERENCES

VEDAS

1) Le Mee J, Gruttner I. Hymns from the ṚgVeda. New York,NY: Alfred A. Knopf; 1975.
2) de Nicolas AT. Meditations through the ṚgVeda: Four Dimensional Man. Boulder, CO and London, UK: Shambhala; 1978.
3) Bhakta MA. Vedic String Theory. BookSurge LLC. www.booksurge.com; 2006.
4) Devi Chand: The Yajur Veda. New Delhi, India: Munshiram Manoharlal Publishers; 1994.
5) Ganapati SV. Sāma Veda. Delhi, India: Motilal Banarasidāss Publishers; 1992.
6) Devi Chand: The Atharva Veda. New Delhi,India: Munshiram Manoharlal Publishers; 1980.
7) Śri Chandrasekharendra Saraswati. The Vedās. Mumbai, India: Bharatiya Vidyā Bhavan; 2006: 7th edition.

UPANIṢADS

1) Sharmā S. ed. 108 Upaniṣ ad: Brahmavidyā, Jñāna and Sādhanā Khaṇ ḍ a. Mathura, India: Yuga Nirmāṇ a Yojanā; 2005.
2) Radhākrishnan S. The Principal Upaniṣ ads. New Delhi, India: Harper Collins Publishers; 1994.
3) Mahādevan TMP. Upaniṣ ads. New Delhi. India: Arnold-Heinemann Publishers; 1975.
4) Madhavānanda S. Minor Upaniṣ ads. Kolkata, India: Advaita Āṣ rama; 1980.
5) Deshmukh VD. Turīya: The Fourth State of Consciousness and the STEP Model of Self-Consciousness. Journal of Interdisciplinary Crossroads, Dec 2004, 1(3): 551-560.

Bhagvad Gītā

1) Swarūpānanda S. Shrimad Bhagvad Gītā. Kolkata, India: Advaita Āṣ rama; 1967.
2) Radhākrishnan S. The Bhagavadgītā. New Delhi, India: Harper Collins Publishers; 2004.
3) de Nicolas AT. The Bhagavad Gītā: The ethics of Decision Making, Berwick, Maine: Nicolas-Hays; 1990.

Brahma Sūtra and Vedānta

1) Ghabhirānanda S. Brahma Sūtra Bhaṣ ya of Śankarāchārya. Kolkata, India: Advaita Āṣ rama; 1996.
2) Tattvānanda S. The Quintessence of Vedānta. kerala, India: Sri Ramakrishna Advaita Āṣ rama, Kalady; 1991.
3) Nikhilānanda S. Vedāntasāra or The Essence of Vedānta of Sadānanda Yogindra. Kolkata, India: Advaita Āṣ rama; 1978.
4) Vimuktānanda S. Aparokshānubhūti or Self-Realization. Kolkata, India: Advaita Āṣ rama; 1966.
5) Parthasārathy A. Ātmabodha: Knowledge of Self. Mumbai, India: Vedānta Life Institute; 1986.
6) Samvid. Prabodha Sudhākara: The Nectar Ocean of Enlightenment. Chennai, India: Samata Books, 1987.
7) Tejomayānanda S. Tattvabodhaḥ of Śri Ādi Śankarāchārya, Mumbai, India: Central Chinmaya Mission Trust; 2002.
8) Madhavānanda S. Vivekcudāmaṇ i of Śri Śankaracharya. Kolkata, India: Advaita Āṣ rama; 1970.
9) Jagadānanda S. Upadeśa Sāhasrī of Śri Śankaracharya. Chennai, India: Sri Ramakrishna Math, Mylapore; 1970.
10) Ashokānanda S. Avadhūta Gītā: Song of the Free. Chennai, India: Sri Ramakrishna Math, Mylapore; 1981.
11) Bhagwat LB: Śri Jñānadeva's Amṛ itānubhava with Cāngadeva Pāsaṣ ṭ hi. Chennai, India: Samata Books and Sri Mira Trust; 1997.
12) Ādiṣ varānanda S. The Vedānta Way to Peace and Happiness. Woodstock, VT: Skylight Paths Publishing; 2004.
13) Huxley A. The Perennial Philosophy. New York, NY:Harper Collins Publishers; 2004.

Yoga

1) Leggett T. Śankara on the Yoga Sūtrās. Delhi, India: Motilal Banārasidāss Publishers, 1992.
2) Taimni IK. The Science of Yoga: The Yoga Sūtrās of Pātañjali. Wheaton, IL: The Theosophical Publishing House; 1961.

3) Kolhatakar KK. Indian Psychology: Pātañjala Yoga-Darśana, (in Marathi). Mumbai, India: Keśava Bhikaji Dhavale; 1982, 5th edition.
4) Venkateśānanda S The Supreme Yoga: A New Translation of Yoga Vāsiṣ ṭ ha. Volumes I and II. Shivānandanagar, Uttarānchal, India: The Divine Life Society; 2003, 4th edition.
5) Desāi A. Amṛ ita Yoga: Explore,Expand, Experience. The Spiritual Depth of Yoga. Salt Springs, FL: Amṛ ita Yoga Institute; 2004.
6) Deshmukh VD. Presence: The Key to Mental Excellence. Jacksonville, FL: Sunanda V Deshmukh, MD; 1990.
7) Akers BD. The Hatha Yoga Pradīpikā of Swātmārāma. Woodstock, NY: YogaVidya.com; 2002.
8) Dinakar LG. (in Marathi). Yoga Yājñavalkya. Pune, India: Dinakar LG; 2006.
9) Paramānanda S. Silence as Yoga. Cohasset, MA: Vedanta Center Publishers; 1974.
10) Vivekānanda S, Translation and commentary. The Yoga Sūtrās of Pātañjali. London, UK: Watkins Publishing; 2007.
11) Guṇ de DG. Yoga and Health (in Marathi). Kolhapur, India: GJG Yoga Academy; 1988.
12) Shannahoff-Khalsa DS. Kuṇ ḍ alini Yoga Meditation: Techniques specific for psychiatric disorders, couple therapy and personal growth. New York, NY: WW Norton and Company; 2006.

PRĀṆĀYĀMA

1) Nāgendra HR. Prāṇ āyāma: The Art and Science. Bangalore, India: Vivekānanda Kendra Yoga Prakāśana; 1998.
2) Rāmdev S. Prāṇ āyāma: Its Philosophy and Practice. Haridwar, India: Divya Prakāśan; 2005.
3) Kuvalayānanda S. Prāṇ āyāma. Mumbai, India: Popular Prakaśan; 1966.

MEDITATION AND CONSCIOUSNESS

1) Ādiśwarānanda S. Meditation and Its Practices: A Definitive Guide to Tachniques and Traditions of Meditation in Yoga and Vedānta. Mayavati, Champwat, India: Advaita Ashram; 2004.
2) Chinmayānanda S. Meditation and Life. Chennai, India: Govindass Parekh for Chinmaya Publication Trust; 1962.
3) Tejomayānada S, Śantānanda S, eds. Living in the Present. Langhorne, PA: Chinmaya Publications; 2008.
4) Bhikkhu Bodhi: In the Buddha's Words. Boston, MA: Wisdom Publications; 2005.
5) Guṇ aratana BH. Mindfulness in Plain English. Boston, MA: Wisdom Publications; 2002.
6) Rosenberg L. Breath by Breath: The Liberating Practice of Insight Meditation. Boston, MA: Shambhala; 1999.

7) Krishnamurti J. The Meditative Mind. Ojai, CA: Krishnamurti Foundation of America; 1989.
8) Deshmukh VD. Neuroscience of Meditation. TSW Holistic Health and Medicine 2006, 1: 275-289.
9) Tolle E. The Power of Now: A Guide to Spiritual Enlightenment. Novato, CA: New World Library and Vancouver, Canada: Namaste Publishing; 2004.
10) Siegel DJ. The Mindful Brain: Reflection and Attunement in the Cultivation of Well-Being. New York, NY: W. W. Norton and Company; 2007.
11) Kak SC. The Architecture of Knowledge: Quantum Mechanics, Neuroscience, Computers and Consciousness.

Kashmir Śaivism

1) Singh J. Śiva Sūtras: The Yoga of Supreme Identity. Motilal Banarasidass Publishers, Delhi, India. 1979, reprint 2008.
2) Singh J. Pratyabhijñāhṛ dayam: The Secret of Self-Recognition. Motilal Banarasidass Publishers, Delhi, India. 1963, reprint 2011.
3) Singh J. Spanda-Kārikās: The Divine Creative Pulsation. Motilal Banarasidass Publishers, Delhi, India. 1980, reprint 2009.
4) Singh J. Vijñānabhairava or Divine Consciousness. Motilal Banarasidass Publishers, Delhi, India. 1979, reprint 1999.

REFERENCES

[1] VandenBos GR, ed. APA Dictionary of Psychology. Washington, DC: *Am. Psychol. Assoc.,* 2007.

[2] Ventegodt S, Kandel I, Merrick, J. *Principles of Holistic Medicine: Quality of Life and Health.* New Hyde Park, NY: Hippocrates Scientific Publications, 2005: 32.

[3] Hall CS and Lindzey G. Lewin's Field Theory. *In Theories of Personality.* 3rd ed. New York NY: John Wiley and Sons, 1978:383-435.

[4] Deshmukh, VD. *Presence as a new mode of human attention.* Society for Neuroscience Abstracts, 1982 November:8.

[5] Deshmukh, VD: *Presence: The Key to Mental Excellence.* Jacksonville, Florida: Sunanda V Deshmukh, MD; 1990.

[6] Gunaratana BH. *Mindfulness in Plain English.* Boston, MA:Wisdom Publications, 2002.

[7] Krishnamurti J. Is one concerned with the total human existence. *In The Flame of Attention,* Chapter 7, 1st Public Talk at Ojai, 1st May 1982.

[8] Vimuktananda, S. *Aparoksnaubhuti or Self-Realization of Śaṅkarāchārya. Kolkata,* India: Advaita Ashram, 1966.

[9] Ramanan VS, ed. *Talks with Sri Ramaṇa Maharṣi.* Tiruvannamalai, India: Sri Ramanashramam, 1955:Talk 98:96.

[10] Bhikkhu Bodhi, ed. Teachings of the Buddha in the Buddha's Words: *An Anthology of Discourses from the Pali Canon.* Boston:Wisdom Publications, 2005:366.

[11] Mark Lee RE, ed. *The Book of Life: Daily Meditations with Krishnamurti.* New York, NY: HarperSanFrancisco, 1995: June 6.

[12] Sri Aurobindo. *The Mother.* Pondicherry, India: Sri Aurobindo Ashram, 2002:22-30.

[13] Micozzi MS, and Singh D. Yoga. In: Micozzi MC. *Fundamentals of Complimentary and Integrative Medicine*, Third edition. Saunders Elsevier, St. Louis, Missouri, USA: 2006: 508-17.

[14] Pressman MD. Energetic Healing. In: Micozzi MC. *Fundamentals of Complimentary and Integrative Medicine,* Third edition. Saunders Elsevier, St. Louis, Missouri, USA: 2006: 313-25.

[15] Shannahoff-Khalsa DS. *Kuṇḍalini Yoga Meditation: Techniques specific for Psychiatric Disorders, Couples Therapy and Personal Growth.* New York. London: W. W. Norton and Company, 2006: 6-7 and 31-32.

[16] Jung CG. *The Psychology of Kuṇḍalini Yoga*: Notes of the Seminar given in 1932 by CG. Jung. Edited by Shamdasani S. Princeton University Press, Princeton New Jersey, USA. 1996: 76-78.

[17] Deshmukh VD. Oscillatory Neural Ectoderm (ONE): the "ONE" hypothesis for human holo-encephalon and behavior. *Medical Hypotheses* 1987, 23: 107-108.
[18] Deshmukh VD. A chain of supra-segmental neuro-oscillatory circuits: A human brain theory. *Clinical Electroencephalography*, 1988, 19(1): 7-13.
[19] Deshmukh VD. *Neurophysiological Interpretation of Ida, Pingala, and Sushumna.* Neurology India, 1991; 39:125-31.
[20] Buzsáki G. *Rhythms of the Brain.* New York, NY: 2006.
[21] Arthur Avlon (Sir John Woodroffe). The Serpent Power: *The Secrets of Tantric and Śaktic Yoga including the translation of Śat-Cakra-Nirupaṇa and Paduka-Pancaka.* New York: Dover Publications, Inc. 1974.
[22] Mookerjee A. *Kuṇḍalini: The Arousal of the Inner Energy*. New York: Destiny Books, 1983.
[23] Rele VG. *The Mysterious Kuṇḍalini: The physical basis of the Kuṇḍalini yoga in terms of Western anatomy and physiology.* Mumbai, India. D. B. Taraporevala Sons and Company, 1960.
[24] Gopi Krishna. *Three Perspectives on Kuṇḍalini*. New Delhi, India. UBS Publishers' Distributers Ltd. 1994.
[25] Saraswati SS. *Kuṇḍalini Tantra.* Munger, Bihar, India. *Yoga Publications Trust,* 1984: 81-85.
[26] Guḷ awani WD. *Mahāyoga Vijñān.* (Sanskrit and Marathi) Pune, India. *Shri Vāsudeva Niwās Prakāshan*, 2nd printing 1996.
[27] Tambe SB, *Cakra-Sudarśana.* 2nd edition. (in Sanskrit and Marathi) Pune, India: *Balaji Tambe Foundation*, 2007.
[28] Deshmukh VD. Limbic-autonomic arousal: its physiological classification and review of the literature. *Clinical Electroencephalography* 1991, 22(1):46-60.
[29] Deshmukh VD. Physiological classification of sleep-wake states: based on tri-vesicular (3V) model of the brain. *Clinical Electroencephalography* 1991, 22(4):225-235.
[30] Deshmukh, VD. Turiya: The fourth state of consciousness and the STEP model of self-consciousness. *Journal of Interdisciplinary Crossroads* 2004 Dec:1, 3, 551-60.
[31] Lutz A, Dunne JD, Davidson RJ. Meditation and the Neuroscience of Consciousness: An Introduction. In Zelazo PD, Moscovitch M, Thompson E, eds. T*he Cambridge Handbook of Consciousness.* Cambridge MA: Cambridge University Press, 2007:499-551.
[32] Holzel BK, Carmody J, Evans KC, Hoge EA, Dusek JA, Morgan L, Pitman RK, Lazar SW. Stress reduction correlates with structural changes in the amygdala. *SCAN* 2010:5,11-17.
[33] Bærentsen KB, Stødkilde-Jørgensen H, Sommerlund B, Hartmann T, Damsgaard-Madsen J, Fosnæs M, Green AC. An investigation of brain processes supporting meditation. *Cogn. Process* 2010;11:57–84.
[34] Delamillieure P, Douceta G, Mazoyera B, Turbelina MR, Delcroixa N, Melleta E, Zagoa L, Crivello F, Petit L, Tzourio-Mazoyera N, Joliot M. The resting state questionnaire: An introspective questionnaire for evaluation of inner experience during the conscious resting state. *Brain Research Bulletin.* 2010; 81:565–573.
[35] Pagnoni G, Cekic M, GuoY. *"Thinking about Not-Thinking": Neural Correlates of Conceptual Processing during Zen Meditation*. PLoS ONE 2008; 3(9): e3083.
[36] Johnstone T, van Reekum CM, Oakes TR and Davidson RJ. The voice of emotion: an FMRI study of neural responses to angry and happy vocal expressions. *Soc. Cogn. Affect. Neurosci.* 2006 December; 1(3): 242–249.

[37] Farb NAS, Segal ZV, Mayberg H, Bean J, McKeon D, Fatima Z, Anderson AK. Attending to the present: mindfulness meditation reveals distinct neural modes of self-reference. *Soc. Cogn. Affect. Neurosci.* 2007 December; 2(4): 313–322.
[38] Davidson RJ; Lutz A. Buddha's Brain: Neuroplasticity and Meditation. *IEEE Signal Process Mag*. 2008 January 1; 25(1): 176–174.
[39] Deshmukh VD. Neuroscience of Meditation. *TSW Holistic Health and Medicine.* 2006:1, 275-89.
[40] Austin JH. Selfless Insight: *Zen and the Meditative Transformations of Consciousness.* Cambridge, MA: The MIT Press; 2009.
[41] Shear J, ed. The Experience of Meditation: *Experts Introduce the Major Traditions.* Princeton, NJ: The Infinity Foundation; 2006.
[42] Deshmukh VD. *Introduction to Vedānta.* In Tattva: An International online monthly magazine for Hindu youth 2009. Available from: URL: www.hinduyuva.org/tattva. Tononi G; Laureys S. The Neurology of Consciousness: An Overview. In Laureys S, Tononi G, Eds. The Neurology of Consciousness: *Cognitive Neuroscience and Neuropathology*. Burlington, MA: Elsevier Ltd; 2009:375-412.
[43] James W. *The Principles of Psychology.* Vol. 1. New York, NY: Cosimo classics; 1890-2007:296-299.
[44] Kneisl CR and Trigoboff E. *Contemporary Psychiatric-Mental Health Nursing*. 2nd ed. New Jersey: Pearson Education, Inc. 2009.
[45] Krishnamurti J. *Daily Quotes. The Book of Life 145.* Available from URL: JKrishnamurti.org.
[46] Raichle ME and Snyder AZ. Intrinsic Brain Activity and Consciousness. In Laureys S, Tononi G, eds. The Neurology of Consciousness: *Cognitive Neuroscience and Neuropathology*. Burlington, *MA:Elsevier* Ltd; 2009:81-88.
[47] Panksepp J, Northoff G. The trans-species core SELF: The emergence of active cultural and neuro-ecological agents through self-related processing within subcortical-cortical midline networks. *Consciousness and Cognition* 2009, 18:193–215.
[48] Posner MI, Rothbart MK. Toward a physical basis of attention and self regulation. *Phys. Life Rev.* 2009 Jun;6(2):103-20.
[49] Deshmukh VD. A Poet's Walk: *A collection of Poems, Essays, and Photographs.* Jacksonville, Florida: Sunanda V Deshmukh;2002:26.
[50] Radhakrishnan, S, ed. and trans. *The Principal Upaniṣads.* New Delhi, India: HarperCollins Publishers; 1994.
[51] Taimani, I.K. *The Science of Yoga.* Wheaton, IL: The Theosophical Publishing House; 1961.
[52] Krishnamurti J. *Meditations*. San Francisco, CA: Harper and Row Publishers;1979:4.
[53] Heilman KM. *Matter of Mind: A Neurologist's View of Brain-Behavior Relationships.* New York, NY: Oxford University Press; 2002.
[54] Zeman A. *Consciousness: a User's Guide*. New Haven CT: Yale University Press; 2002.
[55] Libet B. *Mind Time: The Temporal Factor in Consciousness*. Cambridge, MA: Harvard University Press; 2004.
[56] Zelazo PD, Moscovitch M, Thopson E, Eds. *The Cambridge Handbook of Consciousness.* New York, NY: Cambridge University Press; 2007.
[57] Koch C. *The Neurobiology of Consciousness*. In Gazzaniga MS, ed. *The Cognitive Neurosciences,* 4th ed. A Bradford Book, Cambridge, MA: The MIT Press; 2009:1137-1149.

[58] Deshmukh VD. Functional Brain Model: A Nested Hierarchical and Parallel Organization during Development and Evolution. *Journal of Alternative Medicine Research* 2010:1(1) 5-13.
[59] Panksepp, J. Affective Neuroscience: *The Foundations of Human and Animal Emotions*. New York, NY: Oxford University Press; 1998.
[60] Bleck, T. P. Levels of Consciousness and Attention. In Goetz CG, ed. *Textbook of Clinical Neurology*, 3rd ed. Saunders-Elsevier; 2007.
[61] Pfaff, D. *Brain Arousal and Information Theory: Neural and Genetic Mechanisms*. Cambridge, MA: Harvard University Press; 2006.
[62] Waxman SG. *Clinical Neuroanatomy*. 26th ed. Lange, New York, NY: McGraw Hill; 2010.
[63] Schiff ND. Recovery of Consciousness after Brain Injury: An Integrative Research Paradigm for the Cognitive Neuroscience of Consciousness. In Laureys S, Tononi G, eds. The Neurology of Consciousness: *Cognitive Neuroscience and Neuropathology*. Burlington, MA: Elsevier Ltd; 2009:1123-1136.
[64] Miller BL, Cummings, JL, eds. *The Human Frontal Lobes: Functions and Disorders*. 2nd ed. New York, NY: The Guildford Press; 2007.
[65] Ben-Yehudah, G. and Fiez, J. A. Development of Verbal Memory. In Coch D, Fischer KW, Dawson G, eds. *Human Behavior, Learning, and the Developing Brain: Typical Development*. New York, NY: The Guildford Press; 2007:301-328.
[66] Mesulam, M. M. *Principles of Behavioral Neurology*. Philadelphia, PA: F. A. Davis Company;1985:125-168.
[67] LeDoux JE, Schiller D, and Cain C. Emotional reaction and Action: From Threat Processing to Goal-Directed Behavior. In Laureys S and Tononi G, eds. The Neurology of Consciousness: *Cognitive Neuroscience and Neuropathology*. Burlington, MA: Elsevier Ltd;2009:905-924.
[68] Deshmukh VD. The Multistream Self: Biophysical, Mental, Social, and Existential. *TheScientificWorldJOURNAL*: 2008;(8):331-41.
[69] Prabhavānanda, S. *The Spiritual Heritage of India*. Hollywood, California: Vedanta Press; 1979:208-225.
[70] Madhavānanda, S. *Minor Upaniṣads: Angiras' Ātmopaniṣad*. Calcutta, India: Advaita Ashram; 1980:11-16.
[71] Akhilānada, S. *Hindu Psychology: Its Meaning for the West*. London, UK: Routledge and Kegan Paul Ltd; 1965:54-77.
[72] Radhākrishnan, S. The Bhagavadgitā. New Delhi, India: HarperCollins Publishers; 2004:355-356.
[73] Kandel ER. *In Search of Memory: The Emergence of a New Science of Mind*. New York, NY: W. W. Norton and Company; 2006:374.
[74] Kircher, T. and David A. *The Self in Neuroscience and Psychiatry*, Cambridge, University Press:2003;445-75.
[75] Deshmukh, VD. *Presence: The Key to Mental Excellence*, Jacksonville, Florida: Sunanda V Deshmukh; 1990:119-21.
[76] Bleck T. *Levels of Consciousness and Attention*. In Goetz CG, ed. Textbook of Clinical Neurology, 3rd ed. Saunders-Elsevier: 2007; 3-19.
[77] Baars BJ, Banks WP, and Newman JB, eds. *Essential Sources in the Scientific Study of Consciousness*. Cambridge, MA: The MIT Press; 2003.
[78] Goerner S, and Combs A. Consciousness as a Self-Organizing Process*: An Ecological Perspective, Bio-Systems*, 1998, 46,123-27.
[79] Tononi G. and Edelman GM. *Consciousness and Complexity*. Science, 4 December 1998, 282, 1846-51.

[80] Tononi, G and Balduzzi D. *Toward a Theory of Consciousness*. In Gazzaniga MS, ed. The Cognitive Neurosciences. Cambridge, MA: The MIT Press; 2009:1201-1217.
[81] Balkin TJ, et al. The Process of Awakening: *A PET Study of Regional Brain Activity Patterns Mediating the Re-establishment of Alertness and Consciousness, Brain*, 2002, 125, 2308-19.
[82] Purkey WW and Stanley PH. *The Self in Psychotherapy*. In Cain DJ and Seeman J, *eds. Humanistic Psychotherapies.* Washington. D.C: American Psychological Association; 2002.
[83] Damasio AR. *The Feelings of What Happens*. New York, NY: Hartcourt Brace and Company; 1999.
[84] Damasio AR and Meyer K. *Consciousness: An Overview of the Phenomenon and its Possible Neural Basis*. In Laureys S and Tononi G, eds. The Neurology of Consciousness: Cognitive Neuroscience and Neuropathology. Burlington, MA: *Elsevier Ltd;* 2009; 3-14.
[85] Prabhakaran VK, Narayanan, Zhao Z and Gabriel JDE. Integration of Diverse Information in Working Memory within the Frontal Lobe. *Nature neuroscience,* 2000 January, 3, 1: 85-90.
[86] Miller EK and Cohen JD. An Integrative Theory of Prefrontal Cortex Function. *Annu. Rev. Neurosci*, 2001; 24:167-202.
[87] Fuster JM. Synopsis of Function and Dysfunction of Frontal Lobe. *Acta psychiatr. Scand.*, 1999, 99 (suppl. 395):51-57.
[88] Stuss DT, Knight RT, eds. *Principles of Frontal Lobe Function.* Oxford University Press:2002.
[89] Llinas RR. *I of the vortex: from neurons to self.* Cambridge, MA: The MIT Press; 2001; 21-23 and 127-128.
[90] Jagadananda S. *Upadesha-Sāhasrī: A Thousand Teachings of Sri Shankarāchārya.* Chennai, India: Sri Ramakrishna Math; 1970.
[91] Parthasārathy A. *Ātmabodha: Knowledge of Self by Śri Ādi Śankarāchārya. Mumbai*, India: Vedānta Life Institute; 1971.Ś
[92] Maslow AH. *Toward a Psychology of Being.* 2nd ed. New York, NY: Van Nostrand; 1968.
[93] Yalom, I.D. *Existential Psychotherapy.* New York, NY: Basic Books; 1980.
[94] Newton DS. Erik H. *Erikson.* In Sadock BJ and Sadock VA, eds. *Kaplan and Sadock's Comprehensive Textbook of Psychiatry.* 8th ed. Philadelphia, PA: Lippincott Williams and Wilkins; 2005;1:751.
[95] Meissner WW. *Classic psychoanalysis*. In Sadock BJ and Sadock VA, eds. *Kaplan and Sadock's Comprehensive Textbook of Psychiatry*. 8th ed. Philadelphia, PA: Lippincott Williams and Wilkins; 2005;1: 733.
[96] Haken H. Synergetics of Brain Function. *Int. J. Psychophysiol,* 2006, 60, 110-124.
[97] Scott Kelso JA. Dynamic Patterns: *The Self-Organization of Brain and Behavior.* Cambridge, MA: The MIT Press; 1995.
[98] Scott Kelso JA and Engstrom DA. *The Complementary Nature*. Cambridge, MA: The MIT Press; 2006.
[99] West JB. Ed. Best and *Taylor's Physiological Basis of Medical Practice.* 12th ed. Baltimore, MD: Williams and Wilkins; 1992.
[100] Shneerson JM. Physiological basis of sleep and wakefulness. *In Sleep Medicine: A Guide to Sleep and its Disorders*. 2nd ed. Oxford: Blackwell; 2005; 2:22–53.
[101] Kandel ER, Schwartz JH and Jessell TM, Eds. *Essentials of Neuroscience and Behavior*. Norwalk, CT: Appleton and Lang; 1995:324–346.

[102] Pfaff D. Brain *Arousal and Information Theory: Neural and Genetic Mechanisms*. Cambridge, MA: Harvard University Press; 2006.
[103] Seeley WW, Sturm VE. *Self-representation and the frontal lobes*. In Miller BL, Cummings JL, eds. *The Human Frontal Lobes:Functions and Disorders*. 2nd ed. New York, NY: The Guilford Press; 2007: 317–334.
[104] Arzy S, Thut G, Mohr C, Michel CM, Blanke O. Neural basis of embodiment: distinct contributions of temporo-parietal junction and extrastriate body area. *J. Neurosci.* 2006, 26, 31, 8074–8081.
[105] Carruthers G. A model of the synchronic self. *Conscious. Cogn*. 2006, 16, 2, 533–550.
[106] Cavanna AE, Trimble MR. The precuneus: a review of its functional anatomy and behavioral correlates. *Brain.* 2006, 129, 564–583.
[107] Damasio AR. How the brain creates the mind. In Bloom FE, ed. *Best of the Brain from Scientific American*. New York, NY: Dana Press; 2007: 58–67.
[108] Lou HC, Nowak M, Kjaer TW. The mental self. *Prog. Brain Res.* 2005, 150, 197–204.
[109] Gazzaniga MS. Forty-five years of split-brain research and still going strong. *Nat. Rev. Neurosci*. 2005, 6, 653–659.
[110] Zhu J. Locating volition. *Conscious. Cogn.* 2004, 13, 302–322.
[111] Zimmer C. *The neurobiology of self.* In Bloom FE, ed. Best of the Brain from Scientific American. New York, NY: Dana Press; 2007: 47–57.
[112] Georgalis N. The Primacy of the Subjective: *Foundations for a Unified Theory of Mind and Language.* Cambridge, MA: The MIT Press; 2006.
[113] Zahavi D. Subjectivity and Selfhood: *Investigating the First-Person Perspective*. Cambridge, MA: The MIT Press;2005.
[114] Pred R. Onflow: *Dynamics of Consciousness and Experience.* Cambridge, MA: The MIT Press; 2005.
[115] Huxley A. *The Perennial Philosophy: An Interpretation of the Great Mystics, East and West.* New York, NY: Harper and Brothers; 1945.
[116] Deshmukh VD. Ipseity, Atman and consciousness. In the Proceedings of the Fifth *International Conference of World Association of Vedic Studies*. Washington, DC: 2004 July; 9–11.
[117] Austin JH. Zen and the Brain: *Toward an Understanding of Meditation and Consciousness. Cambridge, MA*: The MIT Press; 1998.
[118] Guyton AC and Hall JE. Textbook of Medical Physiology. 11th ed. *Elsevier-Saunders;* 2006.
[119] Thompson RA and Nelson CA. Developmental science and the media: early brain development. *Am. Psychol.* 2001, 56, 5–15.
[120] Richter SB, Howard BJ and Sturner R. *Normal infant and childhood development*. In McMillan JA, Feigin RD, DeAngelis C, Jones MD, eds. Oski's Pediatrics: Principles and Practice. Philadelphia, PA: Lippincott Williams and Wilkins; 2006; 96:593–601.
[121] Graven S. Sleep and brain development. *Clin. Perinatol.* 2006, 33, 693–706.
[122] Pujol J, Soriano-Mas C, Ortiz H, et al. Myelination of language-related areas in the developing brain. *Neurology* 2006, 66, 339–343.
[123] Fuhrman BP, Zimmerman JJ. Pediatric Critical Care. 3rd ed. Mosby-Elsevier: 2006.
[124] Als H, Butler S. Neurobehavioral development of the preterm infant. In Martin RJ, Fanaroff AA, Walsh MC, eds. Fanaroff and Martin's Neonatal-Perinatal Medicine: Diseases of the Fetus and Infant. 8th ed. *Mosby-Elsevier*; 2006:Chap. 41.
[125] Stern P, Hines PJ. Neuroscience: systems-level brain development. *Science* 2005;310:801–823.
[126] Johnson MH, Munakata Y. Processes of change in brain and cognitive development. *Trends Cogn. Sci*. 2005;9(3):152–158.

[127] Sarnat, H.B. *The new embryology*. In Menkes JH, Sarnat HB, Maria BL, eds. Child Neurology. 7th ed. Philadelphia, PA: Lippincott, Williams and Wilkins; 2005, Chap. 4 (1):259–284.

[128] Cunningham FG, Leveno KJ, Bloom SL, Hauth JC, Gilstrap L, Wenstrom KD, eds. Williams Obstetrics. 22nd ed. New York, NY McGraw-Hill; 2005:106.

[129] Rivkees SA. Emergence and influences of circadian rhythmicity in infants. *Clin. Perinatol*. 2004, (31):217–228.

[130] Schaal, B., Hummel, T., and Soussignan, R. (2004) Olfaction in the fetal and premature infant: functional status and clinical implications. *Clin. Perinatol.* 31, 261–285.

[131] Graven SN. Early neurosensory visual development of the fetus and the newborn. *Clin. Perinatol*. 2004, 31, 199–216.

[132] Greenspan SI, Curry JF. Extending Jean Piaget's approach to intellectual functioning. In Sadock BJ, Sadock VA, eds. *Kaplan and Sadock's Comprehensive Textbook of Psychiatry*. 8th ed. Vol. 1. Philadelphia, PA: Lippincott, Williams and Wilkins; 2005(3.2):528–540.

[133] Newton DS. Erik H. Erikson. In Sadock BJ, Sadock VA, eds. *Kaplan and Sadock's Comprehensive Textbook of Psychiatry*. 8th ed. Vol. 1. Philadelphia, PA: Lippincott, Williams and Wilkins; 2005(6.2):746–755.

[134] Kraft U. Unleashing creativity. In Bloom FE, ed. *Best of the Brain from Scientific American*. New York, NY: Dana Press; 2007: 9–19.

[135] Monnier M. General conclusions. In Monnier M, Meulders M, eds. Functions of The Nervous System: Psycho-Neurobiology. Vol. 4. Amsterdam: *Elsevier;* 1983: 693–698.

[136] Goodale MA, Cant JS, Kroliczak G. Grasping the past and present: when does visuo-motor priming occur? In Ogmen H, Breitmeyer BG, eds. The First Half Second: *The Microgenesis and Temporal Dynamics of Unconscious and Conscious Visual Processes*. Cambridge, MA: The MIT Press; 2004:51–71.

[137] Moore CM, Woolfe JM. Getting beyond the serial/parallel debate in visual search: a hybrid approach. In Shapiro K, ed. The Limits of Attention: *Temporal Constraints in Human Information Processing*. Oxford, UK: Oxford University Press; 2001:178–198.

[138] Young JZ. Philosophy and the Brain. Oxford, UK: Oxford University Press; 1987:11.

[139] Churchland PS. Brain-Wise: *Studies in Neurophilosophy*. Cambridge, MA: The MIT Press; 2002.

[140] Cariani P. Regenerative process in life and mind. *Ann. N. Y. Acad. Sci.* 2000, 901, 26–34.

[141] Jarvilehto T. Theory of the organism-environment system. IV. The problem of mental activity and consciousness. Integr. *Physiol. Behav.l Sci*. 2000, 35(2), 35–57.

[142] Arthem P, Liljenstrom H. On the co-evolution of cognition and consciousness. *J. Theor. Biol.* 1997, 187(4), 601–612.

[143] Hermansen TD, Ventegodt S, Rald E, Clausen B, Nielsen ML, Merrick J. Human development I: twenty fundamental problems of biology, medicine, and neuropsychology related to biological information. *TheScientificWorldJOURNAL* 2006, 6, 747–759.

[144] Ventegodt S, Hermansen TD, Nielsen ML, Clausen B, Merrick J. Human development II: we need an integrated theory of matter, life and consciousness to understand life and healing. *TheScientificWorldJOURNAL* 2006, 6, 760–766.

[145] Ventegodt S, Hermansen TD, Rald E, Flensborg-Madsen T, Nielsen ML, Clausen B, Merrick J. Human development III: bridging brain-mind and body-mind. Introduction to "deep" (fractal, poly-ray) cosmology. *TheScientificWorldJOURNAL* 2006, 6, 767–776.

[146] Ventegodt S, Hermansen TD, Flensborg-Madsen T, Nielsen ML, Clausen B, Merrick J. Human development IV: the living cell has information-directed self-organization. *TheScientificWorldJOURNAL* 2006, 6, 1132-1138.
[147] Posner MI, Rothbart MK. Attention, self-regulation and consciousness. *Philos. Trans. R. Soc. Lond. B Biol. Sci.* 1998, 353(1377): 1915–1927.
[148] Posner MI, Ed. *Cognitive Neuroscience of Attention*. New York, NY: The Guilford Press; 2004.
[149] Manly T, Robertson IH, Galloway M, Hawkins K. The absent mind: further investigations of sustained attention to response. *Neuropsychologia*. 1999, 37, 661–670.
[150] Assmus A, Marshall JC, Ritzl A, Noth J, Zilles K, Fink GR. Left inferior parietal cortex integrates time and space during collision judgements. *Neuroimage*. 2003, 20 (Suppl 1), S82–88.
[151] Robertson IH, Garavan H. Vigilant Attention. *In Gazzaniga MS, ed. The Cognitive Neurosciences.* 3rd ed. A Bradford Book. Cambridge, MA: The MIT Press; 2004; 631–640.
[152] Garavan H, Ross TJ, Stein EA. Right hemispheric dominance of inhibitory control: an event-related functional MRI study. *Proc. Natl. Acad. Sci. U. S. A.* 1999, 96, 8301–8306.
[153] Mendez MF, Gershfield DN. Delirium. In Bradley WG, Daroff RB, Fenichel GM, Jankovic J, eds. Neurology in Clinical Practice: *Principles of Diagnosis and Treatment*. 4th ed. Philadelphia, PA: Butterworth-Heinemann; 2004; 29–41.
[154] Luck SJ, Vogel EK. In Shapiro K, ed. The Limits of Attention: *Temporal Constraints in Human Information Processing*. Oxford, UK: Oxford University Press; 2001;125–140.
[155] Mathews G, Zeidner M, Roberts RD. Emotional Intelligence. *A Bradford Book.* Cambridge, MA: The MIT Press; 2002.
[156] Goleman D. *Working with Emotional Intelligence*. Bantam Books, New York, NY: 1998.
[157] Bar-On R, Tranel D, Denburg NL, Bechara A. Exploring the neurological substrate of emotional and social intelligence. *Brain* 2003, 126, 1790–1800.
[158] Panksepp J. *Affective Neuroscience: The Foundations of Human and Animal Emotions*. Oxford University Press, New York, NY: 1998.
[159] Pritchard TC, Alloway KD. *Neural Regulation of Emotional Behavior*. Madison, CN: Fence Creek Publication; 1999.
[160] Rauch SL, Shin LM, Dougherty DD, Alepert NM, Orr SP, Lasko M, et al. Neural activation during sexual and competitive arousal in healthy men. *Psychiatry Res.* 1999, 91(1), 1–10.
[161] Beauregard M, Levesque J, Bourgouin P. Neural correlates of conscious self-regulation of emotion. *J. Neurosci.* 2001, 21(18), RC165.
[162] Baron-Cohen S, Ring H, Wheelwright S, Bullmore ET, Brammer MJ, Simmons A, Williams SC. Social intelligence in the normal and autistic brain: an fMRI study. *Eur. J. Neurosci.* 1999, 11(6), 1891–1898.
[163] Best M, Williams JM, Coccaro EF. Evidence for a dysfunctional prefrontal circuit in patients with an impulsive aggressive disorder. *Proc. Natl. Acad. Sci. U. S.* A. 2002, 99(12), 8448–8453.
[164] Wild B, Rodden FA, Grodd W, Ruch W. Neural correlates of laughter and humor. *Brain* 2003, 126, 2121–2138.
[165] Heller W, Koven NS, Miller GA. Regional brain activity in anxiety and depression, cognition-emotion interaction, and emotion regulation. In Hugdahl K, Davidson RJ, eds. The Asymmetrical Brain. *A Bradford Book.* Cambridge, MA: The MIT Press; 2000; 533–564.

[166] Llinas RR. i of the vortex: From Neurons to Self. *A Bradford Book.* Cambridge, MA: The MIT Press; 2001.

[167] Wegner, D.M. The Illusion of Conscious Will. *A Bradford Book.* Cambridge, MA: The MIT Press; 2002.

[168] Wegner DM, Sparrow B. Authorship processing. In Gazzaniga MS, ed. The Cognitive Neurosciences. 3rd ed. *A Bradford Book.* Cambridge, MA: The MIT Press; 2004; 1201–1209.

[169] Miller BL, Seeley WW, Mychack P, Rosen HJ, Mena I, Boone K. Neuroanatomy of the self: evidence from patients with fronto-temporal dementia. *Neurology* 2001, 57(5), 817–821.

[170] Johnson SC, Baxter LC, Wilder LS, Pipe JG, Heiserman JE, Prigatano GP. Neural correlates of self-reflection. *Brain* 2002, 125, 1808–1814.

[171] LeDoux J. The self: clues from the brain. *Ann. N. Y. Acad. Sci.* 2003, 1001, 295–304.

[172] Ramachandran VS. A Brief Tour of Human Consciousness: *From Imposter Poodles to Purple Numbers.* New York, NY: PI Press; 2004.

[173] Samson D, Apperly IA, Kathirgamanathan U, Humphreys GW. Seeing it my way: a case of a selective deficit in inhibiting self-perspective. *Brain* 2005, 128, 1102–1111.

[174] Turk DJ, Heatherton TF, Macrae N, Kelly WM, Gazzaniga MS. Out of contact, out of mind: the distributed nature of the self. *Ann. N. Y. Acad. Sci.* 2003, 1001, 65–78.

[175] Vaillant GE. Mental health. *Am. J. Psychiatry* 2003, 160, 1373–1384.

[176] Klamut MK. The promotion of happiness. *Ann. Univ. Mariae Curie Sklodowska* [Med.] 2002, 57(1), 1–9.

[177] McGrath A. Spirituality and wellbeing: some recent discussions. *Brain* 2006, 129, 278–282.

[178] de Nicolas AT. *The Bhagvad Gitā: The Ethics of Decision-Making*. Berwick, ME: Nicolas-Hays; 2004.

[179] Swarūpānanda, S. *Shrimad Bhagvad Gītā.* Calcutta, India: Advaita Ashram; 1967.

[180] Lazar SW, Bush G, Gollub RL, Fricchione GL, Khalsa G, Benson H. Functional brain mapping of the relaxation response and meditation. *NeuroReport* 2000, 11(7), 1581–1585.

[181] Newberg AB, Iversen J. The neural basis of the complex mental task of meditation: neurotransmitter and neurochemical considerations. *Med. Hypotheses* 2003, 61(2), 282–291.

[182] McCraty R, Atkinson M, Bradley RT. Electrophysiological evidence of intuition (part 1): the surprising role of the heart. *J. Altern. Complement. Med.* 2004, 10(1), 133–143.

[183] Andreasen NC. The Creating Brain: *The Neuroscience of Genius.* New York, NY: Dana Press; 2005.

[184] Dietrich A. The cognitive neuroscience of creativity. *Psychon. Bull. Rev.* 2004, 11(6), 1011–1026.

[185] Cahn BR, Delorme A, Polich J. Occipital gamma activation during Vipassana meditation. *Cogn. Process.* 2010, 11(1):39-56.

[186] Vialatte FB, Bakardjian H, Prasad R, Cichocki A. EEG paroxysmal gamma waves during Bhrāmari Prānāyāma: a yoga breathing technique. *Conscious Cogn.* 2009, 18(4):977-988.

[187] Kjaer TW, Bertelsen C, Piccini P, Brooks D, Alving J, Lou HC. Increased dopamine tone during meditation induced change of consciousness. *Brain Res. Cogn. Brain Res.* 2002, 13(2):255-259.

[188] Travis F, Pearson C. Pure Consciousness: Distinct phenomenal and physiological correlates of "Consciousness Itself." *Int. J. Neurosci.* 1999, 100(1-4):77-89.

[189] Baerentsen KB, Stodkilde-Jorgensen H, Sommerlund B, Hartman T, Damsgaard-Madsen J, Fosnaes M, Green AC. An investigation of brain processes supporting meditation. *Cogn. Process.* 2010, 11(1):57-84.
[190] Travis F, Haaga DA, Hagelin J, Tanner M, Arenander A, Nidich S, Gaylord-King C, Grosswald S, Rainforth M, Schneider RH. A self-referential default brain state: patterns of coherence, power, and eLoreta sources during eyes-closed rest and transcendental meditation practice. *Cogn Process.* 2010, 11(1):21-30.
[191] Hodgins HS, Adair KC. Attentional processes and meditation. *Conscious Cogn.* 2010, April 27. [Epub ahead of print].
[192] Williams JM. Mindfulness and psychological process. *Emotion*. 2010, 10(1):1-7.
[193] Luders E, Toga AW, Lepore N, Gaser C. The underlying anatomical correlates of long-term meditation: larger hippocampal and frontal volumes of gray matter. *Neuroimage* 2009, 45(3):672-678.
[194] Vestergaard-Poulsen P, van Beek M, Skewes J, Bjarkam CR, Stubberup M, Bertelsen J, Roepstorff A. Long-term meditation is associated with increased gray matter density in the brain stem. *NeuroReport* 2009, 20(2):170-174.
[195] Pagnoni G, Cekic M, Guo Y. "Thinking about not-thinking": neural correlates of conceptual processing during Zen meditation. *PLoS One*. 2008, 3(9):e3083.
[196] Streeter CC, Jensen JE, Perlmutter RM, Cabral HJ, Tian H, Terhune DB, Ciraulo DA, Renshaw PF. Yoga asana sessions increase brain GABA levels: a pilot study. *J. Altern. Complement Med*. 2007, 13(4):419-426.
[197] Csikszentmihaly M. Flow: *The Psychology of Optimal Experience*. New York, NY: HarperPerrenial; 1990.
[198] Krishnamurti J. *The Meditative Mind.* In Quinn WD, ed. Ojai, CA: Krishnamurti Foundation of America; 1989.
[199] Freeman WJ. Mesoscopic neurodynamics: from neuron to brain. *J. Physiol.* (Paris) 2000, 94, 303–322.
[200] Hickman CP Jr, Roberts LS. *Biology of Animals*, 6th edition. Dubuque, IA: Wm C Brown Communications, Inc; 1994:197-221.
[201] West JB, ed. Best and Taylor's Physiological Basis of Medical Practice, 12th edition. Baltimore, MD: Williams and Wilkins; 1991:1061-67.
[202] Damasio AR. *The Feeling of What Happens: Body and Emotion in the Making of Consciousness.* New York, NY: *Harcourt Brace and Company*; 1999: 260 and 303.
[203] Damasio AR, Meyer K. Consciousness: An Overview of the Phenomenon and its Possible Neural Basis. In Laureys S, Tononi G, eds. The Neurology of Consciousness: *Cognitive Neuroscience and Neuropathology*. Burlington, MA: Elsevier Ltd; 2009:3-14.
[204] Soodak H, Iberall A. A physical science for complex systems. *Science* 18;201(4356)Aug 1978:579-82.
[205] Iberall AS and Soodak H. A Physics for Complex Systems. In Yates FE, Garfinkel A, Walter DO, Yates GB eds. Self-Organizing Systems: *The Emergence of Order*. New York, NY: Plenum Press; 1987:499-520.
[206] Iberall AS, Soodak H. Primer on Homeokinetics: *A physical Foundation for Complex Systems*. Laguna Woods, CA: Cri-de-Coeur Press; 1998:1-24.
[207] Iberall AS. The Physics, Chemical Physics, and Biological Physics of the Origin of Life on Earth. *Ecological Psychology*, 13(4), 2001:315-27.
[208] Ramakrishna Rao K. Prologue: Introducing Indian Psychology. In Ramakrishna Rao K, Paranjpe AC, Dalal AK, eds. Handbook of Indian Psychology. New Delhi, India: *Foundation Books,* Cambridge University Press India Pvt. Ltd; 2008:1-18.

[209] Paranjpe AC, Ramakrishna Rao K. Psychology in the Advaita Vedanta. In Ramakrishna Rao K, Paranjpe AC, Dalal AK, eds. *Handbook of Indian Psychology*. Foundation Books, New Delhi, India: Cambridge University Press India Pvt. Ltd; 2008:253-85.
[210] Jha AK. Personality in Indian Psychology. In Ramakrishna Rao K, Paranjpe AC, Dalal AK, eds. Handbook of Indian Psychology. New Delhi, India: *Foundation Books,* Cambridge University Press India Pvt. Ltd; 2008:348-60.
[211] Swarupānanda S. *Shrimad Bhagavad Gitā.* Calcutta, India: Advaita Ashrama; 1967.
[212] Gambhirananda S. Brahma-Sutra Bhashya of Shankaracharya. Calcutta, India: *Advaita Ashrama;* 1996, 6th impression.
[213] Tononi G, Laureys S. *The Neurology of Consciousness: An Overview*. In Laureys S, Tononi G, eds. the Neurology of Consciousness: Cognitive Neuroscience and Neuropathology. Burlington, MA: *Elsevier* Ltd; 2009:375-412.
[214] Bleck T. Levels of Consciousness and Attention. In Goetz CG, ed. *Textbook of Clinical Neurology*, 3rd ed. Saunders-Elsevier; 2007:3-19.
[215] Homma I, Masaoka Y. Breathing rhythms and emotions. *Exp. Physiol.* 2008, 93.9:1011-21.
[216] Nagendra HR. *Prāṇāyāma: The art and science*. Bangalore, India: Vivekananda Kendra Yoga Prakashan; 1998.
[217] Swanson LW. Anatomy of the soul as reflected in the cerebral hemispheres: neural circuits underlying voluntary control of basic motivated behaviors. *The Journal of comparative neurology,* 2005, 493:122-31.
[218] Haggard P. Human volition: toward a neuroscience of will. *Nature Reviews/Neuroscience*. 9, Dec 2008: 934-45.
[219] Hallett M. Volitional control of movement: the physiology of free will. *Clinical Neurophysiology* 2007, 118:1179-92.
[220] Pred R. Onflow: *dynamics of consciousness and experience.* Cambridge, MA: The MIT Press; 2005:300-03.
[221] Schafer L. Non-empirical reality: *transcending the physical and spiritual in the order of the one*. Zygon. June 2008, 43(2): 329-51.
[222] Hume RE, translator. *The Thirteen Principal Upaniṣads*, 2nd edition. Oxford, UK: Oxford University Press; 1877-1968.
[223] Radhakrishnan S, ed. and trans. *The Principal Upaniṣads*. New Delhi, India: HarperCollins; 2004: 13th impression.
[224] Deussen, P. *The Philosophy of the Upaniṣads*. New York: Dover publications, Inc; 1966.
[225] Goodall, D. Hindu Scriptures. Berkeley, LA: University of California Press; 1996.
[226] Mahadevan TMP. Upanishads: *The Selections from 108 Upaniṣads*. New Delhi: Arnold-Heinemann; 1975.
[227] Jones BE. The neural basis of consciousness across the sleep-waking cycle. In Jasper HH, Descarries L, Castellucci VF, Rossignol S, eds. *Consciousness At The Frontiers of Neuroscience, Advances in Neurology*, New York, NY: Lippincott-Raven; 1998: vol. 77.
[228] Nikhilanand S. The Upaniṣads. London: George Allen and Unwin, Ltd; 1963.
[229] Bhanu CG, ed. *Maṇdukyopaniṣad with Commentary and Translation.* Mumbai: Damodar Savalaram and Mandali; 1913.
[230] Apte, VS *The Student's Sanskrit-English Dictionary*. Delhi, India: Motilal Banarsidass; 1970.
[231] Fischer-Schreiber I, Ehrhard F-K, Friedrichs K, Diener, MS, eds. *The Encyclopedia of Eastern Philosophy and Religion.* Boston, MA: Shambhala Press; 1989.

[232] Deshmukh VD. *Mental Excellence.* Self-published and registered with the Library of Congress: 1988.
[233] Taimani, I.K. The Science of Yoga. Wheaton, IL: *The Theosophical Publishing House;* 1961.
[234] Austin JH. *Zen and the Brain*. Cambridge, MA: The MIT Press; 1998.
[235] Walsh RN. Meditation. Chapter 35, in Corsini R, ed. *Handbook of Innovative Therapy,* 2nd edition. New York, NY: John Wiley and Sons; 2001.
[236] Bucksbazen JD. To Forget the Self: *An Illustrated Guide to Zen Meditation.* Los Angeles, CA: The Zen Center of Los Angeles; 1977.
[237] Miller JJ, Fletcher K, Kabat-Zinn J. Three-year follow-up and clinical implications of a mindfulness meditation-based stress reduction intervention in the treatment of anxiety disorders. *General Hospital Psychiatry*1995, 17: 192–200.
[238] Epstein M. Attention in analysis. *Psychoanalysis Contemporary Thought*1988, 11: 171–89.
[239] Freud S. Recommendations to Physicians Practicing Psychoanalysis. Standard ed., London, UK: Hogarth Press; 1912-1955: Vol. 12.
[240] Mapstone M, Rosler A, Hays A, Gitelman DR, Weintraub S. Dynamic allocation of attention in aging and Alzheimer disease. *Archives of Neurology* 2001, 58(9): 1443–47.
[241] Barrett AM, Crucian GP, Schwartz R, Nallamshetty H, Heilman KM. Seeing trees but not the forest: Limited perception of large configurations in Parkinson disease. *Neurology* 2001, 56(6): 724–29.
[242] Csikszentmihalyi M. Flow: *The Psychology of Optimal Experience.* New York, NY: Harper and Row Publishers, Inc; 1990.
[243] Knight RT, Staines RW, Swick D, Chao LL. Prefrontal cortex regulates inhibition and excitation in distributed neural networks. Acta Psychologica 1999, 101: 159–78.
[244] Miller EK, Cohen JD. An integrative theory of prefrontal cortex function. *Annual Review of Neuroscience* 2001, 24: 167–202.
[245] Bunge SA, Ochsner KN, Desmond JE, Glover GH, Gabrieli JDE. Prefrontal regions involved in keeping information in and out of mind. *Brain* 2001, 124: 2074–86.
[246] Fernandez-Duque D, Posner MI. Brain imaging of attentional networks in normal and pathological states. *Journal of Clinical and Experimental Neuropsychology* 2001, 23(01): 74–93.
[247] Deshmukh VD. 1994. *The quiescent brain and consciousness.* Poster presentation in the conference on "Toward a Scientific Basis for Consciousness," Tucson, Arizona April 12-17, 1994.
[248] Zeman A. *Consciousness: An invited review*. Brain 2001, 124: 1263–89.
[249] Deshmukh VD. Vedic Psychology: A Science of Wisdom. *J. Altern. Med. Res.* 2011;3(1): (in print).
[250] Ramkrishna Rao K, Paranjpe AC, Dalal AK, eds. *Handbook of Indian Psychology.* New Delhi, India: Foundation Books, Cambridge University Press; 2008.
[251] VandenBos GR, ed. APA Dictionary of Psychology. Washington, DC: *American Psychological Association*; 2007.
[252] Sadock BJ, Sadock VA. *Kaplan and Sadock's Synopsis of Psychiatry: Behavioral Sciences/Clinical Psychiatry*, 10th ed. Philadelphia, PA: Wolters Kluwer | Lippincott Williams and Wilkins, Health; 2007: 207-213.
[253] Sadock BJ, Sadock VA. *Kaplan and Sadock's Synopsis of Psychiatry: Behavioral Sciences/Clinical Psychiatry*, 10th ed. Philadelphia, PA: Wolters Kluwer | Lippincott Williams and Wilkins, Health; 2007: 12-18.

[254] Gaw AC. *Cultural Issues.* In Hales RE, Yudofsky SC, Gabbard GO, eds. The American Psychiatric Publishing Textbook of Psychiatry. 5th ed. Washington, DC: *American Psychiatric Publishing,* Inc; 2008: 1529-1547.
[255] Yalom ID. *Existential Psychotherapy*. New York, NY: Basic Books; 1980.
[256] Ghosh S. *The Original Yoga*. New Delhi: Munshiram Manoharlal; 1999.
[257] Krishnamurti J. *Meditations*. San Francisco, CA: Harper and Row Publishers; 1979:4.
[258] Brodal Per. The Central Nervous System: Structure and Function. 3rd edition, New York, NY: Oxford University Press; 2004.
[259] Hales RE, Yudofsky SC, Gabbard GO, eds. Textbook of Psychiatry, 5th edition. *The American Psychiatric Publishing*; 2008.
[260] Trimble MR, *The Soul in the Brain: The Cerebral Basis of Language, Art, and Belief.* Baltimore, MD: The Johns Hopkins University Press; 2007.
[261] Brusca RC, Brusca GJ. *Invertebrates*. 2nd edition. Sunderland, MA: Sinauer Associates; 2003.
[262] Mosier K, Berenznaya I. Parallel cortical networks for volitional control of swallowing in humans. *Exp. Brain Res.* Oct 2001;140(3): 280-89.
[263] Herman JP et al. Central mechanisms of stress integration: hierarchical circuitry controlling Hypothalamo-pituitary-adrenocortical responsiveness. *Front Neuroendocrinol.* Jul 2003;24(3): 151-80.
[264] Haber SN. The primate basal ganglia: parallel and integrative networks. *J. Chem. Neuroanat. Dec.* 2003;26(4): 317-30.
[265] Lerner Y, Hendler T, Ben-Bashat D, Harel M, Malach R. A hierarchical axis of object processing stages in the human visual cortex. *Cereb. Cortex* Apr 2001;11(4): 287-97.
[266] Wessinger CM et al. Hierarchical organization of the human auditory cortex revealed by functional magnetic resonance imaging. *J. Cogn. Neurosci. Jan.* 1 2001; 13(1):1-7.
[267] Eskenasy AC, Clarke S. Hierarchy within human SI: supporting data from cytochrome oxidase, acetylcholinesterase and NADPH-diaphorase staining patterns. *Somatosens Mot. Res.* 2000; 17(2):123-32.
[268] Nyffler T et al. Time-dependent hierarchical organization of spatial working memory: a transcranial magnetic stimulation study. *Eur. J. Neurosci. Nov.* 2002;16(9):1823-27.
[269] Davis MH, Johnsrude IS. Hierarchical processing in spoken language comprehension. *J. Neurosci*. Apr 15 2003;23(8):3423-31.
[270] O'Rahilly R, Muller F. *The Embryonic Human Brain.* 2nd edition. New York, NY: Wiley-Liss; 1999:100-01 and 442-49.
[271] Graham A. Development of the pharyngeal arches. *Am. J. Med. Genetics* 2003;119A:251-56.
[272] Santagati F, Rijli FM. Cranial neural crest and the building of the vertebrate head. *Nature Reviews/Neuroscience,* 2003;vol 4 Oct:806-18.
[273] Chandrasekhar A. Turning heads: Development of vertebrate branchio-motor neurons. *Developmental Dynamics* 2004;229:143-161.
[274] Romer AS, Parsons TS. *The Vertebrate Body.* Orlando, FL: Saunders College Publishing 1986:35.
[275] Ertekin C, Aydogdu I. Neurophysiology of swallowing. *Clin. Neurophysiol. Dec.* 2003; 114(12):2226-44.
[276] Sawczuk A, Mosier KM. Neural control of tongue movement with respect to respiration and swallowing. *Crit. Rev. Oral Biol. Med.* 2001;12(1):18-37.
[277] Pagliardini S, Ren J, Greer JJ. Ontogeny of the pre-Botzinger complex in perinatal rats. *J. Neurosci*. 2003 Oct 22; 23(29): 9575-84.

[278] Barman S. *Brainstem control of cardiovascular function.* In Klemm WR, Vertes RP, eds. Brainstem mechanisms of behavior. New York, NY: John Wiley and Sons. 1990:353-381.
[279] Drew T, Prentice S, Schepens B. Cortical and brainstem control of locomotion. *Prog. Brain Res.* 2004;143:251-61.
[280] Brocard F, Dubuc R. Differential contribution of reticulo-spinal cells to the control of locomotion induced by the Mesencephalic locomotor region. *J. Neurophysiol.* 2003 Sep; 90(3):1714-27.
[281] Noga BR et al. Mechanism for activation of locomotor centers in the spinal cord by stimulation of the Mesencephalic locomotor region. *J. Neurophysiol.* 2003 Sep; 90(3):1464-78.
[282] Sasaki S, Yoshimura K, Naito K. The neural control of orienting: role of multiple-branching reticulospinal neurons. *Prog. Brain Res.* 2004;143:383-389.
[283] Horn AK, Helmchen C, Wahle P. GABAergic neurons in the rostral Mesencephalon of the macaque monkey that control vertical eye movements. *Ann. N Y Acad. Sci.* 2003 Oct; 1004:19-28.
[284] Enderle JD. Neural control of saccades. *Prog. Brain Res.* 2002;140:21-49.
[285] Waitzman DM et al. Contribution of the superior Colliculus and the Mesencephalic reticular formation to gaze control. *Ann. N Y Acad. Sci.* 2002 Apr; 956: 111-29.
[286] Jurgens U. Neural pathways underlying vocal control. *Neurosci. Biobehav. Rev.* 2002 Mar; 26(2):235-258.
[287] Siebert S, Jurgens U. Vocalization after Periaqueductal grey inactivation with GABA agonist muscimol in the squirrel monkey. *Neurosci. Lett.* 2003 Apr 10; 340(2):111-14.
[288] MacWhinney B. Models of the emergence of language. *Annu. Rev. Psychol.* 1998; 49:199-227.
[289] Butler AB, Hodos W. Comparative Vertebrate Neuroanatomy: *Evolution and Adaptation*. New York, NY: Wiley-Liss. 1996:104-105.
[290] Horn G. Pathways of the past: The imprint of memory. *Nature Reviews/Neuroscience* 2004;5:108-20.
[291] Panksepp J. Affective Neuroscience: *The foundations of human and animal emotions.* New York, NY: Oxford University press; 1998.
[292] Davis M, Whalen PJ. The amygdala: vigilance and emotion. *Molecular Psychiatry* 2001; 6:13-34.
[293] Benson DF. *The Neurology of Thinking.* New York, NY: Oxford University Press; 1994.
[294] Fuster JM. Frontal lobe and cognitive development. *J Neurocytol.* 2002 Mar-Jun; 31(3-5):373-85.
[295] Haxby JV, Hoffman EA, Gobbini MI. Human neural systems for face recognition and social communication. *Biol. Psychiatry*. 2002 Jan 1; 51(1):59-67.
[296] Nofzinger EA et al. Human regional cerebral glucose metabolism during non-rapid eye movement sleep in relation to waking. *Brain.* 2002 May; 125(Pt 5):1105-15.
[297] Balkin TJ et al. The process of awakening: a PET study of regional brain activity patterns mediating the re-establishment of alertness and consciousness. *Brain.* 2002 Oct; 125(Pt 10):2308-19.
[298] Jones BE. Arousal systems. *Front Biosci.* 2003 May 1; 8, s438-451.
[299] Heilman KM, Gonzalez Rothi LJ. *Treatment of disorders of cognition: An Introduction*. In Noseworthy JH, ed. Neurological Therapeutics. New York, NY: Martin Dunitz. 2003:2717-19.
[300] Swanberg MM et al. Executive Dysfunction in Alzheimer's disease. *Arch. Neurol.* 2004 Apr; vol 61:556-60.

[301] Sternberg RJ, Lubart TI. *The Concept of Creativity: Prospects and Paradigms*. In Sternberg RJ, ed. Handbook of Creativity. Cambridge, UK: Cambridge University Press;1999:3-15.
[302] Dietrich A. The cognitive neuroscience of creativity. *Psychonomic Bulletin and Review*, 2004;11(6):1011-26.
[303] Andreasen NC. The Creating Brain: *The Neuroscience of Genius.* New York – Washington, DC: Dana Press; 2005.
[304] Freeman WJ. Mesoscopic neurodynamics: from neuron to brain. *J. Physiol. Paris.* 2000 Sep-Dec;94(5-6):303-22.
[305] Christoff K, Ream JM, Geddes LP, Gabrieli JD. Evaluating self-generated information: anterior prefrontal contribution to human cognition. *Behav. Neurosci.* 2003 Dec;117(6):1161-68.
[306] Heilman KM, Nadeau SE, Beversdorf DO. *Creative innovation: possible mechanisms. Neurocase.* 2003 Oct; 9(5), 369-379.
[307] Faw B. Consciousness, motivation, and emotion: Biopsychological reflections. In Ellis RD, Newton N, eds. *The Caldron of Consciousness: Motivation, affect and Self-Organization* – An Anthology. Philadelphia, PA: John Benjamins Publishing Company; 2000: 55-90.
[308] Forehand CJ. *Integrative Functions of the Nervous System.* In Rhoades RA, Bell DR. (2009) Medical Physiology: Principles for Clinical Medicine. 3rd ed. Philadelphia, PA: Wolters Kluwer | Lippincott Williams and Wilkins; 2009: 122-139.
[309] Stern Y. *Neuropsychological evaluation.* In Rowland LP, Pedley TA. (2010) Merritt's Neurology. 12th ed. Philadelphia, PA: Wolters Kluwer | Lippincott Wlliams and Wilkins; 2010: 118-121.
[310] James W. The varieties of Religious Experience: A study in human nature. New York, NY: *Barnes and Noble Classics;* 2004:329-330.
[311] Lamb R. Sacred. In Mittal S, Thursby G, eds. Studying Hinduism: *Key Concepts and Methods*. New York, NY: Routledge; 2008: 339-353.
[312] Kneisl CR, Trigoboff E. *Contemporary Psychiatric-Mental Health Nursing*. 2nd ed. New Jersey: Pearson-Prentice Hall; 2009.
[313] Sansone RA, Sansone LA. Psychotherapy: What's metaphysical got to do with it? *Psychiatry (Edgemont),* 2009, 6(12):26-31.
[314] Farb NA, Segal ZV, Mayberg H, Bean J, McKeon D, Fatima Z, Anderson AK. Attending to the present: mindfulness meditation reveals distinct neural modes of self-reference. *Soc. Cogn. Affect. Neurosci.* 2007, 2(4):313-322.
[315] Travis F and Shear J. Focused attention, open monitoring, and automatic self-transcending: Categories to organize meditations from Vedic, Buddhist, and Chinese traditions. *Conscious Cogn.* Feb 2010, 16 [Epub ahead of print].
[316] Teixeira ME. Self-transcendence: a concept analysis for nursing praxis. *Holist. Nurs.* Pract. 2008, 22(1):25-31.
[317] Walach H, Kohls N, Belschner W. Transpersonal Psychology – Psychology of Consciousness: chances and problems. *Psychother. Psychosom. Med. Psychol.* 2005, 55(9-10):405-415.
[318] Lincoln V. Eco-spirituality: A pattern that connects. *J. Holist. Nurs*. 2000, 18(3):227-244.
[319] Cloninger CR. Evolution of Human Brain Function: the Functional structure of Human Consciousness. *Aust N Z J Psychistry* 2009, 43(11):994-1006.
[320] Chandler E. Spirituality. *Hosp. J.* 1999, 14(3-4):63-74.
[321] Bulkeley K. The Wondering Brain: *Thinking about Religion with and beyond Cognitive Neuroscience.* Routledge, New York, NY: 2005.

[322] Panksepp J. The neuroevolutionary and neuroaffective psychobiology of the prosocial brain. In Dunbar RIM, Barrett L. eds. *Oxford Handbook of Evolutionary Psychology.* New York, NY: Oxford University Press; 2007: 145-162.
[323] Solms M, Turnbull O. *The brain and the inner world: An introduction to the neuroscience of subjective experience.* New York, NY: Other Press; 2002.
[324] Gendlin ET. The 'Mind'/'Body' problem and first-person process: Three types of concepts. In Ellis RD, Newton N. eds. *The Caldron of Consciousness: Motivation, affect and Self-Organization* – An Anthology. Philadelphia, PA: John Benjamins Publishing Company; 2000: 109-118.
[325] Locke Simeon. Consciousness, *Self-Consciousness, and the Science of Being Human.* Westport, CT: Praeger; 2008.
[326] Toews DW, Kay JJ, Lister NME, eds. *The Ecosystem Approach: Complexity, Uncertainty, and Managing for Sustainability.* New York, NY: Columbia University Press; 2008.
[327] Fuchs T. Ecology of the Brain: *A Systemic view for Psychiatry and Psychotherapy.* Nervenarzt. 2005, 76(1):1-10.
[328] Panksepp J. Affective consciousness in animals: perspectives on dimensional and primary process emotion approaches. *Proc. Biol. Sci.* 2010 Oct 7;277(1696):2905-7.
[329] Schiff ND. Central thalamic contributions to arousal regulation and neurological disorders of consciousness. *Ann. N Y Acad. Sci.* 2008;1129:105-18.
[330] Manna A, et al., Neural correlates of focused attention and cognitive monitoring in meditation, *Brain Res. Bull.* 2010, doi:10.1016/j.brainresbull.2010.03.001
[331] Shergill SS, Brammer MJ, Fukuda R, Bullmore E, Amaro E, Jr., Murray RM, McGuire PK. *Hum. Brain Mapping 16*:219–227, 2002.
[332] Rubia K, Smith AB, Woolley J, Nosarti C, Heyman I, Taylor E, Brammer M. Progressive increase of frontostriatal brain activation from childhood to adulthood during event-related tasks of cognitive control. *Hum Brain Mapp.* 2006 Dec;27(12):973-93.
[333] Berman R, Negishi M, Vestal M, Spann M, Chung MH, Bai X, Purcaro M, Motelow JE, Danielson N, Dix-Cooper L, Enev M, Novotny EJ, Constable RT, Blumenfeld H. Simultaneous EEG, fMRI, and behavior in typical childhood absence seizures. *Epilepsia.* 2010 Jul 1. doi: 10.1111/j.1528-1167.2010.02652.x. [Epub ahead of print]
[334] Feinberg TE. The nested neural hierarchy and the self. *Conscious Cogn.* 2010 Oct 14. [Epub ahead of print].
[335] Dehaene S, Naccache L. Towards a cognitive neuroscience of consciousness: basic evidence and workspace framework. *Cognition.* 2001 Apr;79(1-2):1-37.
[336] Silva S, Alacoque X, Fourcade O, Samii K, Marque P, Woods R, Mazziotta J, Chollet F, Loubinoux I. Wakefulness and loss of awareness: Brain and brainstem interaction in the vegetative state. *Neurology®* 2010;74:313–320.
[337] Vandekerckhove M, Panksepp J. The flow of anoetic to noetic and autonoetic consciousness: a vision of unknowing (anoetic) and knowing (noetic) consciousness in the remembrance of things past and imagined futures. *Conscious Cogn.* 2009 Dec;18(4):1018-28. Epub 2009 Aug 26.
[338] Northoff G, Panksepp J. The trans-species concept of self and the subcortical-cortical midline system. *Trends Cogn Sci.* 2008 Jul;12(7):259-64. Epub 2008 Jun 12.
[339] Panksepp J, Northoff G. The trans-species core SELF: the emergence of active cultural and neuro-ecological agents through self-related processing within subcortical-cortical midline networks. *Conscious Cogn.* 2009 Mar;18(1):193-215.
[340] Kak SC. Active agents, intelligence and quantum computing. *Information Sciences.* 2000, 128: 1-17.

[341] Kak SC. On science of consciousness in ancient India. *Indian Journal of History of Science*. 1997, 32: 105-120.
[342] Kak SC. The Gods Within: On the Vedic understanding of mind and neuroscience. *Adyar Library Bulletin*. 2000, 64: 7-55.
[343] Kak SC. The three languages of the brain: quantum, reorganizational, and associative. In Pribram K. and King J. eds. *Learning as Self-Organization*. Lawrence Erlbaum Associates 1996: 185-219.
[344] Damasio A. Self Comes to Mind: Constructing the Conscious Brain. New York, NY: *Pantheon Books*; 2010: 21.
[345] Sporns O. Networks of the Brain. Cambridge, MA: The MIT Press; 2011: p. 181 & 205-206.
[346] Bhikkhu Bodhi, ed. *Teachings of the Buddha in the Buddha's Words: An Anthology of Discourses from the Pali Canon.* Boston, MA: Wisdom Publications; 2005: 262-263.
[347] Squire LR, Bloom FE, McConnell SK, Roberts JL, Spitzer NC, and Zigmond MJ. (2003). Fundamental Neuroscience. 2nd ed. Academic Press, An Inprint of Elsevier Science, San Diego, CA:1353-1394.
[348] Deshmukh VD. Cascading morpho-regulatory energy and the biological form: Theory and Reality. *Medical Hypotheses* 1991, 35: 59-67.
[349] Harel BT, and Tranel D. Functional Neuroanatomy: Neuropsychological correlates of cortical and subcortical damage. In Yudofsky SC, and Hales RE. (eds.). *The American Psychiatric Publishing Textbook of Neuropsychiatry and Behavioral Neurosciences*, 5th ed. Washington DC. American Psychiatric Publishing, Inc. 2008: 45-91.
[350] Cohen RA, Salloway S, and Sweet LH. Neuropsychiatric Aspects of Disorders of Attention. In Yudofsky SC, and Hales RE. (eds.). *The American Psychiatric Publishing Textbook of Neuropsychiatry and Behavioral Neurosciences*, 5th ed. Washington DC. American Psychiatric Publishing, Inc. 2008: 405-44.
[351] Bleck TP. Levels of Consciousness and Attention. In Goetz CG. (ed.) Textbook of Clinical Neurology. 3rd ed. Philadelphia. *Saunders Elsevier.* 2007: 3-19.
[352] Stevens S. and Hening WA. Sleep and Wakefulness. In Goetz CG. (ed.) Textbook of Clinical Neurology. 3rd ed. Philadelphia. *Saunders Elsevier*. 2007: 21-33.
[353] Friedman JH, and Chou KL. Mood, Emotion. And Thought. In Goetz CG. (ed.) Textbook of Clinical Neurology. 3rd ed. Philadelphia. *Saunders Elsevier*. 2007: 35-54.
[354] Brewer JB, Gabrieli JDE, Preston AR, Vaidya CJ, and Rosen AC. Memory. In Goetz CG. (ed.) Textbook of Clinical Neurology. 3rd ed. Philadelphia. *Saunders Elsevier.* 2007: 63-78.
[355] Swanberg MM, Nasreddine ZS, Mendez MF, and Cummings JL. Speech and Language. In Goetz CG. (ed.) Textbook of Clinical Neurology. 3rd ed. Philadelphia. *Saunders Elsevier.* 2007:79-98.
[356] Doty RL, and Bromley SM. Cranial Nerve I: Olfactory Nerve. In Goetz CG. (ed.) Textbook of Clinical Neurology. 3rd ed. Philadelphia. *Saunders Elsevier*. 2007: 99-112.
[357] Goodwin J. Cranial Nerve III, IV, and VI: The Oculomotor System. In Goetz CG. (ed.) Textbook of Clinical Neurology. 3rd ed. Philadelphia. *Saunders Elsevier.* 2007: 133-64.
[358] Hain TC. Cranial Nerve VIII: The Vestibulocochlear System. In Goetz CG. (ed.) Textbook of Clinical Neurology. 3rd ed. Philadelphia. *Saunders Elsevier.* 2007: 199-215.
[359] Hermanowicz N. Cranial Nerve IX (Glossopharyngeal) and X (Vagus). In Goetz CG. (ed.) Textbook of Clinical Neurology. 3rd ed. Philadelphia. *Saunders Elsevier*. 2007: 217-29.

[360] Benarroch E, Freeman R, and Kaufmann H. Autonomic Nervous System. In *Goetz CG.* (ed.) Textbook of Clinical Neurology. 3rd ed. Philadelphia. *Saunders Elsevier.* 2007: 383-404.
[361] Stebbins GT. Neuropsychological Testing. In Goetz CG. (ed.) Textbook of Clinical Neurology. 3rd ed. Philadelphia. *Saunders Elsevier.* 2007: 539-57.

Reviews and Comments by Readers

"Great stuff...the idea is excellent and the material extraordinary. I like the cover and the illustrations. You are a man of great talent!"

Henry J. Mankin, M.D.
Edith M. Ashley Professor of Orthopedics Emeritus, Harvard Medical School,
Former Chief of Orthopedic Surgery, Massachusetts General Hospital, Boston, MA. USA

"This book is quite remarkable and fascinating. It is, not just a scholarly exposition of Vedānta based on current researches of neuroscience by an accomplished neuroscientist, but a moving account of Vedānta by a great seeker of Vedānta. I believe the reader will be transported to great heights reading Vinod Ji's soul-stirring poems and his clear analysis of many great mystics' accounts. I am sure this book is going to be a powerful instrument of dispelling the darkness of ignorance."

Swami Shantanand
Shānti Temple, Montrose, Philadelphia, USA

"This energy perspective is unique, beautiful and to the point. I love articles with Sanskrit in them."

Prof. Antonio de Nicolas PhD
Emeritus SUNY at Stony Brook, New York,
Director of Biocultural Research Institute, St Augustine, Florida

"Dr. Deshmukh delivers a brilliant union of neuroscience, spiritualism, and creativity. He brings a depth and breadth of wisdom and insight applicable to a beginner's mind as well as for a seasoned spiritualist."

Jana Whiddon, PhD, LMHC
Jana Whiddon Counseling, Inc
190 Fitzgerald Rd. Suite #1
Lakeland, FL 33813

"I enjoyed reading this book which fills an important niche by bringing together and juxtaposing two closes, yet far apart, disciplines; Vedanta and Neuroscience. One is ancient and well established; the other is cutting edge science and still evolving. One is based on intuitive insights gained through introspection; the other is based on brain imaged while performing its functions. Yet, the author shows in this book, using his expertise as a neuroscientist and knowledge as a Vedantin, how the two disciplines complement each other in producing an understanding of the very basic stuff of life: Consciousness and Self. This is a book which will be valued by scientists and philosophers alike."

Raju Chidambaram, PhD.
Author of "Law of Love and the Mathematics of Spirituality"

"The holistic understanding of consciousness, brain and mind has a lot to gain from the classical teaching of Self-Consciousness in Vedānta Philosophy, as it was taught by great masters like Sri Ramana Maharshi, his students Papaji, Sri Nanna Garu, and their students teaching the philosophy today, like Mooji.

Consciousness cannot be understood without direct experience; it has no meaning to think about consciousness. Only Self-inquiry can reveal the depth of its mystery for us. Words cannot really describe the experience of Consciousness and the Self. Writing a book on the subject is therefore an extreme challenge. Vinod Deshmukh has done a good job in this regard; you might not understand consciousness completely from reading this book but you will get an important pointing to the direct experience of it, making the understanding of brain, mind and awareness within your own reach. I warmly recommend the book to all researchers in this field."

Søren Ventegodt MD, EU-MSc-CAM.
Director of the Quality of Life Research Center, Copenhagen, and student of Mooji

INDEX